T0175648

PEDIATRIC SLEEP PEARLS

Lourdes M. DelRosso, MD, FAASM

Assistant Professor of Pediatrics
Associate Director, Pediatric Sleep Laboratory
University of California, San Francisco School of Medicine
UCSF Benioff Children's Hospital
San Francisco/Oakland, California

Richard B. Berry, MD

Professor of Medicine
University of Florida
Medical Director
University of Florida Health Sleep Center
Gainesville, Florida

Suzanne E. Beck, MD

Professor of Clinical Pediatrics
University of Pennsylvania Perelman School of Medicine
Medical Director, Sleep Laboratory
Children's Hospital of Philadelphia
Philadelphia, Pennsylvania

Mary H. Wagner, MD

Associate Professor
Department of Pediatrics
University of Florida
Gainesville, Florida

Carole L. Marcus, MBBCh

Distinguished Endowed Chair in Pediatrics
Professor of Pediatrics
University of Pennsylvania
Director, Sleep Center
Children's Hospital of Philadelphia
Philadelphia, Pennsylvania

ELSEVIER

ELSEVIER

1600 John F. Kennedy Blvd.
Ste 1800
Philadelphia, PA 19103-2899

PEDIATRIC SLEEP PEARLS   ISBN: 978-0-323-39277-8

Copyright © 2017 by Elsevier, Inc. All rights reserved.

No part of this publication may be reproduced or transmitted in any form or by any means, electronic or mechanical, including photocopying, recording, or any information storage and retrieval system, without permission in writing from the publisher. Details on how to seek permission, further information about the Publisher's permissions policies and our arrangements with organizations such as the Copyright Clearance Center and the Copyright Licensing Agency, can be found at our website: www.elsevier.com/permissions.

This book and the individual contributions contained in it are protected under copyright by the Publisher (other than as may be noted herein).

Notices

Knowledge and best practice in this field are constantly changing. As new research and experience broaden our understanding, changes in research methods, professional practices, or medical treatment may become necessary.

Practitioners and researchers must always rely on their own experience and knowledge in evaluating and using any information, methods, compounds, or experiments described herein. In using such information or methods they should be mindful of their own safety and the safety of others, including parties for whom they have a professional responsibility.

With respect to any drug or pharmaceutical products identified, readers are advised to check the most current information provided (1) on procedures featured or (2) by the manufacturer of each product to be administered, to verify the recommended dose or formula, the method and duration of administration, and contraindications. It is the responsibility of practitioners, relying on their own experience and knowledge of their patients, to make diagnoses, to determine dosages and the best treatment for each individual patient, and to take all appropriate safety precautions.

To the fullest extent of the law, neither the Publisher nor the authors, contributors, or editors assume any liability for any injury and/or damage to persons or property as a matter of products liability, negligence or otherwise, or from any use or operation of any methods, products, instructions, or ideas contained in the material herein.

Library of Congress Cataloging-in-Publication Data
Names: DelRosso, Lourdes M., author. | Berry, Richard B., 1947- author. |
  Beck, Suzanne E., author. | Wagner, Mary H., author. | Marcus, Carole L.,
  author.
Title: Pediatric sleep pearls / Lourdes M. DelRosso, Richard B. Berry,
  Suzanne E. Beck, Mary H. Wagner, Carole L. Marcus.
Description: Philadelphia, PA : Elsevier, [2017] | Includes bibliographical
  references.
Identifiers: LCCN 2016024652 | ISBN 9780323392778 (pbk. : alk. paper) | ISBN
  9780323428330 (Online)
Subjects: | MESH: Sleep Wake Disorders--diagnosis | Sleep Wake
  Disorders--therapy | Child | Adolescent | Polysomnography | Case Reports
Classification: LCC RJ506.S55 | NLM WL 108 | DDC 618.92/8498--dc23 LC record
available at https://lccn.loc.gov/2016024652

Content Strategist: Kellie J. Heap/Russell Gabbedy
Content Development Specialist: Lisa M. Barnes
Publishing Services Manager: Hemamalini Rajendrababu
Project Manager: Shereen Jameel
Design Direction: Ryan Cook
Marketing Manager: Michele Milano

Printed in United States of America

Last digit is the print number: 9 8 7 6 5 4 3

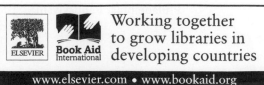

Working together to grow libraries in developing countries

www.elsevier.com • www.bookaid.org

I want to dedicate this book to my mother, Violeta, and my husband, Ken,
for their encouragement and support.

Lourdes M. DelRosso

Dedicated to my wife, Cathy, and my children, David and Sarah.

Richard B. Berry

This book is dedicated to the patients who live with sleep disorders and to my colleagues
and mentors who have taught me to understand and treat sleep disorders in children.
It is truly rewarding to help these children sleep.

Suzanne E. Beck

For my family, Barry, Daniel, and Analiese, who are everything to me!

Mary H. Wagner

Dedicated to my patients.

Carole L. Marcus

Preface

The goal of this book is to use the Pearls format to present information that we feel will be useful for sleep medicine physicians who care for pediatric patients, as well as for pediatricians who often have patients with challenging sleep problems without the ready availability of a specialist experienced in caring for infants and children. The case-based format with short chapters, each making a few important points, is a good way for physicians to acquire information easily in small portions. The need for this book grew out of feedback concerning *Sleep Medicine Pearls*, focused primarily on adults. More material on pediatric sleep problems was desired by a number of readers. In addition, we wanted to provide information about some less common pediatric sleep disorders seen at large referral centers (Children's Hospital of Philadelphia and UF Health Shands Children's Hospital).

The Editors

Acknowledgments

Angele Arthur MD, Methodist Charlton Medical Center, Dallas, TX, contributed to Case 93. Priya S. Prashad MD, MSCE, from New York Medical College, Valhalla, NY; and Lawrence W. Brown MD, Dennis J. Dlugos MD, Tamara Feygin MD, Brian N. Harding FRCPath, Gregory G. Heuer MD, PhD and Thornton B. Alexander Mason MD, PhD, all from The Children's Hospital of Philadelphia and the University of Pennsylvania, Philadelphia, PA, contributed to Case 67, which was previously published in Pediatric Neurology.

The authors thankfully acknowledge Joel Traylor, BS, RPSGT, for technical support.

We thank our team of sleep technologists and staff at the Children's Hospital of Philadelphia and at the University of Florida Health Sleep Center.

We thank the staff at Elsevier.

Last but not least, we would like to express our gratitude to our patients and their families, without whom this book would never have been possible.

Contents

PART 1

Introduction to Pediatric Sleep Medicine

CASE 1

Pediatric sleep history: A 4 year-old with snoring, gasping and witnessed apneas

Lourdes M. DelRosso

CASE PRESENTATION

A 4-year-old boy presented for evaluation of loud snoring, gasping during sleep, witnessed apnea, and increased work of breathing during sleep. The parents noted that the child often sleeps with his neck hyperextended. During the daytime, he is active and playful. He goes to bed at 8 PM and falls asleep within 15 minutes. He does not wake up during the night. He wakes up spontaneously at 8 AM. During the day, he takes a 1-hour nap at noon. He does not have any medical problems and does not take any medication. The review of systems was noncontributory.

QUESTION

Can you diagnose this child with obstructive sleep apnea syndrome (OSAS) based on history alone?

ANSWER

No. History is helpful in screening patients for OSAS and determining which need further evaluation, but polysomnography (PSG) is the gold standard for the diagnosis of pediatric OSAS.

DISCUSSION

Multiple studies have demonstrated that clinical history alone fails to accurately predict OSAS in children. Although snoring is the most common symptom in children who are diagnosed with OSAS, not all children who snore have OSAS. Indeed, although about 10% of young children snore every night,[1] only 1% to 4% of children have OSAS.[2] A study of 222 children with symptoms suggestive of OSAS demonstrated that snoring for more than five nights a week had a sensitivity of 77% and a specificity of 48% in detecting pediatric OSAS[3]; other studies have had similar findings. The American Academy of Pediatrics recommends screening children for snoring at each well-child visit.[1] Children who snore every night and have additional symptoms or signs suggestive of OSAS should be evaluated further (Box 1-1). Clinical history alone does not discriminate between habitual snorers and patients with OSAS.[4] Other nocturnal symptoms of OSAS include gasping, neck hyperextension, mouth breathing, diaphoresis, sleeping sitting up, and secondary enuresis (bedwetting in a child who was previously dry at night). Parents often describe that the child has increased work of breathing during sleep, with retractions and paradoxical breathing (parents notice the chest caving in or the abdomen moving forcefully). Diurnal symptoms may include inattention, hyperactivity, daytime sleepiness, morning headaches, and poor academic performance.[1] Witnessed apneas have a sensitivity of 42% and a specificity of 88%, whereas mouth breathing has a sensitivity of 84% and specificity of 23% in detecting OSAS.[3] If symptoms suggestive of OSAS are present, the American Academy of Pediatrics recommends nocturnal PSG or further evaluation by a sleep medicine specialist.[1] PSG is the gold standard for the diagnosis of OSAS.

Although clinical history does not predict the presence or severity of OSAS in children, a detailed clinical history aids in screening for sleep disorders in children (Table 1-1), and with some other diagnoses, history alone can provide a diagnosis. Sleep disorders that can usually be diagnosed by history alone include insomnia, restless legs syndrome, sleepwalking, night terrors, and disorders of circadian rhythm.

The pediatric history should include past medical history. The past medical history aids in screening patients at higher risk of sleep disorders (see cases in "Sleep in medical conditions"). Medication

---

BOX 1-1   SYMPTOMS AND SIGNS OF OSAS
History
Frequent snoring (≥3 nights/wk)
Labored breathing during sleep
Gasps or snorting noises or observed episodes of apnea
Sleep enuresis (especially secondary enuresis)[a]
Sleeping in a seated position or with the neck hyperextended
Cyanosis
Headaches on awakening
Daytime sleepiness
Attention-deficit hyperactivity disorder
Learning problems
Physical Examination
Underweight or overweight
Tonsillar hypertrophy
Adenoid facies
Micrognathia and retrognathia
High-arched palate
Failure to thrive
Hypertension

[a]Enuresis after at least 6 months of continence.
(Marcus CL, Brooks LJ, Draper KA, et al. Clinical Practice Guideline: Diagnosis and management of childhood obstructive sleep apnea syndrome. *Pediatrics.* Sep 2012;130(3):e714-e755.)

TABLE 1-1. Pediatric sleep history

Evaluation	Sample Question and/or Symptom	Sleep Disorder Screened
Sleep initiation	Does the child sleep in his own room? Does the child sleep in his own bed? Are there electronics in the bedroom? Is there a bedtime routine? Are there pets in the room?	Poor sleep hygiene
	Caffeine use Medications	Medication side effects
	Does the child fall asleep independently? How long does it take for the child to fall asleep? Uncomfortable feelings in the legs Urge to move the legs	Insomnia Circadian rhythm disorder Restless legs syndrome
Sleep maintenance	Snoring Witnessed apnea or gasping Increased work of breathing Enuresis Neck hyperextension	OSAS
	Sleepwalking Nightmares Night terrors	Parasomnias
	Frequent awakenings Hypnagogic hallucinations Sleep paralysis	Insomnia Sleep deprivation Narcolepsy
Daytime symptoms	Excessive daytime sleepiness Cataplexy	Narcolepsy
	Excessive daytime sleepiness Inattention and hyperactivity Irritability Cognitive deficits	OSAS Periodic limb movement disorder Insufficient sleep

Symptoms and signs of OSA (copyright PEDIATRICS Volume 130, Number 3, September 2012 Page 579).

lists must be updated at every sleep medicine visit because there are many medicines that adversely affect sleep (see "Drug effects on sleep"). Just as in other medical fields, the pediatric sleep history should also include past surgical history and family and social history.

Our patient was referred for PSG and OSAS was diagnosed.

CLINICAL PEARLS

1. Clinical history alone can be used to diagnose some pediatric sleep disorders, but not OSAS.
2. Clinical history can provide clues for patients at high risk of sleep disorders.
3. PSG is the gold standard for the diagnosis of pediatric OSAS.

REFERENCES

1. Marcus CL, Brooks LJ, Draper KA, et al. Clinical practice guideline: diagnosis and management of childhood obstructive sleep apnea syndrome. *Pediatrics*. Sep 2012;130(3):e714–e755.
2. Lumeng JC, Chervin RD. Epidemiology of pediatric obstructive sleep apnea. *Proc Am Thorac Soc*. Feb 15 2008;5(2):242–252.
3. Kang KT, Weng WC, Lee CH, et al. Detection of pediatric obstructive sleep apnea syndrome: history or anatomical findings? *Sleep Med*. May 2015;16(5):617–624.
4. Carroll JL, McColley SA, Marcus CL, Curtis S, Loughlin GM. Inability of clinical history to distinguish primary snoring from obstructive sleep apnea syndrome in children. *Chest*. Sep 1995;108(3):610–618.

A 6-year-old girl with tonsillar hypertrophy, high-arched palate, and snoring

Lourdes M. DelRosso

CASE PRESENTATION

A 6-year-old girl was referred for evaluation of snoring. The parents did not notice gasping or witness apnea. The family denied excessive daytime sleepiness, inattention, or hyperactivity. The patient did not have any other medical problems and did not take any medications.

PHYSICAL EXAM

Physical exam revealed a cooperative, alert girl, who was developmentally normal. Her height and weight were at the 50th percentile. Pulse was 80 beats/min, respiratory rate 14 breaths/min, and blood pressure 90/60 mm Hg. She did not have an adenoid facies. Her nasal mucosa and turbinates were normal. Her jaw was normal. Her oral airway exam revealed a high-arched palate (Figure 2-1), oropharynx that was Mallampati grade IV, and tonsil size 3+. The cardiopulmonary and neurologic exams were normal.

QUESTION

Should this child be diagnosed with obstructive sleep apnea syndrome (OSAS)?

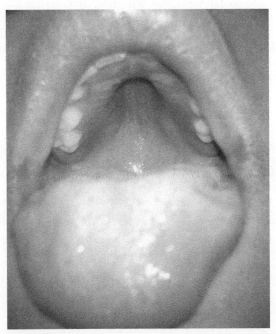

FIGURE 2-1 ■ Oral airway exam revealed high-arched palate.

ANSWER

No. OSAS is not diagnosed by history or physical exam. The child needs to be referred for polysomnography.

DISCUSSION

The physical exam on a pediatric sleep patient, just like in any other specialty, begins with observation of the patient. Genetic, neuromuscular, or neurodevelopmental conditions that predispose the patient to sleep disorders should be noted (see Section 14: Sleep in medical conditions and Sleep in neurologic conditions). The patient's level of alertness, affect, cooperation, and interaction can give clues to comorbidities that affect sleep (see Sleep in psychiatric conditions and Sleep and neurodevelopmental disorders). The child's anatomy must be carefully noted. The facial appearance includes noting syndromic features, adenoid facies, midface hypoplasia, micrognathia, or retrognathia. Scoliosis and other chest wall abnormalities must be noted. A thorough physical exam includes height, weight, and vital signs. The nasal exam includes evaluation of the nares, septum, nasal polyps, and turbinates. Inspection of the teeth, tongue, palate, tonsil size, and Mallampati score (for children old enough to cooperate; Table 2-1) follows. Initially, the Mallampati score was developed to predict difficult tracheal intubation.[1] It consisted of three grades assessed with the patient sticking out his or her tongue. The Mallampati score later was modified by Dr. Friedman, to apply it to patients with sleep-disordered breathing.[2] The Mallampati-Friedman score is assessed with the tongue in the neutral position inside the mouth. A fourth grade was added, as described in Table 2-1.[2] All the pearls in this book refer to the modified Mallampati-Friedman grade.

Studies have demonstrated a limited utility of tonsil size and Mallampati score as predictors of OSAS.[3] In fact, the positive predictive value of the physical exam to diagnose OSAS is 45%.[2] For this reason the American Academy of Pediatrics recommends objective testing with polysomnography.[4] Reasons for the low predictive value of physical exam include the fact that the tonsils may extend superiorly beyond what can be appreciated on physical exam, the inability to assess the adenoid on routine physical exam, and the effect of neuromotor factors on upper airway collapsibility during sleep.

Similar to the physical exam, the utility of imaging in the diagnosis of OSAS is limited. Lateral neck radiography can visualize the tonsils, adenoid, upper airway caliber, and neck soft tissue. However, this is not needed routinely to manage therapy in a typical child with OSAS and tonsillar hypertrophy on physical exam, because the otolaryngologist will directly visualize adenoidal size during surgery. Lateral neck radiographs or endoscopy may be useful in assessing for adenoidal regrowth in children with recurrence of OSAS and a history of prior adenoidectomy. Computed tomography and magnetic resonance imaging provide a more detailed view of the upper airway; however, these studies are not recommended as diagnostic tools for routine care of patients with OSAS.[5]

Our patient was referred for overnight polysomnography, which did not show obstructive sleep apnea.

TABLE 2-1.	Description of Brodsky tonsil size[6] and modified Mallampati-Friedman grade[1,2]		
Tonsil Size	**Description of Tonsils**	**Mallampati-Friedman**	**Description (Visible)**
0	Within the tonsillar fossa	I	Faucial pillars, soft palate, and uvula
1+	≤25% of the oropharyngeal width	II	Faucial pillars and soft palate visualized but uvula masked by the base of the tongue
2+	26%-50% of the oropharyngeal width	III	Only soft palate visible
3+	51%-75% of the oropharyngeal width	IV	Soft palate not visible
4+	>75% of the oropharyngeal width		

CLINICAL PEARLS

1. The physical exam has limited utility in the diagnosis of childhood OSAS.
2. Polysomnography is the gold standard tool in the diagnosis of pediatric OSAS patients.

REFERENCES

1. Mallampati SR, Gatt SP, Gugino LD, et al. A clinical sign to predict difficult tracheal intubation: a prospective study. *Can Anaesth Soc J.* Jul 1985;32(4):429–434.
2. Friedman M, Ibrahim H, Bass L. Clinical staging for sleep-disordered breathing. *Otolaryngol Head Neck Surg.* Jul 2002;127(1):13–21.
3. Mitchell RB, Garetz S, Moore RH, et al. The use of clinical parameters to predict obstructive sleep apnea syndrome severity in children: the Childhood Adenotonsillectomy (CHAT) study randomized clinical trial. *JAMA Otolaryngol Head Neck Surg.* Feb 2015;141(2):130–136.
4. Marcus CL, Brooks LJ, Draper KA, et al. Diagnosis and management of childhood obstructive sleep apnea syndrome. *Pediatrics.* Sep 2012;130(3):e714–e755.
5. Slaats MA, Van Hoorenbeeck K, Van Eyck A, et al. Upper airway imaging in pediatric obstructive sleep apnea syndrome. *Sleep Med Rev.* Jun 2015;21:59–71.
6. Brodsky L. Modern assessment of tonsils and adenoids. *Pediatr Clin North Am.* Dec 1989;36(6):1551–1569.

A 10-year-old girl with an unusual finding on physical exam

Lourdes M. DelRosso

CASE PRESENTATION

A 10-year-old girl was referred for evaluation of snoring. The parents noted that snoring started 3 weeks earlier, during a recent upper airway infection, but had resolved in the last week. The parents did not notice gasping or witness apnea. The family denied excessive daytime sleepiness, restless legs, or parasomnias. The patient did not have any other medical problems and did not take any medications. Her past surgical history was positive for tonsillectomy and adenoidectomy at age 6, for recurrent tonsillitis. The review of systems was negative for fever, sore throat, and difficulty swallowing.

PHYSICAL EXAM

Physical exam revealed a cooperative girl, afebrile. Her height and weight were at the 35th percentile. She did not have an adenoid facies. Her nasal mucosa and turbinates were normal. She did not have a high-arched palate. Her oral airway exam is seen in Figure 3-1. The remainder of the cardiovascular and neurologic exam was normal.

LABORATORY AND SLEEP FINDINGS

Soft-tissue lateral neck x-ray did not show adenoid hypertrophy.

QUESTIONS

In Figure 3-1, what does the white arrow point to? What is the next step in the care of this patient?

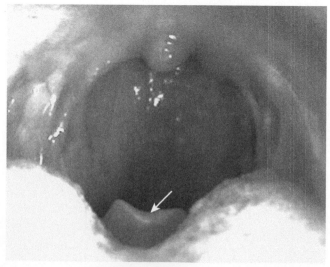

FIGURE 3-1 ■ Oral airway exam.

ANSWERS

The white arrow points at the epiglottis. The patient is currently asymptomatic, and no further intervention is recommended.

DISCUSSION

A visible epiglottis is a normal finding in children. The epiglottis derives from the third and fourth embryonic brachial arches.[1] In infants, the tip of the epiglottis is positioned at the level of the first cervical vertebra (C1). The proximity of the epiglottis to the soft palate allows the infant to feed and breathe at the same time by sealing off the nasal airway. The epiglottis starts descending after 6 months of age.[2] By 24 months, the tip of the epiglottis is at the middle of the body of the second cervical vertebra (C2). By 10 years of age, the tip of the epiglottis is anterior to the lower plate of C2. During adolescence and adulthood, the tip of the epiglottis lies anterior to the intervertebral disc space between C2 and C3.[3] Congenital abnormalities of the epiglottis are rare and include hypoplastic, bifid, and rudimentary epiglottis.

The oropharyngeal Mallampati grade was introduced in 1983 as a predictor of difficult airway intubation. It consists of four different grades (I-IV), with the lower grades representing a less crowded oropharyngeal anatomy. Later on, a Mallampati class 0 was added when the epiglottis was visible on mouth opening or tongue protrusion. In a study of 764 adults, Mallampati class 0 was seen in 1.18% of patients, and, incidentally, all were female.[4]

Our patient was asymptomatic. Her snoring was associated with an acute respiratory illness, and it resolved. A polysomnography was not recommended. The parents were educated on the signs and symptoms of obstructive sleep apnea.

CLINICAL PEARLS

1. The epiglottis can be visible during examination of the oropharynx in children.
2. The epiglottis may be visible in 1% of adults, predominantly in women.
3. Mallampati grade 0 can be cited in cases where the epiglottis is visible.

REFERENCES

1. Jamaluddin Ahmed F, Shinohara AL, Bonifecio da Silva SM, Andreo JC, Rodrigues Ade C. Visible epiglottis in children. *Int J Clin Pediatr Dent*. Sep-Dec 2014;7(3):223–224.
2. Alamri Y, Stringer MD. A high-rising epiglottis: a benign anatomical variant. *Clin Anat*. Jul 2011;24(5):652–654.
3. Schwartz DS, Keller MS. Maturational descent of the epiglottis. *Arch Otolaryngol Head Neck Surg*. Jun 1997;123(6):627–628.
4. Ezri T, Warters RD, Szmuk P, et al. The incidence of class "zero" airway and the impact of Mallampati score, age, sex, and body mass index on prediction of laryngoscopy grade. *Anesth Analg*. Oct 2001;93(4):1073–1075. table of contents.

Overview of pediatric polysomnography: A newborn infant with snoring and witnessed apnea

Lourdes M. DelRosso

CASE PRESENTATION

A newborn infant with micrognathia was referred for inpatient polysomnogram (PSG) during her neonatal intensive care unit admission for evaluation of snoring and witnessed apnea. The infant was born via normal spontaneous vaginal delivery at 40 weeks gestational age. Apgar scores were 7 at 1 minute and 9 at 5 minutes after birth. Soon after birth, the patient was noted to have breathing pauses. There was no other pertinent medical history.

PHYSICAL EXAM

Physical exam while awake revealed an active infant in no distress awake. Her vital signs were normal. Her weight was at the 45th percentile, length was at the 30th percentile, and head circumference was at the 60th percentile. She had micrognathia but was not otherwise dysmorphic. Her eyes, ears, and nose were normal. Oral exam revealed a normal palate. Her lungs were clear to auscultation bilaterally, with no retractions while awake. Neurologic exam was normal. As the infant fell asleep, there was gasping and witnessed apneas.

QUESTIONS

Can PSG be performed in a newborn infant?

ANSWERS

Yes, PSG can be performed in children of all ages.

DISCUSSION

PSG is the gold standard tool in the diagnosis of sleep-disordered breathing in children. The American Academy of Sleep Medicine (AASM) Practice Parameters for the respiratory indications of PSG in children recommends PSG for the diagnosis of obstructive sleep apnea, among other respiratory indications (Table 4-1),[1] and PSG is often used to evaluate obstructive apnea, central apnea, or hypoxemia in the newborn. Nap PSG is not recommended for the diagnosis of obstructive sleep apnea syndrome (OSAS). The nonrespiratory indications for PSG (usually in older children) include evaluation of periodic leg movement disorder, evaluation of suspected narcolepsy (followed by a multiple sleep latency test), nocturnal seizure disorder, atypical parasomnias, and suspicion of restless legs syndrome.[2] PSG is not indicated for evaluation of bruxism or typical, noninjurious parasomnias.

PSG should be performed according to the AASM Manual for the Scoring of Sleep and Associated Events. Sleep architecture is scored differently in infants <2 months of age, and criteria for infant sleep stage scoring are now included in the manual. Respiratory events are scored differently for children <18 years of age (optional for children aged >13 years); these differences are outlined in the manual. The parameters reported for pediatric PSGs are similar to those reported for adult patients, except that the AASM recommends reporting periodic breathing and hypoventilation during the diagnostic PSG. Portable sleep study devices are currently not recommended for use in children.

Our patient underwent PSG in the neonatal intensive care unit. Severe OSAS was diagnosed. The patient was evaluated by the plastic surgery team for mandibular distraction.

TABLE 4-1. **Respiratory indications for polysomnography in children**	
Diagnosis	**Management**
1. Obstructive sleep apnea 2. Congenital central hypoventilation 3. Sleep-related hypoventilation 4. Primary sleep apnea of infancy	1. After adenotonsillectomy, for evaluation of residual obstructive sleep apnea 2. Continuous positive airway pressure titration 3. After craniofacial surgery for OSAS 4. OSAS treated with oral appliances 5. Prior to tracheostomy decannulation

CLINICAL PEARLS

1. PSG is useful in children of all ages.
2. PSG in children is used for the evaluation of respiratory and nonrespiratory conditions.
3. Hypoventilation and periodic breathing are reported in pediatric PSGs.

REFERENCES

1. Aurora RN, Zak RS, Karippot A, et al. Practice parameters for the respiratory indications for polysomnography in children. *Sleep*. Mar 2011;34(3):379–388.
2. Aurora RN, Lamm CI, Zak RS, et al. Practice parameters for the non-respiratory indications for polysomnography and multiple sleep latency testing for children. *Sleep*. Nov 2012;35(11):1467–1473.

A 2-week-old infant with some challenging epochs on polysomnography

Lourdes M. DelRosso

CASE PRESENTATION

The sleep technician asks your opinion about stage scoring on an infant's polysomnography (PSG). The study was performed on a 2-week-old infant because of parental concern for breathing pauses. A representative epoch is shown in Figure 5-1.

QUESTION

What stage is seen in this epoch?

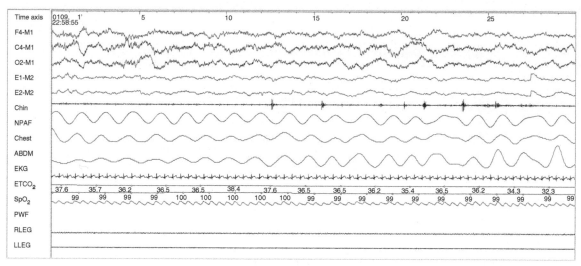

FIGURE 5-1 ■ Representative epoch during which the infant is quiet, not moving, and with his eyes closed.

ANSWER

The epoch has features of NREM sleep, such as closed eyes, regular respiration, and absence of rapid eye movements. There are also features of REM sleep: low-baseline chin electromyogram (EMG) with transient muscle activity and low-voltage mixed-frequency electroencephalogram (EEG). The stage is transitional sleep (Stage T).

DISCUSSION

The American Academy of Sleep Medicine (AASM) Manual for the Scoring of Sleep and Associated Events version 2.2, section IV, states the scoring criteria for sleep staging in children (infants older than 2 months to children younger than 18 years) and infants (full-term birth to 2 months of age).[1] Section VIII of the manual describes the scoring criteria for respiratory events in children. The criteria are summarized in Tables 5-1 and 5-2. Scoring of stages and respiratory events differs between children and adults. Pediatric scoring rules for respiratory events are recommended for use in children younger than 13 years old and are optional for children between 13 and 18 years of age.

The physiologic parameters measured in pediatric PSG are similar to those measured in adults, with a few exceptions, mainly capnography. Although recording hypoventilation is "optional" in adults, it is "recommended" in children. For a more detailed explanation of capnography, see Clinical Pearls

TABLE 5-1.   Summary of pediatric sleep staging (see the manual for full criteria)

Stage	Infants 0-2 mo Post Term	Infants and Children Older Than 2 mo Post Term
Wakefulness (Stage W)	Any of the following are present: 1. Eyes open 2. Vocalization or feeding 3. Eyes open intermittently or scanning eye movements **plus** sustained chin EMG tone with bursts of muscle activity **plus** irregular respiration **plus** low-voltage irregular or mixed-voltage EEG	Any of the following are present: 1. >50% posterior dominant rhythm (PDR) 2. Eye blinks, scanning eye movements, or rapid eye movements with increased chin tone
NREM 1	N/A	PDR <50% of epoch If no PDR, any of the following: 1. EEG: 4-7 Hz with slowing of >1-2 Hz from stage W 2. EEG: High-amplitude 3-5 Hz 3. Slow eye movements 4. Vertex sharp waves 5. Hypnagogic hypersynchrony
NREM 2	N/A	Same as adult (K complexes and sleep spindles)
NREM 3	N/A	Same as adults (>20% slow wave activity)
NREM	>4 of the following are present: 1. Eyes closed (no eye movements) 2. Chin tone in chin EMG 3. Regular respiration 4. EEG: Trace alternant, high-voltage slow or sleep spindles Few body movements	NREM without recognizable spindles, K complex, or slow waves
REM	>4 of the following are present: 1. Low chin EMG 2. Eyes closed (at least one rapid eye movement) 3. Irregular respiration 4. Sucking, twitches, or brief head movements Continuous EEG without spindles	Same as adult
Transitional (Stage T)	Either 3 NREM and 2REM or 2 NREM and 3 REM characteristics	N/A

TABLE 5-2.   **Comparison between pediatric and adult respiratory scoring rules (all criteria must be met)[1]**

Event	Pediatric Scoring Criteria for Children <18 yr Old (Optional for Children ≥13 yr)	Adult Scoring Criteria For Adults >18 yr Old (Optional for Children ≥13 yr)
Obstructive apnea	≥90% drop in oronasal thermal sensor Minimum of two breaths duration Presence of respiratory effort during the event	≥90% drop in oronasal thermal sensor Minimum of 10 sec duration Presence of respiratory effort during the event
Central apnea	≥90% drop in oronasal thermal sensor Absence of respiratory effort during the event Event lasts ≥20 sec **or** is shorter (minimum of two breaths duration) but is associated with **either**: 1. Arousal 2. ≥3% desaturation 3. For infants <1 yr: decrease in heart rate to <50 beats/min for at least 5 sec or <60 beats/min for 15 sec	≥90% drop in oronasal thermal sensor Absence of respiratory effort during the event Event lasts ≥10 sec
Mixed apnea	≥90% drop in oronasal thermal sensor Minimum of two breaths duration Absence of effort in one portion of the event and presence of effort in another portion of the event	≥90% drop in oronasal thermal sensor Minimum of 10 sec duration Absence of effort in the beginning of the event and presence of effort in the second part of the event
Hypopnea	≥30% drop in nasal pressure transducer signal ≥3% desaturation **or** arousal Minimum of two breaths duration	≥30% drop in nasal pressure transducer signal ≥3% desaturation **or** arousal Minimum of 10 sec duration
Obstructive hypopnea (optional)	Meets criteria for hypopnea and **any** of the following: 1. Snoring 2. Increased flattening of the nasal pressure transducer signal 3. Chest-abdomen paradoxing	Meets criteria for hypopnea and **any** of the following: 1. Snoring 2. Increased flattening of the nasal pressure transducer signal 3. Chest-abdomen paradoxing
Central hypopnea (optional)	Meets criteria for hypopnea and **none** of the following is present: 1. Snoring 2. Increased flattening of the nasal pressure transducer signal 3. Chest-abdomen paradoxing	Meets criteria for hypopnea and **none** of the following is present: 1. Snoring 2. Increased flattening of the nasal pressure transducer signal 3. Chest-abdomen paradoxing
Respiratory-effort-related arousal (optional)	Minimum of two breaths duration Does not meet hypopnea criteria but has increased effort, flattening of nasal pressure, or elevation of $ETCO_2$ associated with an arousal	Minimum of 10 sec duration Does not meet hypopnea criteria but has increased effort or flattening of nasal pressure associated with an arousal
Hypoventilation	Recommended PCO_2 >50 mm Hg for >25% of Total Sleep Time	Optional Either: 1. Arterial PCO_2 >55 mm Hg for ≥10 min 2. Elevation in PCO_2 ≥10 mm Hg during sleep to values above 50 mm Hg for ≥10 min
Periodic breathing or Cheyne-Stokes	Periodic breathing: ≥3 central pauses, lasting >3 sec each, separated by ≤20 sec of normal breathing	Cheyne-Stokes (all must apply): 1. ≥3 central events (apneas or hypopneas) 2. Crescendo-decrescendo pattern of breathing between events 3. Cycle length ≥40 sec 4. ≥5 events over ≥2 h of recording

in Case 6: A 14-year-old with an abnormal $ETCO_2$ waveform during polysomnography. Reporting periodic breathing is also "recommended" in children, unlike in adults (who are more likely to have Cheyne-Stokes respiration than periodic breathing). The montage, sampling rates, and filter settings for each channel are found in the AASM scoring manual.

For indications for PSG in children, see Clinical Pearls in Case 4: Overview of pediatric polysomnography.

CLINICAL PEARLS

1. The rules for scoring sleep stages and respiratory events are found in the AASM Manual for the Scoring of Sleep and Associated Events.
2. Sleep stages for full-term infants from 0 to 2 months of age are wakefulness, NREM, REM, and Stage T.
3. Sleep stages for children and infants older than 2 months are wakefulness, NREM, NREM1, NREM2, NREM3, and REM sleep.
4. Scoring rules for respiratory events in children are different from those for adults.

REFERENCE

1. Berry RB, Gamaldo CE, Harding SM, Lloyd RM, Marcus CL, Vaughn BV. *The AASM Manual for the Scoring of Sleep and Associated Events: Rules, Terminology and Technical Specifications, Version 2.2*. Darrien, IL: American Academy of Sleep Medicine; 2015.

A 14-year-old with an abnormal end-tidal CO_2 waveform during polysomnography

Lourdes M. DelRosso

CASE PRESENTATION

A 14-year-old boy presented for evaluation of snoring. The patient snored loudly and breathed through his mouth. He did not have any other sleep-related concerns and did not have any other medical problems. His past surgical history was significant for tonsillectomy and adenoidectomy for recurrent tonsillitis at age 4.

PHYSICAL EXAM

Physical exam revealed an alert, cooperative, and obese boy. His vital signs were within the normal range. His height was at the 45th percentile, and his weight was at the 95th percentile. He had a slightly adenoid facies. He did not have enlarged turbinates. The oropharynx was Mallampati grade III. Tonsils were surgically absent. He did not have micrognathia or retrognathia. The remainder of the exam was normal.

LABORATORY AND SLEEP FINDINGS

The polysomnography (PSG) revealed a sleep efficiency of 87%, with normal sleep-stage distribution. The apnea–hypopnea index was 1/h. The mean SpO_2 was 97%, with a nadir of 95%. There was no evidence of hypoventilation (end-tidal CO_2 was <50 torr for the entire study). The Periodic leg movement index (PLMI) was 0/h. You review the study (sample epoch is seen in Fig. 6-1).

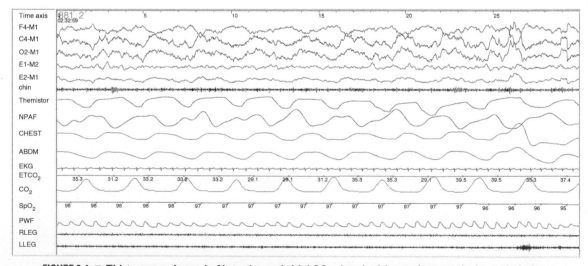

FIGURE 6-1 ■ Thirty-second epoch. Note the end-tidal CO_2 signal without plateaus during exhalation.

QUESTION

What causes the end-tidal CO$_2$ waveforms seen in Figures 6-1 and 6-2? How reliable is the CO$_2$ value?

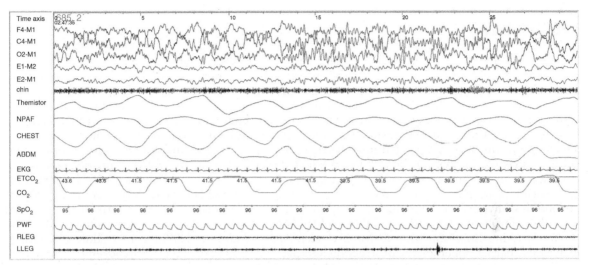

FIGURE 6-2 ■ Thirty-second epoch with end-tidal CO$_2$ signal with notched appearance.

ANSWER

The end-tidal signal CO$_2$ waveform shows triangular peaks and notched waveforms rather than the end-tidal plateaus associated with low CO$_2$ values. These artifacts can be seen in patients with nasal obstruction and mouth breathing and in patients receiving supplemental oxygen through the cannula. A notched appearance may be due to moisture in the tubing.

DISCUSSION

An arterial blood gas is the gold standard test for assessment of oxygenation and ventilation. Unfortunately, the test requires an invasive arterial puncture that can be associated with significant side effects including pain and rarely infection or damage to the blood vessel. Further, the blood gas provides information for only one moment in time (unless an indwelling catheter is used), and the child is often crying and hyperventilating during the procedure. Noninvasive monitoring of oxygenation by pulse oximetry and ventilation by capnography (end-tidal CO$_2$ monitoring) or transcutaneous CO$_2$ monitoring is recommended in pediatric polysomnography as alternative measures of oxygenation and ventilation during PSG. These methods are advantageous in that they provide continuous monitoring during nocturnal PSG.[1] The American Academy of Sleep Medicine (AASM) Manual for the scoring of sleep and associated events recommends the use of end-tidal CO$_2$ or arterial PCO$_2$ for detection of hypoventilation during a diagnostic PSG. Monitoring for hypoventilation is optional for adults but recommended for children. This is because hypoventilation is common in children, particularly in association with obstructive sleep apnea syndrome. Children may show a pattern of persistent, partial upper airway obstruction associated with hypercapnia and hypoxemia, rather than cyclic, discrete obstructive apneas; this has been termed *obstructive hypoventilation*.[2] According to the AASM manual, the use of transcutaneous PCO$_2$ or arterial PCO$_2$ monitoring during a titration PSG study is optional, but transcutaneous PCO$_2$ monitoring is often performed in pediatric patients (in addition to monitoring of end-tidal PCO$_2$).

The end-tidal PCO$_2$ and transcutaneous PCO$_2$ values must be interpreted carefully. A valid end-tidal PCO$_2$ wave must have an end-tidal plateau (Figs. 6-3 and 6-4). Signals without plateaus (see Figs. 6-1 and 6-2) might provide a falsely low end-tidal PCO$_2$ value and often occur in patients with nasal obstruction, mouth breathing, those receiving supplemental oxygen via cannula, or because of technical issues with placement of the cannula or secretions or condensate collecting in the tubing. The capnography waveform consists of four phases (see Fig. 6-3). Phase 1 represents the exhaled anatomic dead space and should not contain CO$_2$ (except in cases of rebreathing). Phase 2 represents a mixture of anatomic and alveolar dead space. Phase 3 represent the alveolar CO$_2$. The end of phase 3 is the peak end-tidal CO$_2$ value, which is the value to be reported. This plateau has a slight uptick. Phase 4 represents inspiration.

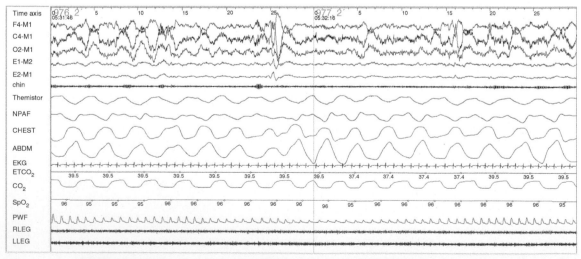

FIGURE 6-3 ■ Sixty-second epoch with accurate end-tidal CO$_2$ signal (with plateau).

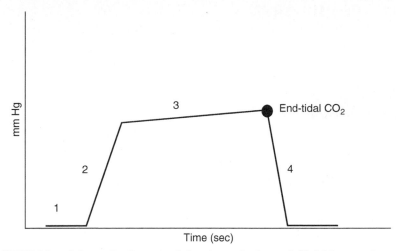

FIGURE 6-4 ■ **Schematic diagram of the phases in the end-tidal CO$_2$ waveform.**

Transcutaneous PCO$_2$ uses different technology than that used to measure end-tidal PCO$_2$. The transcutaneous monitor measures an approximation of arterial CO$_2$ by warming the skin via heated electrochemical sensors to "arteriolize" the skin capillary blood flow. The signal usually lags behind the end-tidal CO$_2$ changes by 2 minutes or more and is, therefore, more useful in detecting trends than breath-to-breath changes. The sensors must be moved during the night to avoid skin burns and must be regularly re-membraned and calibrated.[3] It cannot be used in patients with extensive skin damage, for example, severe eczema, or in patients with poor perfusion and might not work well in very obese patients. New transcutaneous PCO$_2$ equipment can use lower skin temperature, and probes are less likely to cause burns.

There are pros and cons to each type of CO$_2$ measurement.[4] End-tidal CO$_2$ provides breath-by-breath values, showing brief hypercapnic episodes associated with obstructive apnea, and it is also useful as an ancillary sensor to detect apnea. During PSG, end-tidal CO$_2$ monitoring can be performed using a specialized cannula that also provides nasal pressure monitoring. However, the technologist must be diligent about purging the cannula if it fills with secretions, as well as placement of the cannula, which may need to be repositioned over the mouth if the child is mouth breathing. End-tidal values can be falsely low in patients with severe chronic obstructive lung disease, such as cystic fibrosis, because of long and variable time constants (resistance × compliance of the alveolar units) in these patients. Transcutaneous monitoring provides steady-state measurements, which are particularly helpful in patients receiving continuous positive airway pressure (CPAP) or supplemental oxygen, when it could be difficult to acquire a good end-tidal waveform.

The sleep study in our patient did not show obstructive sleep apnea. Weight loss was recommended, along with otolaryngology evaluation for possible nasal obstruction causing snoring and mouth breathing.

CLINICAL PEARLS

1. Arterial blood gas reading is the gold standard for assessment of oxygenation and ventilation.
2. Arterial PCO$_2$, end-tidal CO$_2$, and transcutaneous CO$_2$ are recommended in diagnostic PSG for pediatric patients.
3. The presence of a plateau on the end-tidal CO$_2$ waveform indicates a valid signal.

REFERENCES

1. Beck SE, Marcus CL. Pediatric polysomnography. *Sleep Med Clin*. Sep 2009;4(3):393–406.
2. Standards and indications for cardiopulmonary sleep studies in children. American Thoracic Society. *Am J Respir Crit Care Med*. Feb 1996;153(2):866–878.
3. Eberhard P. The design, use, and results of transcutaneous carbon dioxide analysis: current and future directions. *Anesth Analg*. Dec 2007;105(6 Suppl):S48–S52.
4. Redline S, Budhiraja R, Kapur V, et al. The scoring of respiratory events in sleep: reliability and validity. *J Clin Sleep Med*. Mar 15 2007;3(2):169–200.

CASE 7

A 3-year-old boy with rhythmic activity on electroencephalogram

Lourdes M. DelRosso

CASE PRESENTATION

A 3-year-old boy presented for evaluation of snoring. The parents stated that snoring started 3 months earlier, but they had not noticed gasping or witnessed pauses. His sleep schedule was consistent without nocturnal awakenings, but the child was described as a restless sleeper. The parents denied night terrors, sleepwalking, or nightmares. The child did not have any past medical or surgical history and was not taking any medications. Review of systems was negative for asthma, allergies, or gastroesophageal reflux. He was developing normally. Polysomnography (PSG) was ordered to evaluate snoring.

PHYSICAL EXAM

Physical exam revealed a well-developed child, with normal developmental milestones for age. His vital signs were within normal limits. His height was 87 cm (27th percentile), and his weight was 13 kg (46th percentile). He did not have an adenoid facies or a high-arched palate. The oropharyngeal Mallampati grade was III, and tonsil size was 1+. His lungs were clear to auscultation. The remainder of his exam was normal.

LABORATORY AND SLEEP FINDINGS

Nocturnal PSG revealed the following: total sleep time 430 minutes, total recording time 537 minutes, sleep efficiency 85%, arousal index 10/h, periodic leg movement index 1/h, and apnea–hypopnea index (AHI) 0.9/h. There were frequent epochs showing rhythmic electroencephalogram (EEG) activity as seen in Figure 7-1. These EEG waves were seen during N1 and N2 and during sleep-wake transitions.

QUESTIONS

Is the activity seen in Figure 7-1 normal in this child?

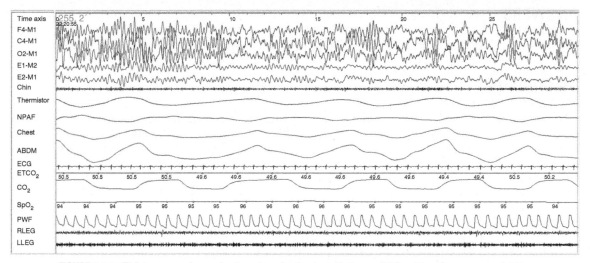

FIGURE 7-1 ■ Thirty-second epoch showing rhythmic activity on EEG with a frequency of 4 Hz.

ANSWERS

Yes, this is a normal finding in children. Figure 7-1 shows hypnagogic hypersynchrony (HH).

DISCUSSION

The scoring manual defines HH as bilateral, rhythmic, and paroxysmal activity consisting of diffuse, high-amplitude (75 to 350 μV) sinusoidal waves with a frequency of 3 to 4.5 Hz. These waves, usually more pronounced in the central derivations, appear in drowsiness and disappear when deeper stages of sleep are achieved. Although described as bilateral and symmetric, asymmetric HH has been described and should not be considered abnormal. HH is seen in 95% of normal infants at 6 months of age, and it decreases with age, seen in only 10% of 11-year-olds. Rarely, a small sharp wave can be seen interspersed between the HH waves, and it should be interpreted with caution because it usually does not represent "spike and wave."[1] Hypersynchronous theta (4 to 7 Hz) and delta (0.5 to 4 Hz) activity have also been described during arousal out of NREM in normal children.[2]

In this patient, an AHI <1.4/h is considered normal, and a diagnosis of primary snoring was made.

CLINICAL PEARLS

1. HH is a normal finding in infants and children.
2. HH is a rhythmic, diffuse, bilateral, and high-amplitude rhythm with a frequency of 3 to 4.5 Hz.
3. A diagnosis of primary snoring is made if a PSG is normal but snoring is present.

REFERENCES

1. Azzam R, Bhatt AB. Mimickers of generalized spike and wave discharges. *Neurodiagn J*. Jun 2014;54(2):156–162.
2. Williams SG, Correa D, Lesage S, Lettieri C. Electroencephalographic hypersynchrony in a child with night terrors. *Sleep Breath*. May 2013;17(2):465–467.

A 3-month-old infant with monomorphic waves on electroencephalogram

Lourdes M. DelRosso

CASE PRESENTATION

A 3-month-old infant is referred for evaluation of breathing pauses. The infant was born full term, without complications. The parents noticed brief breathing pauses during sleep and soft snoring. The parents denied gasping or episodes of cyanosis. The infant was born full term via normal spontaneous vaginal delivery from a G3P2 mother; there were no complications at birth. There was no other contributory medical history or review of systems.

PHYSICAL EXAM

The infant slept comfortably and appeared in no distress. His weight was at the 78th percentile, and his length was at the 63th percentile. There was no nasal obstruction and no cleft palate. The cardio-vascular and neurologic exams were normal.

LABORATORY AND SLEEP FINDINGS

A polysomnography (PSG) revealed a total sleep time of 420 minutes and lights on epoch-lights out epoch (TRT) of 515 minutes; the sleep efficiency was 81%. Sleep stage distribution was normal for age. Apnea–hypopnea index was 0.6 SpO_2; nadir was 96%. A representative epoch during wakefulness is seen in Figure 8-1.

QUESTIONS

Is the electroencephalogram (EEG) normal for his age?

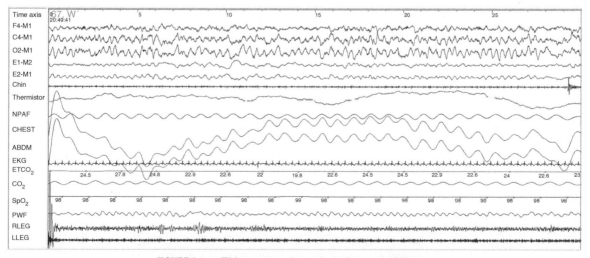

FIGURE 8-1 ■ **Thirty-second epoch during wakefulness.**

ANSWERS

Yes, the EEG is normal, and it demonstrates posterior dominant rhythm (PDR) with a frequency of 3.5 Hz.

DISCUSSION

PDR on EEG, usually called "alpha rhythm" in the mature brain, consists of monomorphic, sinusoidal waves seen in the occipital leads during relaxed wakefulness with the eyes closed. The frequency in adults and children older than 8 years of age is 8 to 13 Hz. Eye opening or stimulation will attenuate the alpha rhythm.

PDR can be distinguished by 3 months of age, and, typically, it consists of waves with a frequency of 3 to 4 Hz.[1,2] The frequency increases with age (Table 8-1). The amplitude of the PDR in adults is usually 15 to 45 μV, and in children, 50 to 60 μV, with 95% of children and 65% of adults having asymmetric amplitude with higher voltages on the right side, possibly because of differences in the thickness of the skull. PDR with lower frequencies than expected for age may represent a pathologic process and, thus, requires further evaluation.[2]

TABLE 8-1. Posterior dominant rhythm frequencies at different ages

Age	Frequency (Hz)
3 mo	3.5
6 mo	6
36 mo	8
9 yr	9
Adult	8-13

CLINICAL PEARLS

1. The PDR can be seen in infants 3 months or older, during relaxed wakefulness with eyes closed. The signal is attenuated with eye opening.
2. The frequency of the PDR increases with age until the adult frequency of 8 to 13 Hz is reached.
3. PDR with lower frequencies than expected for age may represent a pathologic process and, thus, requires further evaluation.

REFERENCES

1. Scraggs TL. EEG maturation: viability through adolescence. *Neurodiagn J*. Jun 2012;52(2):176–203.
2. Laoprasert P. *Atlas of Pediatric EEG*. New York, NY: McGraw-Hill Medical; 2011.

A newborn infant with an alternating electroencephalogram pattern

Lourdes M. DelRosso

CASE PRESENTATION

A newborn infant was referred for polysomnography (PSG) for evaluation of suspected breathing pauses. The infant was born full term without complications. The parents noticed some brief breathing pauses during sleep. The parents denied snoring, gasping, or episodes of cyanosis. There is no other contributory medical history or review of systems.

PHYSICAL EXAM

The patient was a full-term infant with length and weight at the 50th percentile. Physical exam revealed a normal nasal bridge, no retrognathia, and no cleft palate. The remainder of the exam was also normal.

LABORATORY AND SLEEP FINDINGS

PSG revealed a total sleep time of 460 minutes, lights on epoch-lights out epoch of 589 minutes, sleep efficiency 78%, and apnea–hypopnea index of 1.2/h. There were no central apneas, no cardiac arrhythmias, and no periodic limb movements during sleep.

A representative epoch during sleep is shown in Figure 9-1.

QUESTIONS

Is the electroencephalogram (EEG) normal? What is this EEG pattern called?

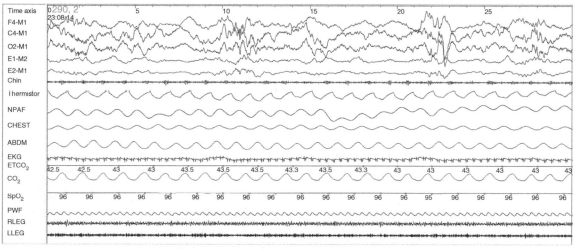

FIGURE 9-1 ■ Thirty-second epoch during sleep.

ANSWERS

Yes, this is a normal EEG in the newborn. The EEG pattern is called *trace alternant*.

DISCUSSION

The EEG of the developing brain has bursts of high-amplitude mixed-frequency waves interspersed with periods of flat, attenuated activity. This pattern is called *trace discontinue*, and it is present until 36 weeks postconceptional age. This rhythm is later replaced by "trace alternant," in which brief bursts of high-amplitude delta waves are interspersed among periods of low-amplitude waves (25 to 50 μV). This pattern can be seen up to 46 weeks postconceptional age. As the neonate matures, the EEG pattern continues evolving into the patterns seen in wake, NREM, and REM sleep. Sleep spindles are usually seen by 2 months of age but might appear as early as at birth in a full-term infant, and K complexes develop by 4 months. Usually, REM and all NREM stages of sleep can be identified by 6 months of age.[1]

CLINICAL PEARLS

1. Trace discontinue and trace alternant are EEG patterns seen in the developing brain.
2. Trace discontinue is usually seen until 36 weeks postconceptional age.
3. Trace alternant can be seen up to 46 weeks postconceptional age.

REFERENCES

1. Scraggs TL. EEG maturation: viability through adolescence. *Neurodiagn J.* Jun 2012;52(2):176–203.

A 2-month-old infant with sleep-onset REM period on polysomnography

Mary H. Wagner

CASE PRESENTATION

A concerned set of first-time parents present to the clinic with their 2-month-old infant. The infant is very sleepy during the day, sleeping 3 to 4 hours, and then maintaining wakefulness for only 1 hour before falling back to sleep again. The parents have noticed that the baby's mouth and face twitch at sleep onset. They have been researching sleep online and are concerned that this is a manifestation of sleep-onset REM (SOREMP), which, combined with the infant's sleepiness, indicates that the baby has narcolepsy. The baby was born full term by normal vaginal delivery with no complications. Family medical history, past medical history, and review of systems were negative.

PHYSICAL EXAM

Cardiopulmonary and neurologic exams were normal.

QUESTION

What is the next step in the care of this infant?

ANSWER

Parental reassurance and education that this baby has a normal sleeping pattern, including SOREMPs.

DISCUSSION

The sleep-wake schedule for infants <3 months of age is characterized by sleep periods lasting 3 to 4 hours, with periods of wakefulness lasting 1 to 2 hours for feeding, which occur around the clock. Three sleep states can be distinguished in newborns: REM sleep, NREM sleep, and transitional stage (see Clinical Pearls in Case 5: A 2-week-old infant with some challenging epochs on polysomnography). During the first year of life, the sleep pattern and distribution of sleep stages change as the infant matures. Entering sleep through stage REM is normal for infants <3 months of age, with a transition to the mature pattern of entering sleep through NREM sleep noted after age 3 months. Schultz showed that infants <3 months of age had REM latencies (REM latency being the time from sleep onset to the first appearance of REM sleep) predominantly <8 minutes.[1] By age 6 months, fewer sleep onsets (about 18%) occur through REM.[2] In adults, REM latency is typically approximately 90 minutes, and *SOREMP* is defined as REM occurring within 15 minutes of sleep onset.[3]

The specific EEG patterns allowing the identification of different stages of NREM sleep begin to appear at age 2 months. By age 6 months, K complexes, spindles, and slow waves have appeared, allowing the identification of different stages of NREM sleep.[3] Over the first year of life, the amount of REM sleep decreases from 50% to 30%,[2] resulting in a change in the ratio of REM to NREM. This shifts from the amount of REM sleep being greater than NREM sleep in newborns to the amount of NREM sleep exceeding the amount of REM sleep in 60% of 3-month-old infants and 90% of 6-month-old infants.[4]

The sleep duration and timing also change during the first year of life. Newborns sleep in 3- to 4-hour stretches, with 1 to 2 hours of wakefulness. In a study by Coons, sleep cycles were noted to lengthen by 6 weeks of age, with further lengthening through age 6 months.[2] This is accompanied by extended periods of wakefulness, which gradually increase to 3 to 4 hours by age 4 months. The timing of sleep periods also shifts, with consolidation of longer sleep periods at night and well-defined daytime naps, usually by age 4 months. During the first 6 months of life, the total sleep duration in infants ranges from a mean of 14.2 hours to the 98% percentile level of 18.1 hours.[5] Further, Iglowstein et al. found that all children nap through age 1 year, with the duration of daytime napping decreasing from 5.4 to 3.4 hours.[5] Nap duration decreases further with age, with most children stopping daytime naps by 5 years of age.

The parents of the infant in this case were reassured that the baby had a normal sleep pattern for age, including entering sleep through stage REM sleep.

CLINICAL PEARLS

1. At term, three sleep states can be identified in infants: REM, NREM, and transitional.
2. Infants normally enter sleep through REM sleep through age 3 months.
3. During infancy, the amount of REM sleep decreases from approximately 50% to 30%.
4. Sleep duration and timing also shift as the infant matures, with consolidation of nocturnal sleep and discrete daytime naps.

REFERENCES

1. Schulz H, Salzarulo P, Fagioli I, Massertani R. REM latency: development in the first year of life. *Electroencephalogr Clin Neurophysiol*. 1983;56(4):316–322.
2. Coons S. Development of sleep and wakefulness during the first 6 months of life. In: Guilleminault C, ed. *Sleep and Its Disorders in Children*. New York: Raven Press; 1987:17–27.
3. Berry RB. *Fundamentals of Sleep Medicine*. Philadelphia: Elsevier Saunders; 2012:224, 82, 70.
4. Sheldon S. Development of sleep in infants and children. In: Sheldon S, Ferber R, Kryer MH, Gozal D, eds. *Principles and Practice of Pediatric Sleep Medicine*. 2nd ed. Philadelphia: Elsevier Saunders; 2014:17–20.
5. Iglowstein I, Jenni OG, Molinari L, Largo RH. Sleep duration from infancy to adolescence: reference values and generational trends. *Pediatrics*. 2003;111(2):302–307.

An infant with high amplitude on an electroencephalogram recording

Mary H. Wagner

CASE PRESENTATION

A sleep technologist new to your center has asked you to review a worrisome electroencephalogram (EEG) recording obtained on an infant aged 10 months. The infant was undergoing a sleep study for mild snoring and restlessness. The infant was born at term, without problems, and has been healthy without significant medical issues. No history of seizures has been reported. The technologist is concerned that the EEG finding may indicate seizure activity because of the high amplitude of the EEG waves. The technologist had been practicing in an adult sleep laboratory for the past 5 years. The EEG from the sleep study is shown in Figure 11-1.

QUESTION

Does this EEG represent an abnormal finding?

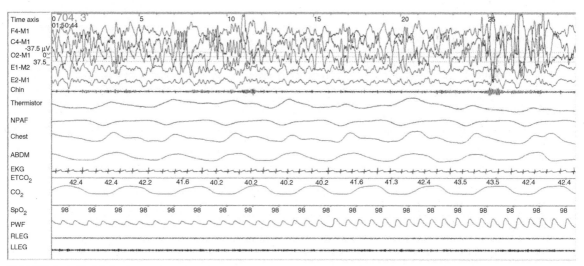

FIGURE 11-1 ■ Multiple channel tracing from the sleep study. F4-M1, C4-M1,O2-M1, E1-M2,E2-M1 are electroencephalogram leads used for sleep staging; NPAF- nasal pressure; ABDM- abdomen; EKG-electrocardiogram; ETCO2- end tidal carbon dioxide; CO2- carbon dioxide; SpO2- oxygen saturation; PWF- pulse wave form; RLEG- right leg electromyogram; LLEG- left leg electromyogram.

ANSWER

No, the EEG demonstrates slow wave activity with the high EEG voltage amplitude characteristically seen in young children.

DISCUSSION

The sleep of normal infants changes dramatically during the first year of life. Changes include the development of EEG waveforms that allow NREM sleep to be divided into stages N1, N2, and N3. Stages N1, N2, and N3 should be identifiable by 5 to 6 months of life,[1] with the identification of sleep spindles by age 3 months and both K complexes and slow wave activity by 6 months. *Slow wave activity* is defined by a frequency of 0.5 to 2 Hz and amplitude >100 μV and is maximal over the frontal scalp regions.[2] As noted in the AASM scoring manual, slow wave activity in children is frequently of high amplitude (100 to 400 μV).[2] Slow wave activity in adults has a similar frequency but a lower peak-to-peak amplitude (>75 μV). In both adults and children, N3 sleep is scored when 20% of an epoch of sleep consists of slow wave activity meeting frequency (0.5 to 2 Hz) and amplitude criteria (>75 μV) in the frontal leads.[2] One potential source of confusion for sleep technologists used to scoring adult records, is the high amplitude of slow waves noted in children. Of note, older people have slow wave activity that is lower in both density and amplitude.[3,4] Dubé has hypothesized that changes in slow wave activity in adults are related to cortical thinning in brain regions thought to be important in slow wave generation.[4]

Figure 11-1 shows a 30-second epoch with high-voltage EEG waves. The amplitude is highest in the frontal leads and slightly lower in the central and occipital leads. In addition, the respiratory pattern is quite regular in depth and frequency, another characteristic of slow wave sleep. There is no evidence of seizure activity.

CLINICAL PEARLS

1. The different stages of NREM sleep can by identified by age 6 months, with the appearance of sleep spindles by age 3 months and both K complexes and slow wave activity by age 6 months.
2. Slow wave activity in infants and children is of similar frequency to that found in adults (0.5 to 2 Hz), but it is of higher amplitude (100 to 400 μV).
3. N3 sleep should be scored when 20% of an epoch of sleep contains slow wave activity.

REFERENCES

1. Grigg-Damberger M, Gozal D, Marcus CL, et al. The visual scoring of sleep and arousal in infants and children. *J Clin Sleep Med.* 2007;3(2):201–240.
2. Berry RB, Brooks R, Gamaldo CE, et al. for the American Academy of Sleep Medicine. *The AASM Manual for Scoring of Sleep and Associated Events; Rules, Terminology and Technical Specifications, Version 2.2.* Darien, IL: American Academy of Sleep Medicine; 2015. Available from: aasmnet.org.
3. Fogel S, Martin N, Lafortune M, et al. NREM sleep oscillations and brain plasticity in aging. *Front Neurol.* 2012;3(article 176):1–6.
4. Dubé J, Lafortune M, Bedetti C, et al. Cortical thinning explains changes in sleep slow waves during adulthood. *J Neurosci.* 2015;35(20):7795–7807.

A 7-month-old infant with a series of central apneas

Lourdes M. DelRosso

CASE PRESENTATION

A 7-month-old infant presented for evaluation of breathing pauses during sleep that occurred during both the night and daytime naps. The infant was born full term without perinatal complications. The parents denied snoring, gasping, or episodes of cyanosis. The infant was developing normally. The parents denied any past medical or surgical history. The infant did not take any medications. Review of systems was negative for emesis or weight loss.

PHYSICAL EXAM

Physical exam revealed a well-developed infant with adequate milestones for age. His vital signs were within normal range. His weight was at the 45th percentile, and his length was at the 38th percentile. He did not have a high-arched palate, and his tonsils were not appreciated. His lungs were clear to auscultation. Neurologic exam was unremarkable. The remainder of the exam was normal.

LABORATORY AND SLEEP FINDINGS

Polysomnography (PSG) revealed a lights on epoch-lights out epoch of 550 minutes, total sleep time (TST) 478 minutes, sleep efficiency 86%, arousal index 14/h, central apnea index 2/h, obstructive apnea index 0/h, and SpO_2 nadir of 91%. End-tidal CO_2 values were <50 torr throughout the night. The pattern of breathing seen in Figure 12-1 was present for 2% of the TST.

QUESTION

What are the events depicted in Figure 12-1?

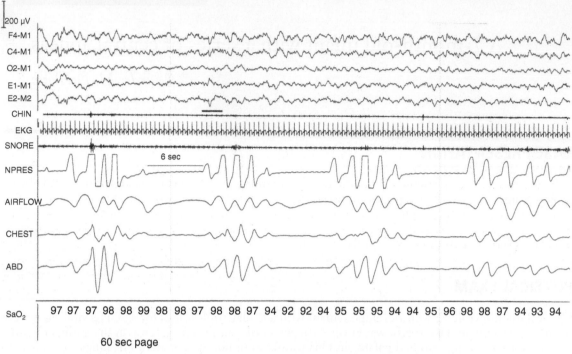

FIGURE 12-1 ■ Series of breathing pauses in a 60-second representative epoch.

ANSWER

Figure 12-1 demonstrates periodic breathing during REM sleep. Some of the individual breathing pauses fit criteria for central apnea, that is, the events last for the duration of two or more breaths and are associated with at least 3% desaturation. Periodic breathing usually occurs during REM sleep in infants.

DISCUSSION

The central control of breathing is located in the brainstem respiratory centers (medulla and pons). These centers integrate information and receive feedback from vagal afferents from the lungs, central chemoreceptors (pH), peripheral chemoreceptors (CO_2 and O_2), and baroreceptors (Fig. 12-2).[1] The system matures during the first year of life. Instability in the control of breathing in infants results in a pattern of hyperventilation followed by hypocapnia and apnea called *periodic breathing*.[2] Factors that predispose infants to respiratory instability include low functional residual capacity, neuronal instability, sleep stage, and lower apneic threshold.[3] In infants, periodic breathing usually occurs during REM sleep, whereas in adults (and some children), it most often occurs during NREM sleep at sleep onset or during periods of sleep-wake transition. The scoring manual defines periodic breathing as three or more episodes of central apneas lasting for at least 3 seconds each and separated by 20 seconds or less of normal breathing.

Periodic breathing in all ages also occurs in the setting of high altitude (above 2500 m). The *International Classification of Sleep Disorders*, third edition (ICSD-3), diagnosis of high-altitude periodic breathing requires the presence of insomnia, sleepiness, morning headache, awakening with shortness of breath, or witnessed apneas. If PSG is performed, the diagnostic criteria require a central apnea index of 5/h or higher. At high altitudes, hypobaric hypoxia stimulates the ventilatory response, resulting in hyperventilation, hypocapnia, and central apnea.

Periodic breathing in the absence of high altitude is considered pathologic if it exceeds 5% TST in a full-term infant or 10% TST in a preterm infant <40 weeks conceptional age. The most common cause of periodic breathing in children is prematurity, but it may also be seen as a developmental phenomenon in a term baby. However, elevated periodic breathing may be a marker of central nervous system pathology; brain tumors and hydrocephalus have been found to affect the respiratory centers, resulting in central apneas and periodic breathing.[4,5]

Our patient's PSG was normal for age. Further follow-up was not needed.

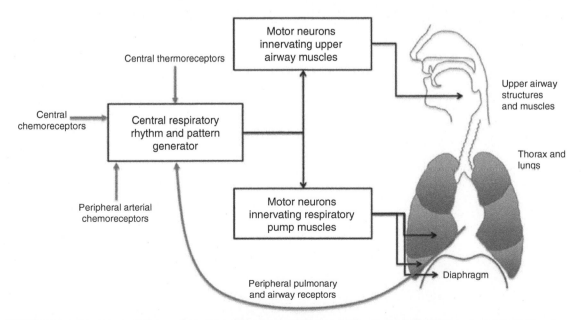

FIGURE 12-2 ■ **Overview of the control of breathing from "Sleep and respiratory physiology in adults."** (Sowho, et al. *Clinical Chest Medicine* 35 2014 page 471 Figure 2.)

CLINICAL PEARLS
1. Periodic breathing is commonly seen in preterm infants. It is considered pathologic if it exceeds 5% of TST in term infants and 10% of TST in preterm infants.
2. Periodic breathing is caused by ventilatory instability and is seen primarily during REM sleep in infants or during sleep-wake transitions and at high altitudes.
3. Periodic breathing can be a sign of central nervous system pathology.

REFERENCES

1. Ross KR, Rosen CL. Sleep and respiratory physiology in children. *Clin Chest Med*. Sep 2014;35(3):457–467.
2. Edwards BA, Sands SA, Berger PJ. Postnatal maturation of breathing stability and loop gain: the role of carotid chemoreceptor development. *Respir Physiol Neurobiol*. Jan 1 2013;185(1):144–155.
3. Khan A, Qurashi M, Kwiatkowski K, Cates D, Rigatto H. Measurement of the CO_2 apneic threshold in newborn infants: possible relevance for periodic breathing and apnea. *J Appl Physiol (1985)*. Apr 2005;98(4):1171–1176.
4. Marcus CL. Images in clinical medicine. Periodic breathing in an infant with hydrocephalus. *N Engl J Med*. Jun 13 1996;334(24):1577.
5. Kuna ST, Smickley JS, Murchison LC. Hypercarbic periodic breathing during sleep in a child with a central nervous system tumor. *Am Rev Respir Dis*. Oct 1990;142(4):880–883.

A 15-month-old with central apnea

Suzanne E. Beck

CASE PRESENTATION

A 15-month-old toddler was referred for overnight polysomnography (PSG) for the evaluation of suspected obstructive sleep apnea syndrome. She had snoring every night and adenotonsillar hypertrophy but no daytime symptoms. She was born full term, had reached all developmental milestones appropriately, and was otherwise healthy. She was on no medications.

PHYSICAL EXAM

Vital signs were normal. Weight, length, and head circumference were at the 50th percentile for age. Physical exam revealed a normal child with tonsils extending beyond the pillars (3+). Her exam was otherwise unremarkable.

LABORATORY AND SLEEP FINDINGS

PSG revealed a total sleep time (TST) of 490 minutes; sleep efficiency of 90%; N1 2% of TST; N2 52%; N3 24%; REM 22%; obstructive apnea–hypopnea index 0/h; central apnea index 1.1/h; arousal index 10.2/h; SpO_2 nadir 95%; and peak end-tidal CO_2 48 mm Hg. Representative tracings of her sleep are shown in Figures 13-1 and 13-2.

QUESTION

Which of the figures has a respiratory event that meets pediatric respiratory scoring criteria for children?

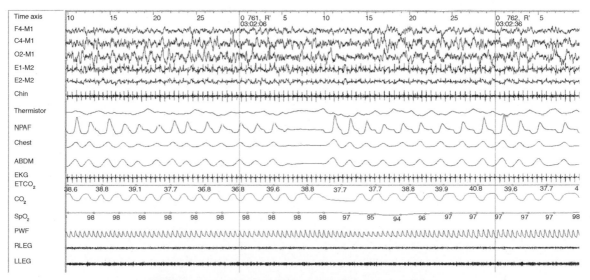

FIGURE 13-1 ■ A representative 60-second epoch of sleep.

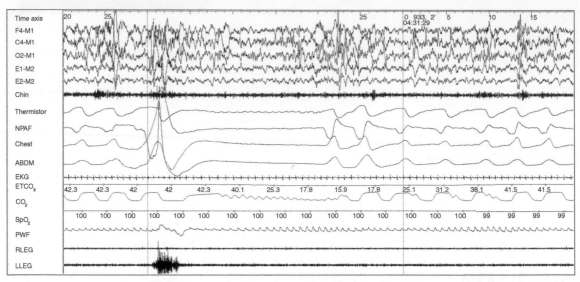

FIGURE 13-2 ■ A representative 60-second epoch of sleep.

ANSWER

Figure 13-1 shows a 6-second central apnea followed by a brief, oxyhemoglobin desaturation that is ≥3%. The child's respiratory rate was 30 breaths/min, so the average duration of 2 breaths was 4 seconds. This central pause exceeds this duration and meets pediatric respiratory scoring criteria. Figure 13-2 shows an 18-second central pause following an arousal. There was no desaturation, arousal, or bradycardia following the central pause so it does not meet pediatric respiratory scoring criteria. Cardiogenic oscillation was noted in the capnography tracings of both figures.

DISCUSSION

According to pediatric respiratory scoring rules, a central apnea is scored when there is a drop in the peak signal excursion by ≥90% of the pre-event baseline using an oronasal thermal sensor, the event is associated with absent inspiratory effort throughout the entire duration, and at least one of the following is met: (1) the event lasts ≥20 seconds or (2) the event lasts at least the duration of two breaths during baseline breathing and is associated with either (i) an arousal, (ii) arterial oxygen desaturation ≥3%, or (iii) in infants <12 months of age, a decrease in heart rate to <50 beats/min for at least 5 seconds or <60 beats/min for at least 15 seconds.[1] In other words, central apneas in children are scored if they are at least two breaths in duration and are associated with a ≥3% desaturation, an arousal or bradycardia, or are ≥20 seconds in duration. This differs from adult criteria for the scoring of central apneas where the duration of the central pause must be ≥10 seconds, and there is no requirement for associated desaturation, arousal, or bradycardia.

Central apneas in infants and in children are common because of a vigorous Hering-Breuer reflex (compensatory central respiratory pauses following the stimulation of pulmonary stretch receptors following a large breath, such as with a sigh or body movement). In addition, young children often have variable breathing during REM sleep, including central apneas. Desaturations following these central apneas are typically brief and usually do not drop below 91%[2] but can drop lower in infants.[3] The central apnea index in children is usually <1/h in normal children,[4] but different authors have used different definitions of *central apnea*, making it difficult to apply meaningful norms. When describing central apneas in pediatric patients, it is important to describe the duration, frequency, and associated physiologic abnormalities that follow each event. This description has more significance than the index does. Children and infants have smaller lungs and a more compliant chest wall than adults do, resulting in a lower functional residual capacity at rest. This explains the tendency for desaturation following brief pauses in breathing. Thus, an isolated central apnea of 15 to 20 seconds duration following a sigh and associated with transient, mild desaturation may be physiologically normal. However, deeper and more frequent desaturations following brief central apneas may indicate decreased pulmonary reserve. This pattern is typical of small infants or children with underlying lung disease (even mild asthma). An isolated longer central apnea longer than 20 seconds may be normal,[5] but central apneas that are of longer duration or very frequent could be pathologic and may indicate central nervous system problems or control of breathing abnormalities.

Our patient had a few central apneas, all of which were brief and associated with only minimal desaturation, as shown in Figure 13-1, and although they met pediatric respiratory scoring criteria, none was considered pathologic or clinically significant. The parents were reassured that no treatment was needed at this time.

CLINICAL PEARLS

1. Central apneas in children are scored if they are at least two breaths in duration and are associated with a ≥3% desaturation, an arousal or bradycardia, or are ≥20 seconds in duration. This differs from adult criteria for the scoring of central apneas where the duration of the central pause must be ≥10 seconds, and there is no requirement for associated desaturation, arousal, or bradycardia.
2. Desaturation with central apneas usually indicates a decreased pulmonary reserve, whereas prolonged central apneas are more likely to indicate a central nervous system abnormality.
3. In infants and children, the duration and frequency of the central events and the associated physiologic abnormalities that follow have more clinical significance than the central apnea index does.

REFERENCES

1. Berry RB, Gamaldo CE, Harding SM, Lloyd RM, Marcus CL, Vaughn BV. *The AASM Manual for the Scoring of Sleep and Associated Events: Rules, Terminology and Technical Specifications, Version 2.2.* Darien, IL: Academy of Sleep Medicine; 2015.
2. Uliel S, Tauman R, Greenfeld M, Sivan Y. Normal polysomnographic respiratory values in children and adolescents. *Chest.* 2004;125(3):872–878.
3. Stebbens VA, Poets CF, Alexander JR, Arrowsmith WA, Southall DP. Oxygen saturation and breathing patterns in infancy. 1: Full term infants in the second month of life. *Arch Dis Child.* 1991;66(5):569–573.
4. Traeger N, Schultz B, Pollock AN, Mason T, Marcus CL, Arens R. Polysomnographic values in children 2-9 years old: additional data and review of the literature. *Pediatr Pulmonol.* 2005;40(1):22–30.
5. Weese-Mayer DE, Morrow AS, Conway LP, Brouillette RT, Silvestri JM. Assessing clinical significance of apnea exceeding fifteen seconds with event recording. *J Pediatr.* 1990;117(4):568–574.

A 19-month-old child with irregular, heavy breathing during sleep

Suzanne E. Beck

CASE PRESENTATION

A 19-month-old child was evaluated because of parental concerns of irregular, heavy breathing during sleep, noticed on a recent family vacation during which they slept in the same room. The child snored occasionally with colds, but the parents did not notice diaphoresis, gasping, apnea, or color changes during sleep. The child was born after a full-term gestation and had no medical problems. The child was developing typically and growing well. He was playful and active during the day, with no change in respiratory pattern, coughing, or shortness of breath. There was no family history of neuromuscular, metabolic, or respiratory conditions.

PHYSICAL EXAM

Physical exam revealed a healthy child with normal vital signs. Growth parameters were at the 40th percentiles for weight and height and the 50th percentile for head circumference. Physical exam was normal.

LABORATORY AND SLEEP FINDINGS

Polysomnography (PSG) revealed a total sleep time of 461 minutes. Sleep efficiency was 87%. The sleep-stage distribution was normal. The obstructive apnea–hypopnea index was 0.1/h. The central apnea index was 0/h. SpO_2 nadir was 92%. The $ETCO_2$ was below 50 Torr for the entire study. The periodic limb movement index was 2.5/h.

QUESTION

Should you be concerned with the change in respiratory patterns seen in Figure 14-1, *A* and *B*?

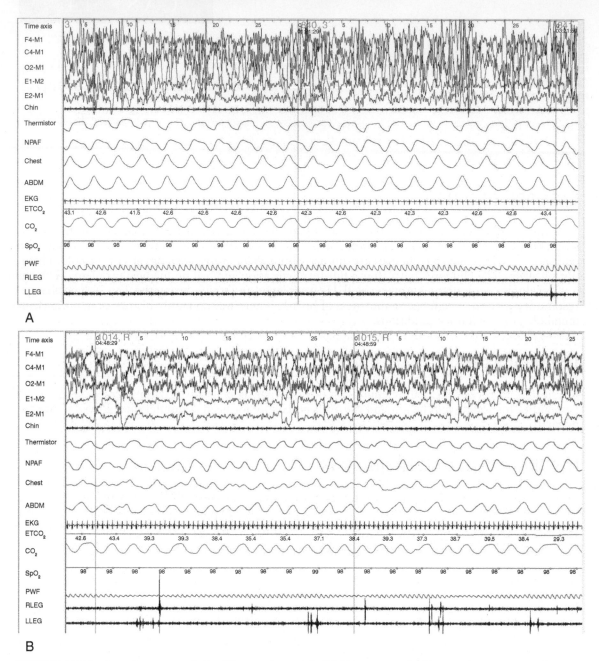

FIGURE 14-1 ■ Tracing of a representative 60-second epoch in N3 (**A**) compared with a respiratory pattern in a 60-second epoch of REM sleep (**B**).

ANSWER

No, the breathing pattern in this child is normal. The respiratory rate is 21 to 25 breaths/min. The respiratory rate and tidal volumes are variable in REM sleep. The respiratory rate in children is increased compared with adults.

DISCUSSION

Respiratory patterns in sleep differ from those during wakefulness and vary according to sleep state. In NREM sleep breathing is regular, whereas in REM sleep, breathing is erratic and shallow, with irregularities in amplitude and frequency synchronous with REM bursts.[1] Respiratory rates during sleep slow during infancy and childhood until reaching adult rates (Table 14-1).[2,3] Smaller, younger infants and children have higher respiratory rates than larger, older children, and the respiratory rate decreases exponentially with increasing body weight.[4] Respiratory rates in newborns and infants are higher during REM compared with NREM sleep.[5] Minute ventilation also decreases with age (from 250 ml/kg/min in newborns to 100 ml/kg/min in adolescents), paralleling maturational changes in respiratory frequency and metabolic demands,[4] and is slightly higher in REM than NREM sleep in newborns and infants.[3] Tidal volume is decreased in both NREM and REM compared with the wakeful state, and it is more variable in REM than in NREM sleep.[1]

To meet ventilatory demands during sleep, it is more energy efficient for the newborn and young child to increase respiratory frequency rather than tidal volume because of the mechanical properties of the lungs and thorax.[6] Paradoxical breathing (i.e., asynchronous or out-of-phase motion of the chest and abdomen) during REM sleep is common in newborns and small children, and it decreases with age.[5] The highly compliant thorax of the infant (required for passage through the birth canal) and child accounts for this; as the chest wall matures (calcification of the ribs and connective tissues), compliance decreases and asynchronous breathing is uncommon.[3]

Our patient's nocturnal PSG was normal. The breathing pattern that the parents observed was normal. The parents were reassured and educated about normal breathing patterns in children.

TABLE 14-1.   Respiratory rates (breaths/min) during sleep in children[3]

	Newborn	Infant 3-9 mo	12 mo	Preschool 2-6 yr	School Age 7-11 yr	Adolescent 12-18 yr
Median	40	27-29	24	20	18	15-18
Interquartile range	34-52	22-30	20-27	14-26	17-19	17-18

CLINICAL PEARLS

1. Respiratory rates are higher in infants and children compared with adults.
2. Minute ventilation decreases with age and is slightly higher in REM than in NREM sleep, consistent with the higher respiratory rates in REM sleep.
3. Paradoxical breathing is common in infants and children, particularly in REM sleep, because of a highly compliant chest wall.

REFERENCES

1. Krieger J. Respiratory physiology: breathing in normal subjects. In: Kryger MH, Roth T, Dement WC, eds. *Principles and Practice of Sleep Medicine.* 5th ed. St. Louis: Saunders; 2011:232–244.
2. Rusconi F, Castagneto M, Gagliardi L, et al. Reference values for respiratory rate in the first 3 years of life. *Pediatrics.* Sep 1994;94(3):350–355.
3. Rosen C. Maturation of breathing during sleep. In: Marcus CL, Carroll JL, Donnelly DF, Loughlin GM, eds. *Sleep and Breathing in Children.* 2nd ed. New York: Informa Healthcare; 2008:118–120.
4. Gagliardi L, Rusconi F. Respiratory rate and body mass in the first three years of life. The working party on respiratory rate. *Arch Dis Child.* Feb 1997;76(2):151–154.
5. Gaultier C, Praud JP, Canet E, Delaperche MF, D'Allest AM. Paradoxical inward rib cage motion during rapid eye movement sleep in infants and young children. *J Dev Physiol.* Oct 1987;9(5):391–397.
6. Polgar G, Weng TR. The functional development of the respiratory system from the period of gestation to adulthood. *Am Rev Respir Dis.* Sep 1979;120(3):625–695.

A 4-week-old infant with jerking movements during sleep

Suzanne E. Beck

CASE PRESENTATION

A 4-week-old infant was referred for evaluation of jerking movements during sleep. The movements began at 2 weeks of age and have occurred almost every night. The movements were described as large twitches of the arms and body that occurred when the baby was asleep and stopped when she awoke. The baby was otherwise healthy, feeding well, and growing. There was no fever, rash, illnesses, or trauma. She was born full term, without complications, to a healthy mother who was not taking medications and did not use illicit drugs. There was no family history of seizure disorder or dysautonomia.

PHYSICAL EXAM

Vital signs were normal. Weight, length, and head circumference were at the 40th percentiles for age. Exam revealed an awake, alert infant whose head was normocephalic and atraumatic, with nondysmorphic facial features. Pupillary light reflexes and eye movements were normal. There was normal range of motion and muscle bulk of the extremities. The infant's spontaneous movements were symmetric and normal while awake. Primitive reflexes, cranial nerves, and deep tendon reflexes were intact. The rest of the exam was normal.

LABORATORY AND SLEEP FINDINGS

Home video recording of events shows that upon falling asleep, the baby demonstrated repetitive, paroxysmal contractions of both upper extremities in clusters of 4 to 5 jerks/min for 10 minutes. Movements were brief (about 1 second) and involved the upper extremities (usually both but sometimes just one), resulting in movement of the entire upper body. The eyes were closed during the movements. There were no generalizing features and no effect on respiration or color. Holding the extremity did not suppress the contractions. Upon waking the infant, the movements stopped.

The baby did fall asleep in the office, demonstrating similar rhythmic jerks of the upper extremities. There was no eye deviation. Upon awaking the infant, the spasms abruptly ceased. The baby appeared normal subsequently.

QUESTION

What is the most likely diagnosis?

ANSWER

The infant's movements during sleep are consistent with benign sleep myoclonus of infancy.

DISCUSSION

Benign sleep myoclonus of infancy, also called benign neonatal sleep myoclonus, first described in 1982 by Coulter and Allen,[1] is a disorder commonly mistaken for seizures during the newborn period. Benign sleep myoclonus of infancy is characterized by repetitive, rhythmic, myoclonic jerks that occur only while the infant is asleep and disappear upon wakefulness, a distinguishing feature of the diagnosis. The movements are often brief, repetitive, bilateral, and massive, typically involving the large muscle groups of the extremities, trunk, or whole body and rarely the face.[2] Benign sleep myoclonus is classified as a sleep-related movement disorder; diagnostic criteria are listed in Box 15-1.[2]

Onset is usually between birth and 1 month; peak expression is between 15 and 35 days of age.[3] In a review of 167 cases, benign sleep myoclonus resolved by 3 months of age in 64% and by 6 months of age in 95% of the infants.[3] The prevalence of the condition is not known. There are no known sequelae and no evidence of increased risk for seizures.[3] The cause is not known but may be related to immature spinal reflexes. Treatment with medications is not indicated.

As the name implies, benign sleep myoclonus of infancy is a benign condition in infants, but it is often mistaken for epilepsy. There are certain features of benign sleep myoclonus of infancy that are distinguishable from epilepsy. First, benign sleep myoclonus of infancy occurs only during sleep and stops abruptly when the infant is woken. Seizures, however, can occur in both wakeful and sleep states. For seizures occurring while awake, the eyes are usually open. If seizure onset is during sleep, the eyes often open at the onset of the seizure. Second, benign sleep myoclonus of infancy usually occurs in otherwise healthy newborns, whereas neonatal seizures often occur in the context of infection, encephalopathy, or metabolic disorders. Infantile spasms (West syndrome) have a different pattern, usually involving flexion of the head and extension of the extremities, and usually occur after the first month of age. The electroencephalogram (EEG) pattern in infantile spasms shows hypsarrhythmia, and in myotonic seizures, shows epileptiform discharges, whereas the EEG pattern in benign myoclonus of infancy is normal.[2] There may be superimposed muscle artifact, but the EEG is without ictal or interictal abnormalities or arousals. Other conditions that occur during wake such as startle disease (hyperekplexia) and myoclonic encephalopathies should be distinguished from benign myoclonus of infancy. Benign myoclonus of infancy has been reported as common in neonatal abstinence syndrome in infants born to mothers addicted to opiates,[4] and it may be considered a subtype.[2]

In contrast to periodic limb movements where the muscle activity occurs in bursts of 0.5 to 10 seconds over longer regular intervals of 20 to 40 seconds, the myoclonic twitches of benign sleep myoclonus of infancy are typically shorter (40 to 300 ms each), occur in more frequent clusters of 4 to 5/min, and occur over 15 to 60 minutes or longer.[2] Benign sleep myoclonus of infancy is not the same as sleep starts, which occur at sleep-wake transitions and are not repetitive.[2]

In most cases, the diagnosis of benign neonatal sleep myoclonus is suspected on clinical grounds alone, and further evaluation is not necessary if the child is otherwise healthy, developmentally normal, and has a normal neurologic exam.[3] Further evaluation is warranted if the infant has risk factors for neurologic disease, signs of metabolic or infectious disease, developmental concerns, abnormal physical exam, or presents in an atypical fashion. If infection or metabolic disturbance is suspected, appropriate studies should be ordered. If epilepsy or seizures are suspected, EEG and brain imaging

---

BOX 15-1 *INTERNATIONAL CLASSIFICATION OF SLEEP DISORDERS, THIRD EDITION, DIAGNOSTIC CRITERIA FOR BENIGN SLEEP MYOCLONUS OF INFANCY*[2]

All of the following must be met
1. Repetitive myoclonic spasms involving the whole body, trunk, or limbs
2. Movements occurring in early infancy, typically from birth to age 6 months
3. Movements must only occur during sleep
4. Movements that stop abruptly and consistently when the child is aroused
5. A disorder that is not better explained by another sleep disorder, by a medical or neurologic disorder, or by medication use

are indicated. Prolonged EEG monitoring may be indicated for infants in whom diagnostic confusion remains.[3] Polysomnography is not indicated.

Our patient was diagnosed with benign sleep myoclonus of infancy, and no further evaluation was performed. The favorable prognosis, expected time course for resolution, and anticipatory guidance (namely not to stimulate the baby out of the episodes) were discussed. Episodes resolved by 4 months of age, and the child was developmentally normal at subsequent follow-up visits.

CLINICAL PEARLS

1. Benign sleep myoclonus of infancy is characterized by repetitive, rhythmic, myoclonic jerks that occur only while the infant is asleep and disappear during wakefulness.
2. Benign sleep myoclonus of infancy usually begins within the first month of age and resolves by age 3 months.
3. In most cases, the diagnosis of benign neonatal sleep myoclonus is suspected on clinical grounds alone, and further evaluation is not necessary if the child is otherwise healthy, is developing normally, and has a normal neurologic exam.

REFERENCES

1. Coulter DL, Allen RJ. Benign neonatal sleep myoclonus. *Arch Neurol.* 1982;39(3):191–192.
2. American Academy of Sleep Medicine. *International Classification of Sleep Disorders.* 3rd ed. Darien, IL: American Academy of Sleep Medicine; 2014.
3. Maurer VO, Rizzi M, Bianchetti MG, Ramelli GP. Benign neonatal sleep myoclonus: a review of the literature. *Pediatrics.* 2010;125(4):e919–e924.
4. Held-Egli K, Ruegger C, Das-Kundu S, Schmitt B, Bucher HU. Benign neonatal sleep myoclonus in newborn infants of opioid dependent mothers. *Acta Paediatr.* 2009;98(1):69–73.

An 8-year-old boy with abnormal capnography on polysomnogram

Suzanne E. Beck

CASE PRESENTATION

An 8-year-old boy with snoring and restless sleep was referred for polysomnography (PSG) because of suspected obstructive sleep apnea syndrome (OSAS). He was overweight but had no other medical problems. He was on no medication. The family history was noncontributory.

PHYSICAL EXAM

The patient was an overweight boy who was alert and interactive. His weight was 38 kg (90th percentile), height was 140 cm (78th percentile), and body mass index 19.4 kg/m² (90th percentile). He had nondysmorphic facial features. His tonsils were 2+. His muscle tone and strength were normal. The rest of his physical exam was normal.

LABORATORY AND SLEEP FINDINGS

PSG revealed a total sleep time (TST) of 508 minutes; 93% sleep efficiency; REM time 146 minutes (28% of TST); obstructive apnea–hypopnea index 0.7/h; central apnea index 0.3/h; SpO_2 nadir 95%; peak end-tidal CO_2 55 mm Hg; end-tidal CO_2 >50 mm Hg for 2% of TST. The capnography displayed an abnormality as shown in Figures 16-1 and 16-2.

QUESTIONS

1. What is the abnormality present on the capnography tracing shown in Figures 16-1 and 16-2?
2. What is the cause of the abnormality?

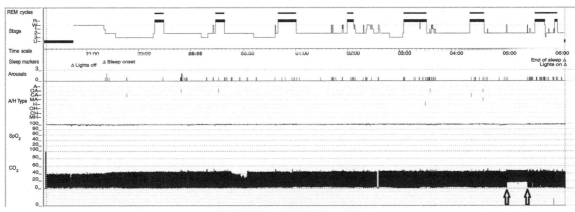

FIGURE 16-1 ■ PSG hypnogram.

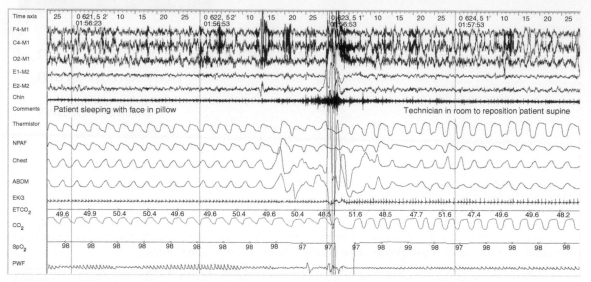

FIGURE 16-2 ■ One hundred and twenty–second epoch of sleep before and after the technician repositioned patient.

ANSWERS

1. The capnography tracing shows a period with elevated inspired CO_2 levels (see Fig. 16-1 between the *arrows*). Figure 16-2 shows the elevated inspiratory CO_2 baseline (note that the inspired CO_2 during atmospheric breathing should be close to zero), without a clear end-expiratory pause. This pattern is typically due to rebreathing of carbon dioxide, for example, in this case, when the child sleeps prone with his face in the pillow (Fig. 16-3).
2. The problem was resolved when the technician repositioned the patient from prone to supine (see Fig. 16-2). This rebreathing of CO_2 may cause elevation of the peak end-tidal CO_2 or an increase in percentage of sleep time with the end-tidal CO_2 above normal. In most cases, it is an incidental finding.

DISCUSSION

Monitoring CO_2 during sleep is an important aspect of pediatric PSG because children are prone to obstructive hypoventilation (long periods of partial obstruction as part of their spectrum of OSAS). The obesity epidemic has also resulted in more children with the obesity hypoventilation syndrome necessitating the need to monitor CO_2. In addition, most pediatric sleep centers care for children with hypoventilation because of various underlying conditions such as chronic lung disease, neuromuscular disease, central nervous system or metabolic problems, craniofacial syndromes, or chest wall anomalies. Further, most pediatric sleep centers monitor CO_2 to guide adjustments in noninvasive ventilation or to monitor for hypoventilation during oxygen titration studies. End-tidal CO_2 can also be used as a backup channel for airflow, but it is oversensitive and is, therefore, recommended as an adjunct signal only for this purpose.[1]

CO_2 can be monitored noninvasively by end-tidal CO_2 or transcutaneous CO_2 sampling, and both have been shown to be useful in pediatric PSG as surrogates of arterial CO_2.[2] For a discussion of CO_2 monitoring technology, see Clinical Pearls in Case 6: A 14-year-old with and abnormal end-tidal CO2 waveform during polysomnography. End-tidal CO_2 is measured by infrared capnometry, and measurements can be affected by secretions, mouth breathing, lung disease, or increased dead space. In our patient, the end-tidal CO_2 was elevated because of an increased inspiratory CO_2, resulting from rebreathing into the pillow.

Normal peak end-tidal CO_2 is ≤53 mm Hg during sleep.[3] Hypoventilation in children is defined by elevation of the CO_2 above 50 mm Hg for >25% of TST.[1] It is common to see a single breath with an elevated end-tidal PCO_2 value, especially after sighs or body movements. Therefore, the percentage of total sleep time with hypercapnia is more important than the peak end-tidal PCO_2 value for the night.[4] However, this reading may be inaccurate if the capnogram does not return to zero at inspiration, the signals are not properly calibrated, or the end-tidal waveforms do not reach a plateau.

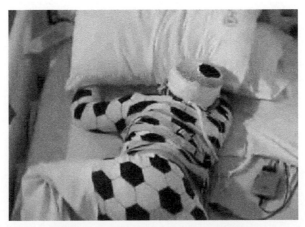

FIGURE 16-3 ■ Patient's sleeping position.

CLINICAL PEARLS

1. *Hypoventilation* in children is defined by elevation of the CO_2 above 50 mm Hg for >25% of TST.
2. It is important to examine the end-tidal CO_2 waveform to determine whether the reported values are accurate and physiologic.
3. Baseline end-tidal CO_2 can be elevated because of positional rebreathing of CO_2.
4. Technicians and parents should be aware that sleeping with one's face in the pillow or with objects over the face may result in rebreathing of CO_2.

REFERENCES

1. Berry RB, Brooks R, Gamaldo CE, et al. *The AASM Manual for the Scoring of Sleep and Associated Events: Rules, Terminology and Technical Specifications, Version 2.2.* Darien, IL: Academy of Sleep Medicine; 2015.
2. Redline S, Budhiraja R, Kapur V, et al. The scoring of respiratory events in sleep: reliability and validity. *J Clin Sleep Med.* 2007;3(2):169–200.
3. Traeger N, Schultz B, Pollock AN, Mason T, Marcus CL, Arens R. Polysomnographic values in children 2-9 years old: additional data and review of the literature. *Pediatr Pulmonol.* 2005;40(1):22–30.
4. Beck SE, Marcus CL. Pediatric polysomnography. *Sleep Med Clin.* 2009;4(3):393–406.

A 13-year-old boy with snoring and abnormal eye movements on polysomnogram

Lourdes M. DelRosso

CASE PRESENTATION

A 13-year-old boy was referred for evaluation of snoring with occasional witnessed apneas. He did not have any other sleep-related concerns. He was diagnosed with obsessive-compulsive disorder at age 12 and had taken fluoxetine 20 mg daily since then. His past surgical history was significant for tonsillectomy and adenoidectomy at age 6.

PHYSICAL EXAM

Physical exam revealed an alert and cooperative boy. His vital signs were within the normal range. His height was at the 40th percentile, and his weight was at the 35th percentile. He did not have an adenoid facies. He did not have enlarged turbinates. The oropharynx was Mallampati grade I. Tonsils were surgically absent. He did not have micrognathia or retrognathia. The remainder of the exam was normal.

LABORATORY AND SLEEP FINDINGS

Polysomnography revealed an apnea–hypopnea index of 1/h, arousal index of 12/h, and SpO_2 nadir of 95%.

A representative epoch is seen in Figure 17-1.

QUESTIONS

What is the mechanism for the eye movements seen in Figure 17-1?

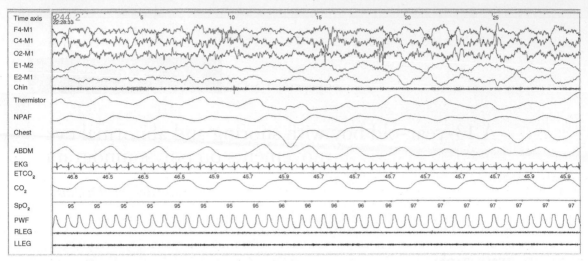

FIGURE 17-1 ■ Thirty-second epoch of N2. Note the eye movements in E1M2 and E2M2.

ANSWERS

Fluoxetine-produced serotonin excess in the brainstem.

DISCUSSION

Fluoxetine-induced eye movements in NREM sleep were first described in the early 1990s. A study of 41 patients taking fluoxetine for either major depressive disorder or obsessive-compulsive disorder and 52 patients receiving tricyclic antidepressants for major depressive disorder or insomnia demonstrated the presence of prominent eye movements during NREM sleep in 48.8% of patients taking fluoxetine and 5.8% of patients taking tricyclic antidepressants. The eye movements persisted after medication discontinuation. The mechanism of the excessive eye movements seen during NREM sleep in patients taking fluoxetine was postulated to be a milder form of serotonin syndrome, where saccadic eye movements were secondary to overactive serotonergic neurons in the brainstem. Serotonin disinhibited the omnipause neurons responsible for the control of saccadic eye movements.[1] This effect on eye movements during sleep has also been reported with other selective serotonin reuptake inhibitors.[2] The number and the amplitude of eye movements during REM and NREM sleep increase in patients taking fluoxetine. Other motor side effects reported in patients taking fluoxetine include dyskinesia, akathisia, bruxism, REM sleep without atonia, and REM behavior disorder.[3,4]

CLINICAL PEARLS

1. Patients taking selective serotonin reuptake inhibitors exhibit excessive eye movements mainly during NREM sleep.
2. This effect may persist after medication discontinuation.
3. Other motor side effects of selective serotonin reuptake inhibitors include REM sleep without atonia, REM behavior disorder, bruxism, akathisia, and dyskinesia.

REFERENCES

1. Schenck CH, Mahowald MW, Kim SW, O'Connor KA, Hurwitz TD. Prominent eye movements during NREM sleep and REM sleep behavior disorder associated with fluoxetine treatment of depression and obsessive-compulsive disorder. *Sleep*. Jun 1992;15(3):226–235.
2. Geyer JD, Carney PR, Dillard SC, Davis L, Ward LC. Antidepressant medications, neuroleptics, and prominent eye movements during NREM sleep. *J Clin Neurophysiol*. Feb 2009;26(1):39–44.
3. Armitage R, Trivedi M, Rush AJ. Fluoxetine and oculomotor activity during sleep in depressed patients. *Neuropsychopharmacology*. Apr 1995;12(2):159–165.
4. Winkelman JW, James L. Serotonergic antidepressants are associated with REM sleep without atonia. *Sleep*. Mar 15 2004;27(2):317–321.

A 3-month-old infant who sleeps with a pacifier

Lourdes M. DelRosso

CASE PRESENTATION

You are reading a polysomnogram from your patient, a 3-month-old infant with maternal report of breathing pauses during sleep. You notice periodic increases in tone in the chin electromyogram (EMG) throughout the study, as seen in Figure 18-1. The sleep study is normal, with a central apnea–hypopnea index (AHI) of 0.1/h and an obstructive AHI of 0.6/h. There were no episodes of desaturation or hypoventilation. The technologist report states "infant slept with pacifier, mother stayed up all night replacing the pacifier." You called the parent to discuss the sleep study results. During your phone conversation, the mother expresses concern about sudden infant death syndrome (SIDS) and states that the pediatrician recommended using the pacifier during nocturnal sleep and daytime naps.

QUESTIONS

1. What do the episodes of increased chin tone seen in Figure 18-1 represent?
2. What recommendations can you give this mother regarding SIDS prevention and pacifier use?

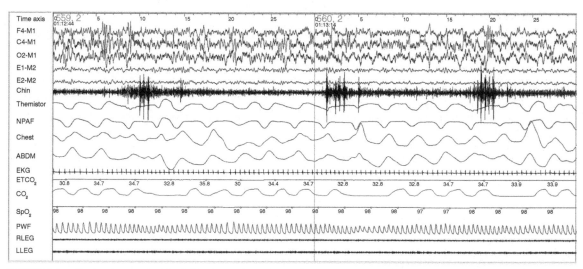

FIGURE 18-1 ■ Two-minute epoch of N2 showing periods of elevated chin EMG tone, which coincide with pacifier sucking.

ANSWERS

1. The elevated tone in the chin EMG leads represents muscle artifact secondary to pacifier sucking.
2. The American Academy of Pediatrics recommends offering infants a pacifier at bedtime and during naps, as one measure to help prevent SIDS. The pacifier does not need to be replaced if it falls out of the infant's mouth. For other SIDS prevention recommendations, see Table 18-1.[1]

DISCUSSION

SIDS is defined as the sudden death of a child <1 year of age that remains unexplained after post mortem and death-scene investigation. The prevalence of SIDS in the USA in 2013 was 39.7 per 100,000 live births (a total of 1563 deaths).[2] The peak of SIDS occurs at 4 months of age; the incidence peaks during winter months; and SIDS occurs more often at high altitudes.[3] Further, 80% of SIDS deaths occur during nighttime sleep.[4]

Modifiable risk factors for SIDS include prone sleep position, maternal smoking, bed sharing, soft sleeping surfaces (e.g., sofas), and overheating (e.g., excessive clothing). Nonmodifiable risk factors for SIDS include male sex, prematurity, low birth weight, young maternal age, and maternal parity (multiparous). Protective factors include supine sleeping, breastfeeding, room sharing, and pacifier use. The primary cause of SIDS is thought to be from rebreathing when the infant is in the prone position, especially when the infant is sleeping on a soft surface or with many bed coverings. For these and other reasons, bed sharing places the infant at risk for SIDS. However, epidemiologic studies have suggested that room sharing *without* bed sharing may be protective. A study of 325 SIDS infants and 1300 age-matched controls revealed that infants who died of SIDS while sleeping alone in a room were more likely to be found with bedclothes covering their heads compared with infants who were room sharing, suggesting a protective effect of having a parent sleeping in proximity to the infant.[4]

There is a strong association between pacifier use and decreased SIDS risk. The mechanism is unknown, but it has been postulated that pacifier use increases arousability, prevents the tongue from obstructing the airway, allows for mouth breathing when the nose is obstructed, reduces gastroesophageal reflux, increases the respiratory drive, and helps maintain the supine position.[5-7] A study of 36 pacifier-using infants showed that 56% of infants lost the pacifier after 30 minutes of sleep, and only 19% of infants kept the pacifier after an hour of sleep.[6] In conclusion, pacifier use has been shown to decrease the risk of SIDS by mechanisms that are not yet completely clear.

TABLE 18-1.   **American Academy of Pediatrics recommendations for safe infant-sleeping environment**[1]

Do	Don't
Place the infant to sleep in the supine position	Place the infant to sleep in the prone or lateral decubitus position
Use a firm mattress covered with a fitted sheet	Allow the infant to sleep on a bed, car seat, stroller, or another sitting device
Place the infant crib or bassinet in the parent's bedroom	Bed-share
Breastfeed	Smoke or use alcohol or drugs
Offer a pacifier at bedtime and nap times	Hang pacifier around the infant's neck
Stay up to date with immunizations	Use apnea monitors to reduce risk of SIDS
Supervised awake tummy time	Use commercially available devices that claim to prevent SIDS (wedges)

CLINICAL PEARLS

1. Protective factors for SIDS include supine sleeping, breastfeeding, room sharing, and pacifier use.
2. Most infants lose the pacifier during the first hour after sleep onset. It is not necessary to replace the pacifier because studies have not shown that this affects SIDS risk. The mechanism of this is unclear.
3. Pacifier use during a polysomnogram can produce an artifact seen in the chin EMG.

REFERENCES

1. Moon RY. SIDS and other sleep-related infant deaths: expansion of recommendations for a safe infant sleeping environment. *Pediatrics*. Nov 2011;128(5):1030–1039.
2. Osterman MJ, Kochanek KD, MacDorman MF, Strobino DM, Guyer B. Annual summary of vital statistics: 2012-2013. *Pediatrics*. Jun 2015;135(6):1115–1125.
3. Mitchell EA, Krous HF. Sudden unexpected death in infancy: a historical perspective. *J Paediatr Child Health*. Jan 2015;51(1):108–112.
4. Blair PS, Platt MW, Smith IJ, Fleming PJ. Sudden infant death syndrome and the time of death: factors associated with night-time and day-time deaths. *Int J Epidemiol*. Dec 2006;35(6):1563–1569.
5. Hauck FR, Omojokun OO, Siadaty MS. Do pacifiers reduce the risk of sudden infant death syndrome? A meta-analysis. *Pediatrics*. Nov 2005;116(5):e716–e723.
6. Hanzer M, Zotter H, Sauseng W, Pfurtscheller K, Muller W, Kerbl R. Pacifier use does not alter the frequency or duration of spontaneous arousals in sleeping infants. *Sleep Med*. Apr 2009;10(4):464–470.
7. Franco P, Scaillet S, Wermenbol V, Valente F, Groswasser J, Kahn A. The influence of a pacifier on infants' arousals from sleep. *J Pediatr*. Jun 2000;136(6):775–779.

A 24-month-old girl with uneventful desaturation

Lourdes M. DelRosso

CASE PRESENTATION

A 24-month-old girl presented for evaluation of snoring. The parents stated that snoring started a month earlier, after a viral infection. The child recovered from the infection, but snoring persisted. The parents denied gasping or witnessing pauses in breathing. Her sleep schedule was consistent, and she did not have nocturnal awakenings or restless sleep. The parents denied night terrors, sleepwalking, or nightmares. The child did not have any past medical or surgical history and was not taking any medications. Review of systems was negative for asthma, allergies, or gastroesophageal reflux disease. She was developing normally.

PHYSICAL EXAM

The child was cooperative and in no distress. She did not have an adenoid facies. Physical exam revealed a normal nasal bridge, no high-arched palate, and no retrognathia. Her tonsils were 2+. The remainder of the exam was normal.

LABORATORY AND SLEEP FINDINGS

Polysomnography revealed a sleep efficiency of 85% and an apnea–hypopnea index of 0.5/h. There were no central apneas, cardiac arrhythmias, or periodic limb movements during sleep. The SpO_2 nadir was 92%, as shown in Figure 19-1.

QUESTIONS

What caused the SpO_2 nadir of 92% seen in this 120-second epoch?

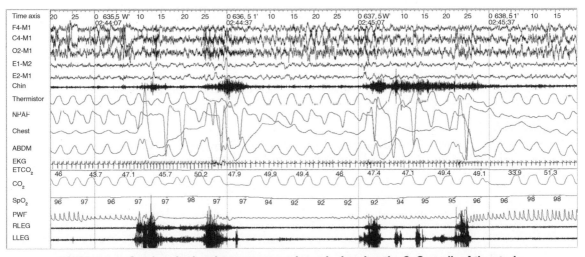

FIGURE 19-1 ■ **One hundred and twenty–second epoch showing the SpO_2 nadir of the study.**

ANSWERS

The SpO$_2$ nadir of 92% seen in this 120-second epoch was caused by a motion artifact on the pulse oximeter. Lead 16 on the image represents the plethysmography wave or pulse wave form (PWF). Note that the PWF decreases in amplitude on epoch 635, corresponding to the artifactually decreased SpO$_2$ reading. The PWF remains flat through epoch 636, and the SpO$_2$ remains low. The PWF resumes a normal amplitude at the end of epoch 637, with normalization of the SpO$_2$ reading.

DISCUSSION

Pulse oximetry estimates arterial hemoglobin oxygen saturation (SpO$_2$) by photoplethysmography (light absorption) of hemoglobin. Oxygenated hemoglobin absorbs infrared light and allows red light to pass through. Deoxygenated hemoglobin absorbs red light and allows infrared light to pass through. The device passes two wavelengths (red [600 to 750 nm] and infrared [850 to 1000 nm]) through a thin body part (finger or earlobe). A photoreceptor on the other side of the finger or earlobe receives the signal and calculates the red/infrared ratio, which is algorithmically converted to a SpO$_2$ value. Most commercial pulse oximeters have an accuracy of 3% to 4% for a single measurement.[1] The performance of pulse oximeters is less accurate when the SpO$_2$ drops below 80%. Because the device recognizes arterial pulsation from background venous blood, skin, soft tissues, and bones, the most common limitation is motion, which is particularly important in pediatric patients. Motion distorts the signal-to-noise ratio and gives lower than true values. Motion is recognized by a distorted plethysmographic waveform as seen in Figure 19-1. Low perfusion, such as in shock, hypothermia, and vasoconstriction, also results in an artifactually low value. The presence of carboxyhemoglobin overestimates SpO$_2$ because light absorption is similar to that of oxyhemoglobin. Methemoglobin absorbs light equally in the red and infrared spectrum and causes underestimation of SpO$_2$. Fetal hemoglobin and hemoglobin S do not interfere with pulse oximetry. Other factors that may affect the accuracy of pulse oximetry include dark skin pigmentation (including bronze baby syndrome), arrhythmia, and synthetic nails and nail polish (especially black blue and green colors). Bilirubin absorbs light in the 450-nm spectrum and, thus, does not affect the pulse oximetry reading, and, therefore, pulse oximetry can be used reliably in infants with jaundice. Probe size and environmental light also play a role. The appropriate probe size must be used in neonates or small infants. When a bigger probe is placed on the tiny finger of an infant, the light may project tangentially and miss the arterial bed, resulting in a lower SpO$_2$ reading. Intense white or infrared light in the room could flood the photodetector and artificially decrease the SpO$_2$ reading.[2]

In summary, pulse oximetry is a valuable tool in polysomnography. Knowledge of its limitations allows the sleep practitioner to accurately identify false signals and potential interference. In our patient, a motion artifact produced the artificially decreased SpO$_2$ nadir of 92%. This section of the oximetry recording was marked as an artifact. The actual SpO$_2$ nadir was 95%.

CLINICAL PEARLS

1. Pulse oximeters are less accurate when the SpO$_2$ drops below 80%.
2. Factors that may affect the accuracy of pulse oximetry include motion, low perfusion, abnormal hemoglobin, dark skin pigmentation, arrhythmia, and synthetic nails and nail polish.
3. The shape and amplitude of the PWF aid in the identification of artifactual SpO$_2$ values.

REFERENCES

1. Nitzan M, Romem A, Koppel R. Pulse oximetry: fundamentals and technology update. *Med Devices (Auckl)*. 2014;7:231–239.
2. Fouzas S, Priftis KN, Anthracopoulos MB. Pulse oximetry in pediatric practice. *Pediatrics*. Oct 2011;128(4):740–752.

A 5-year-old child with unusual leg movements on polysomnography

Mary H. Wagner

CASE PRESENTATION

A sleep technologist asked you to evaluate his scoring of periodic limb movements (PLMs) in a 5-year-old child with a complex medical history including muscle weakness, feeding intolerance, and restless sleep. The technologist shows you the tracing below (Fig. 20-1). You view the video of the sleep study associated with the tracing and see no leg movements.

QUESTION

Does this tracing show PLMs?

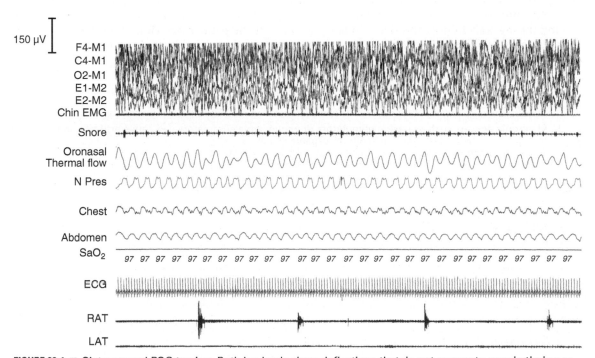

FIGURE 20-1 ■ Sixty-second PSG tracing. Both leg leads show deflections that do not appear to vary in timing or amplitude. F4-M1, C4-M1, O2-M1, E1-M2, E2-M2 are electroencephalogram leads used to stage sleep EMG - electromyogram; N Pres - nasal pressure; SaO2 - oxygen saturation; ECG - electrocardiogram; RAT - right leg electromyogram; LAT - left leg electromyogram.

ANSWER

The tracing shows deflections in both leg leads that are unvarying in frequency and amplitude. These are artifacts caused by a gastric electric stimulator. The regularity and duration of the signals are suspicious for a nonorganic etiology. Review of the history revealed that the child has gastroparesis requiring treatment with a gastric electric stimulator.

DISCUSSION

Gastric electric stimulators are considered for treatment of patients with nausea and vomiting related to gastroparesis who have not responded to medical therapies.[1] A small, battery-powered device is placed under the skin of the lower abdomen. Lead wires are tunneled under the skin to nerves controlling gastric muscles. Timed and controlled electrical impulses are delivered to stimulate gastric contraction and emptying. The device can be adjusted to maximize therapy. Another implanted medical device that can cause artifacts on a polysomnogram (PSG) tracing is a vagus nerve stimulator (see Clinical Pearls in Case 78: 16-year-old boy with intractable seizure disorder and snoring).

PLMs are scored during a sleep study when a series of movements are noted with specific characteristics, which include duration, amplitude, and period of time between movements (see PLM example in Clinical Pearls in Case 68: A 9-year-old boy with snoring and leg movements). The leg movements may be noted in either the left or right leg electromyogram (EMG) lead, with an amplitude of 8 μV above the baseline and a minimum number of four consecutive leg movements for a PLM series. The leg movements must be at least 5 seconds and a maximum of 90 seconds apart, and each movement must have a duration between 0.5 and 10 seconds.[2] A PLM index >5/h is considered abnormal in children, and a PLM index >15/h is considered abnormal in adults.[3] The etiology of periodic limb movements can include uremia, neuropathy, medications (antihistamines, selective serotonin reuptake inhibitors, and metoclopramide), caffeine intake, and low ferritin levels.[4] In this case, the regularity of the deflections in both leg leads is suspicious for being a nonorganic artifact. The deflections were unvarying in amplitude and frequency. In addition, the deflections occurred throughout the tracing during wakefulness and sleep. When the video of the patient was viewed, no leg movements were discernible. The additional history of the patient having a gastric stimulator was obtained from the record, and it explains the artifact seen on this tracing.

CLINICAL PEARLS

1. Electronic devices such as gastric stimulators or vagus nerve stimulators can cause artifacts on PSG tracings that should be distinguished from organic signals.
2. Obtaining a careful history will aid in detection of PSG artifacts.
3. PLMs are scored during sleep when deflections noted in the leg leads meet the specific scoring criteria of a series of four leg movements, 8 μV above the baseline leg EMG, lasting 0.5 to 10 seconds, with intervals between leg movements being at least 5 seconds but not more than 90 seconds long.

REFERENCES

1. Abell T, McCallum R, Hocking M, et al. Gastric electrical stimulation for medically refractory gastroparesis. *Gastroenterology.* 2003;125:421–428.
2. Berry RB, Brooks R, Gamaldo CE, Harding SM, Marcus CL, Vaughn BV for the American Academy of Sleep Medicine. *The AASM Manual for the Scoring of Sleep and Associated Events: Rules, Terminology and Technical Specifications, Version 2.0.* Darien, IL: American Academy of Sleep Medicine; 2012:36.
3. *Periodic Limb Movement Disorder International Classification of Sleep Disorders.* 3rd ed. Darien, IL: American Academy of Sleep Medicine; 2014:292.
4. Berry RB. The restless leg syndrome, periodic limb movements in sleep and the periodic limb movement disorder. In: *Fundamentals of Sleep Medicine.* Philadelphia, PA: Elsevier; 2012:429.

A 16-year-old with snoring and diaphoresis

Lourdes M. DelRosso

CASE PRESENTATION

A 16-year-old boy presented for evaluation of snoring, mouth breathing, and nocturnal diaphoresis. The family denied daytime sleepiness or behavioral problems. He did not have any other sleep-related concerns or medical problems. His past surgical history was negative. The review of systems was negative.

PHYSICAL EXAM

Physical exam revealed an alert and cooperative adolescent. His vital signs were within the normal range. His height was at the 85th percentile, and weight was at the 99th percentile. He did not have micrognathia or retrognathia. The oropharynx was Mallampati grade III. Tonsil size was 1+. The remainder of the exam was normal.

LABORATORY AND SLEEP FINDINGS

Polysomnography (PSG) was performed. The sleep technician saw an artifact in the electroencephalogram (EEG) (Fig. 21-1).

QUESTION

What intervention would be the most appropriate to correct the predominant artifact seen in Figure 21-1?

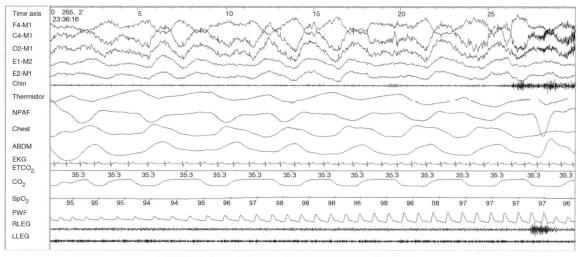

FIGURE 21-1 ■ Thirty-second epoch during N2 sleep.

ANSWER

Figure 21-1 shows sweat artifact in the EEG and eye leads. The technician should cool down the room, remove blankets from the patient, dry the skin, and reapply the electrodes. The ECG artifact is also seen in the EEG leads. For discussion on ECG artifact see Clinical Pearls in Case 22: A polysomnography finding in an 8-year-old with history of seizures.

DISCUSSION

Sweat artifact is commonly seen in PSG. Sodium chloride and lactic acid present in sweat react with the exposed electrodes, producing a chemical reaction that when combined with the skin action potentials produces a low-frequency high-amplitude signal.[1] The most common leads affected by sweat artifact are the EEG and electrooculography (EOG) electrodes, mainly because perspiration on the forehead affects the ground lead that is common to all EEG and EOG channels. Slow movement of the head with each respiration can produce another type of slow-frequency artifact called *respiratory artifact*. This can be easily distinguished from sweat artifact. Respiratory artifact coincides with the signal generated by the respiratory sensors and/or chest and abdominal channels, whereas sweat artifact does not.[2] Figure 21-1 shows slow-frequency, high-amplitude waves on the EEG and EOG channels that do not correlate with respiration.

CLINICAL PEARLS

1. Sweat artifact is common in PSG.
2. Sweat artifact manifests as slow-frequency, undulating waves that are not synchronized with breathing.
3. To correct the artifact, cool the room, dry the skin, and reapply the electrodes.

REFERENCES

1. Siddiqui F, Osuna E, Walters AS, Chokroverty S. Sweat artifact and respiratory artifact occurring simultaneously in polysomnogram. *Sleep Med.* Mar 2006;7(2):197–199.
2. Spriggs WH. *Essentials of Polysomnography: A Training Guide and Reference for Sleep Technicians.* 2nd ed. Burlington: Jones & Bartlett Learning; 2014.

A polysomnography finding in an 8-year-old with history of seizures

Lourdes M. DelRosso

CASE PRESENTATION

You are reading a polysomnogram (PSG) from an 8-year-old boy with a past medical history of seizure disorder controlled on levetiracetam. The sleep study was ordered for evaluation of snoring. As soon as the boy falls asleep, you notice the electroencephalogram (EEG) waves seen in Figure 22-1 (*arrows*).

QUESTION

What causes the waveform seen in Figure 22-1 (*arrows*)?

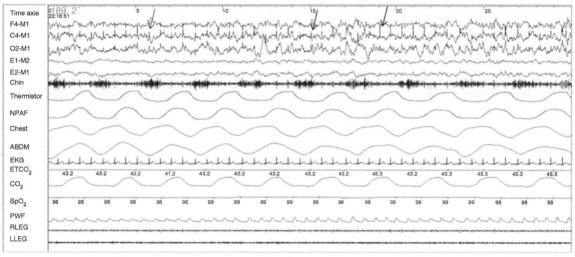

FIGURE 22-1 ■ Thirty-second epoch of N2 showing sharp waveforms (*arrows*).

ANSWER

The arrows point to the artifact caused by the electrocardiogram (ECG). This is easily identified when the ECG is moved next to the EEG leads (Fig. 22-2).

DISCUSSION

The American Academy of Sleep Medicine Manual for the Scoring of Sleep and Associated Events recommends monitoring heart rhythms during PSG using two electrodes applied in a single modified lead II. In standard ECG, lead II is derived from electrodes applied to the right arm and left leg. In PSG, lead II is derived from an electrode placed below the right clavicle and one placed on the left side of the thorax at the fourth intercostal space. The same setup applies for adults and children.

The electrical activity of the heart can propagate through the body and manifest as high-frequency electrical activity on the EEG leads on the scalp (representing the QRS complex). This artifact can be easily identified by superimposing it on the EEG leads.[1] The ECG artifact poses a particular problem for automated interpretation of EEG or PSG.

To minimize the ECG artifact, when present, it is recommended that the two reference electrodes (M1 and M2) be linked. This is also called "double referencing." Linking can be performed physically by connecting the two mastoid electrodes with a jumper cable at the electrode box or by the PSG computer program using derivations where the reference electrode is an average of M1 and M2. This works because if the ECG voltage vector is toward one mastoid, it is away from the other. Therefore, the ECG components of the two signals tend to cancel each other out. This will attenuate or eliminate the ECG artifact on the EEG signals.[2]

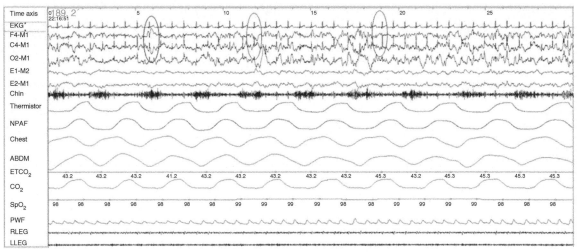

FIGURE 22-2 ■ Same 30-second epoch of N2 with ECG lead moved next to the EEG leads. The sharp waves on the EEG correspond to the QRS complex and represent the ECG artifact (*circles*).

CLINICAL PEARLS

1. The electrical activity of the heart can propagate through the body and manifest as high-frequency electrical activity on the EEG leads on the scalp.
2. To minimize the ECG artifact, when present, it is recommended that the two reference electrodes (M1 and M2) be linked.

REFERENCES

1. Lanquart JP, Dumont M, Linkowski P. QRS artifact elimination on full night sleep EEG. *Med Eng Phys*. Mar 2006;28(2): 156–165.
2. Butkov N, Lee-Chiong TL. *Fundamentals of Sleep Technology*. Philadelphia: Lippincott Williams & Wilkins; 2007. [section 7].

PART 2

Clinical Pediatric Sleep Medicine Pearls

CASE 23

A 14-year-old girl who watches TV to fall asleep

Lourdes M. DelRosso

CASE PRESENTATION

A 14-year-old girl presented with difficulty falling asleep at night and excessive sleepiness during the day for the past 3 months. The symptoms started without any apparent precipitating factor. The patient worked on her homework in her bedroom from 8 PM until 10 PM. During this time, she used a laptop and a smartphone. Once done with her homework, she turned the TV on and left it on until she fell asleep. On most nights she fell asleep by midnight. The parents tried to wake her up from 6 AM until 7 AM. She felt sleepy during the day and dozed off in school and during car rides but did not take scheduled naps. During the weekends, she watched TV until midnight and woke up at 10 AM. She did not report daytime sleepiness on weekends. The family denied snoring, sleepwalking, nightmares, symptoms of restless legs, cataplexy, hypnagogic hallucinations, or sleep paralysis. There were no past medical problems. The review of systems was negative. The physical exam was normal.

LABORATORY AND SLEEP FINDINGS

None

QUESTION

What is the diagnosis in this patient?

ANSWER

The patient has inadequate sleep hygiene (use of electronics in the bedroom before bedtime).

DISCUSSION

Children who have a TV in their bedroom have been found to watch more TV per day compared with children who do not have a TV in their bedroom. Watching TV for more than 2 hours a day has been associated with daytime symptoms of inattention and poor academic achievement; however, some parents erroneously believe that having a TV in the child's bedroom assists with bedtime and sleep.[1]

TV is not the only electronic device used at bedtime. Over the past few years, with the increase in use of portable electronic devices such as smartphones, tablets, and video game consoles, almost all adolescents (97%) have at least one electronic device in their bedroom.[2] These included music players (90%), TV (57%), video game consoles (43%), smartphones (42%) or telephones (34%), and computers (28%).[2] Older adolescents used more devices before bedtime than younger adolescents do. The use of electronics by adolescents in the hour before bedtime has been associated with an increased sleep latency and insufficient sleep. In fact, adolescents who use four devices or more in the hour before bedtime have been found to have a sleep latency longer than 60 minutes and a shorter sleep duration, and they were sleepy during the day and more likely to doze in school.[2,3] Further, 44% of adolescents reported talking on the phone after 9 PM, and 34% reported texting. One third of adolescents reported being woken up by a text message at least once a month. The use of electronic games or computers has been associated with shorter total sleep time and increased daytime fatigue. The use of music at bedtime has also been associated with prolonged sleep latency, decreased total sleep time, and increased tiredness on weekdays.[4]

The use of electronics around bedtime may affect sleep by various mechanisms. Light exposure may delay the circadian clock, the content of electronic devices may increase alertness, and the use of electronic devices may interfere with other healthy activities before bedtime (Fig. 23-1).[4] Our patient and her parents were recommended to remove electronic devices from the bedroom and to institute a consistent bedtime routine.

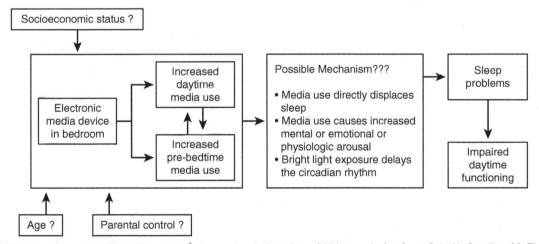

FIGURE 23-1 ■ **Potential effect of the use of electronics during sleep.** (With permission from Cain N, Gradisar M. Electronic media use and sleep in school-aged children and adolescents: a review. *Sleep Med.* Sep 2010;11(8):735-742.)

CLINICAL PEARLS

1. Almost all adolescents use at least one electronic device in their bedroom.
2. Sleep is negatively affected by the use of electronic devices in the hour before bedtime.
3. The effects on sleep may include delayed sleep latency and decreased total sleep time, with subsequent daytime sleepiness.

REFERENCES

1. Crowder JS, Sisson SB, Ramey E, Arnold SH, Richardson S, DeGrace BW. How did the television get in the child's bedroom? Analysis of family interviews. *Prev Med*. Dec 2012;55(6):623–628.
2. National Sleep Foundation. Teens and Sleep. *Sleep in America Poll*. 2006:2006. https://sleepfoundation.org/sites/default/files/2006_summary_of_findings.pdf.
3. Hysing M, Pallesen S, Stormark KM, Jakobsen R, Lundervold AJ, Sivertsen B. Sleep and use of electronic devices in adolescence: results from a large population-based study. *BMJ Open*. 2015;5(1):e006748.
4. Cain N, Gradisar M. Electronic media use and sleep in school-aged children and adolescents: a review. *Sleep Med*. Sep 2010;11(8):735–742.

An 8-year-old with a return to daytime napping

Mary H. Wagner

CASE PRESENTATION

An 8-year-old child presents in the office for evaluation of snoring and school issues. The family reports that the child snores only with upper respiratory tract infections, which occur once or twice a year. The primary care provider is concerned about obstructive sleep apnea. The family reports that the child gave up napping at age 5 years but returned to napping at age 7.5 years. His teachers have reported inattentiveness at school, as well as aggressive behavior during recess. He will often fall asleep on the way home from school, and he takes a nap for at least 1 hour after school. He falls asleep quickly at night but has difficulty getting up in the morning and is not a "morning person." The family admits that the child's bedtime is often delayed until after 10 PM because of family activities, and he must arise at 6 AM to be taken to the precare program at school so his parents can get to work on time. His behavior is not a problem during the summer months when he is able to sleep until 8 AM.

PHYSICAL EXAM

On physical exam the child's height was in the 75th percentile, weight 50th percentile, and body mass index 25th percentile. The child was interactive and alert. He did not have an adenoid facies. The oropharynx was Mallampati 2, with 1 + tonsils. The remainder of the exam was unremarkable.

Polysomnography showed sleep latency 5 minutes; sleep efficiency 95%; normal sleep architecture; apnea–hypopnea index 0.4/h; and periodic limb movements during sleep 0/h.

QUESTION

What is the cause of this child's daytime symptoms?

ANSWER

The cause of this child's daytime symptoms is insufficient sleep, with the child receiving a maximum of 8 hours sleep per night. Daytime symptoms including sleepiness during car rides and difficulty arising in the morning, as well as the inattentiveness and aggressive behavior, were noted in this child. These signs and symptoms can be seen in children who do not get enough sleep at night. Studies of acute sleep restriction demonstrate impaired attentiveness in children compared with children receiving adequate sleep.[1,2] Dahl relates that, although individual children may have a varying response to inadequate sleep, a general pattern of behavior noted in children with insufficient sleep includes irritability, poor focus, and labile emotions.[2] In addition, the family reported fewer symptoms during summer months, when the child was sleeping longer. Thus, the symptoms reported in this child can be attributed to insufficient sleep. Many parents may not appreciate how much sleep their child requires. A 2004 Sleep in America poll on children's sleep demonstrated that a majority of parents reported on one question that their child was getting the correct amount of sleep, while reporting on a separate question that their child's sleep duration is less than the parents think they need.[3]

DISCUSSION

School-age children generally do not take naps, and a return to napping in this age group is a clue that sleep is insufficient or disrupted. Children aged 7 to 10 years should be getting 9 to 12 hours of sleep at night.[4,5] Iglowstein et al. found that sleep duration for normal children ranged from 8.6 to 12 hours in the 7- to 10-year-old age group, with 8-year-olds sleeping 9.1 to 11.7 hours,[4] and Galland et al. found a mean of 9.4 to 9.1 hours over the 7-to 10-year-old age range.[5] In addition, Iglowstein reported that only 0.9% of 7-year-old children were continuing to nap during the day.[4]

Our patient is getting 8 hours of sleep at best, leading to insufficient sleep. The results of the sleep study demonstrated high sleep efficiency, short sleep latency, and no evidence of sleep disruption related to obstructive sleep apnea or leg movements. The family was counseled to extend the child's sleep time to at least 10 hours a night. With this change, the child no longer took daytime naps and had improved attentiveness and behavior at school.

CLINICAL PEARLS

1. A return to daytime napping in children older than 6 years of age indicates insufficient or disrupted sleep.
2. Signs and symptoms of daytime sleepiness in children include aggressive behavior and inattention.
3. Documentation of sleep duration is an important part of the history in children with sleep disorders, as well as those with behavioral and school performance issues.
4. Anticipatory guidance for families should include information about adequate sleep duration for children.

REFERENCES

1. Fallone G, Acebo C, Arnedt JT, Seifer R, Carskadon MA. Effects of acute sleep restriction on behavior, sustained attention, and response inhibition in children. *Percept. Mot Skills.* 2001;93(1):213–229.
2. Dahl R. The impact of inadequate sleep on children's daytime cognitive function. *Semin Pediatr Neurol.* 1996;3(1):44–50.
3. *2004 Sleep in America Poll.* National Sleep Foundation. <https://sleepfoundation.org/sites/default/files/FINAL%20SOF%202004.pdf>; 2004 Accessed 22.01.16.
4. Iglowstein I, Jenni OG, Molinari L, Largo RH. Sleep duration from infancy to adolescence: reference values and generational trends. *Pediatrics.* 2003;11(2):302–307.
5. Galland BC, Taylor BJ, Elder DE, Herbison P. Normal sleep patterns in infants and children: a systematic review of observational studies. *Sleep Med Rev.* 2012;16(3):213–222.

A 10-year-old girl sleeps with her parents and her sister

Lourdes M. DelRosso

CASE PRESENTATION

A 10-year-old girl was referred for evaluation of snoring. She sleeps in the same bed with her parents and with her younger sister, and the parents noted her soft snoring. They stated that they "always slept with their children" and that they are not concerned about it. The mother is currently 38 weeks pregnant with their third child. The family goes to bed at 10 PM in a king-sized bed. The child falls asleep within 10 minutes. She does not have nocturnal awakenings and wakes up in the morning at 7 AM. There is no history of observed apnea, labored breathing during sleep, daytime sleepiness, restless legs, or parasomnias. The remainder of the history was negative.

PHYSICAL EXAM

The child was cooperative and alert. Her vital signs were within the normal range. Weight was at the 30th percentile and height at the 60th percentile. She did not have an adenoid facies or high-arched palate, the jaw was normal, oropharyngeal Mallampati grade was II, and tonsil size was 2+. The remainder of the exam was normal.

LABORATORY AND SLEEP FINDINGS

Polysomnography: total sleep time (TST) 400 minutes; obstructive apnea–hypopnea index (AHI) 1/h; central AHI 0.1/h; SpO_2 nadir 95%; $ETCO_2$ <50 torr for 100% of TST.

QUESTION

What do you advise this family regarding bed sharing?

ANSWER

As the family is expecting another child, they should be educated about the increased risk of sudden infant death syndrome (SIDS) when bed sharing with infants (see Clinical Pearls in Case 18: A 3-month-old infant who sleeps with a pacifier). There are no evidence-based recommendations for bed sharing with older children, and different cultures have different attitudes toward bed sharing.

DISCUSSION

Bed sharing with children has been studied mainly in association with SIDS. Bed sharing has been shown to increase the risk of SIDS and infant death by strangulation and suffocation.[1] For this reason the American Academy of Pediatrics (AAP) recommends room sharing without bed sharing for infants younger than 3 months of age.[2] For older infants, the AAP recommends avoiding bed sharing with a current smoker, with someone who is excessively tired, on sedative medications or substances (e.g., alcohol), with anyone who is not the parent, with multiple persons, or on unsafe sleep surfaces such as sofas.[2] In spite of these recommendations, bed sharing with infants continues to increase in the United States among African Americans and Hispanics.[3] Studies exploring the benefits of bed sharing have shown a positive association between bed sharing and breastfeeding, demonstrating an increased frequency and length of breast feeding when bed sharing.[4] This association, however, does not surpass the risk of SIDS, and the AAP strongly recommends room sharing without bed sharing.

It is important to acknowledge that bed sharing and room sharing practices vary significantly among cultures. A study comparing sleep habits in toddlers (aged 0 to 36 months) from predominantly Asian countries and toddlers from predominantly Caucasian countries showed that children from Asian countries were more likely to sleep in the parents' room or in the parents' bed (Fig. 25-1).[5]

Bed sharing in older children and adolescents has not been thoroughly studied, and the AAP does not have any specific recommendations. Our team educated the family about safe sleep for their future new baby. In particular, we recommended that the baby sleep in a crib in the parents' room but not in the bed with them. No further recommendations were given about co-sleeping with their two older daughters.

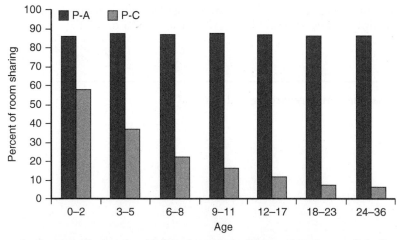

FIGURE 25-1 ■ **Percent of room sharing in children from 0 to 36 months of age.** *P-A,* Predominantly Asian countries; *P-C,* predominantly Caucasian countries. Age is in months. (Used with copyright from Mindell JA, Sadeh A, Wiegand B, How TH, Goh DY. Cross-cultural differences in infant and toddler sleep. *Sleep Med.* Mar 2010;11(3):274-280.)

CLINICAL PEARLS

1. The AAP recommends against bed sharing in infants because of the increased risk of SIDS.
2. Bed sharing varies significantly among cultures, with a higher prevalence in Asian, Hispanic, and African American families
3. The AAP does not have specific recommendations about bed sharing for older children.

REFERENCES

1. Shapiro-Mendoza CK, Kimball M, Tomashek KM, Anderson RN, Blanding S. US infant mortality trends attributable to accidental suffocation and strangulation in bed from 1984 through 2004: are rates increasing? *Pediatrics*. Feb 2009;123(2): 533–539.
2. Moon RY. SIDS and other sleep-related infant deaths: expansion of recommendations for a safe infant sleeping environment. *Pediatrics*. Nov 2011;128(5):1030–1039.
3. Colson ER, Willinger M, Rybin D, et al. Trends and factors associated with infant bed sharing, 1993-2010: the National Infant Sleep Position Study. *JAMA Pediatr*. Nov 2013;167(11):1032–1037.
4. Ball HL. Breastfeeding, bed-sharing, and infant sleep. *Birth*. Sep 2003;30(3):181–188.
5. Mindell JA, Sadeh A, Wiegand B, How TH, Goh DY. Cross-cultural differences in infant and toddler sleep. *Sleep Med*. Mar 2010;11(3):274–280.

A 4-year-old boy with frequent nocturnal awakenings

Lourdes M. DelRosso

CASE PRESENTATION

A 4-year-old boy was evaluated for frequent nocturnal awakenings in the past year. The parents reported a bedtime routine that began at 8 PM and consisted of taking a bath, changing into pajamas, brushing his teeth, and reading a story in his bed. His mother stayed in the room with him until he fell asleep. The patient usually woke up between 3 and 6 times a night, crying. The mother responded by going to his room and lying next to him until he fell back asleep (usually within 5 to 10 minutes). After the third nocturnal awakening, the mother would stay with him for the remainder of the night. The patient woke up at 8 AM. During the day, he took a nap between 1 PM and 3 PM. He snored softly. The family did not report night terrors, sleep talking, or sleepwalking. During the day, the parents noted hyperactivity. Review of systems was negative for anxiety or behavioral problems. He was developmentally appropriate.

PHYSICAL EXAM

Physical exam revealed a cooperative boy in no distress. His vital signs were within normal limits. His weight was at the 45th percentile, and his height was at the 34th percentile. He did not have an adenoid facies or a high-arched palate. His oropharynx was Mallampati grade II. Tonsil size was 1+. He did not have micrognathia or retrognathia. The remainder of the cardiovascular and neurologic exam was normal.

QUESTION

What is the diagnosis in this child?

ANSWER

The diagnosis is chronic insomnia.

DISCUSSION

The *International Classification of Sleep Disorders*, third edition (ICSD-3) criteria for chronic insomnia in children include parental report of either difficulty initiating sleep, maintaining sleep, waking earlier than desired, resistance to going to bed, or difficulty sleeping without parental intervention. Daytime symptoms must be present and may include behavioral problems, hyperactivity, inattention, irritability, or daytime sleepiness. The symptoms must occur at least 3 times a week for at least 3 months.

Previously called *behavioral insomnia of childhood*, chronic insomnia affects up to 30% of children.[1] Chronic insomnia in young children most often results from sleep associations at bedtime (such as being rocked to sleep in the case of an infant or having a parent present until the child falls asleep). This can result in delayed sleep latency. It also results in frequent nocturnal awakenings, which can then interfere with the sleep of the caregiver, and is the usual reason for referral to a sleep clinician. It is normal for children (and individuals of all ages) to have brief awakenings during the night, but usually these are very short, and the child "self-soothes" and falls back to sleep quickly. However, if the child is used to having an association with a caregiver or object at sleep onset, and the caregiver or object is no longer present during the nocturnal awakening, the child may have difficulty falling asleep by himself or herself.

In younger children, the sleep associations are usually parental interventions such as rocking or nursing. Insomnia can also develop when lack of parental limit setting leads to bedtime refusal or resistance (e.g., acquiescing to the child's demands for another drink, another trip to the living room, or more hugs).[1] Other common causes of insomnia in the pediatric age group include anxiety and circadian rhythm disorders.

The American Academy of Sleep Medicine practice parameters for behavioral treatment of bedtime problems and night waking in infants and young children recommend several treatments such as unmodified extinction (see later), graduated extinction (see later), delayed bedtime, and scheduled awakenings as effective interventions for chronic insomnia.[2] As circadian rhythm is not well established in infants until age 3 to 6 months, treatment for insomnia is not usually initiated before 6 months of age, although healthy sleep habits should be encouraged at any age. Interventions should begin with institution of adequate sleep hygiene, including regular bedtime routine, consistent bedtime schedule, and avoidance of electronics and caffeine. Unmodified extinction consists of placing the child in bed and ignoring any negative behavior (crying, yelling, or tantrums). If performed consistently, this usually results in resolution of the insomnia within a few nights. Graduated extinction consists of reducing the parental presence by slowly moving the parent out of the room (e.g., by having the parent sit by the bedroom door for a few nights instead of on the bed). Setting a later bedtime and then slowly moving the bedtime earlier along with implementing positive bedtime routines has also been shown effective in the treatment of insomnia.[3]

The persistence of night waking in the absence of sleep associations may indicate an underlying psychiatric or medical condition (anxiety, gastroesophageal reflux, etc.). Polysomnography is not indicated in the routine evaluation of insomnia, but it is indicated if there is suspicion of obstructive sleep apnea or periodic leg movements. In our patient, graduated extinction was successfully implemented.

CLINICAL PEARLS

1. Chronic insomnia in young children is often secondary to sleep associations or inadequate limit setting.
2. Chronic insomnia in children is manifested by nighttime symptoms (resistance to go to bed, inability to sleep without parental intervention, and frequent awakenings) and daytime symptoms (inattention, hyperactivity, and sleepiness).
3. Interventions for insomnia in children include unmodified extinction, graduated extinction, and delayed bedtime and scheduled awakenings.

REFERENCES

1. Vriend J, Corkum P. Clinical management of behavioral insomnia of childhood. *Psychol Res Behav Manag.* 2011;4:69–79.
2. Morgenthaler TI, Owens J, Alessi C, et al. Practice parameters for behavioral treatment of bedtime problems and night wakings in infants and young children. *Sleep.* Oct 2006;29(10):1277–1281.
3. Moore M. Behavioral sleep problems in children and adolescents. *J Clin Psychol Med Settings.* Mar 2012;19(1):77–83.

A 14-year-old with difficulty falling asleep

Mary H. Wagner

CASE PRESENTATION

A 14-year-old girl presents to the clinic reporting that she has difficulty falling asleep at night, Her mother adds that the mother has difficulty getting her daughter out of bed in the morning and the daughter is frequently late for school. She has had this problem for the past 6 months ever since she was hospitalized for treatment of a broken arm. Her first class starts at 8:45 AM, and she is supposed to wake up at 7:30 AM, but this is quite difficult. She often sleeps through her alarm, and her mother has to "drag" her out of bed at 8 AM. Her daily weekday schedule includes leaving for school at 8:20 AM and getting home from school at 1:30 PM. She has a snack after school, takes a nap from 2 to 4 PM, and then gets up to do her homework. After dinner at 7 PM, she showers and heads to bed at 9 PM. She has her cell phone at her bedside and keeps the TV on at night with the "volume down," to help her fall asleep. She worries about not being able to fall asleep and how it will "ruin her life." She lies in bed for an extended period of time and reports that her mind is often racing until her usual sleep-onset time, which varies from 11 PM to 2 AM. She wishes she could fall asleep earlier but just cannot. Of note, she does report that when she goes to her grandmother's house to visit in a distant state (same time zone), it is much easier for her to fall asleep. Once she falls asleep, she stays asleep for only 2 to 3 hours before waking and having trouble falling asleep again. She has had eight tardy notices at school this semester. While at school she is slightly sleepy in her first class but does not fall asleep at school, and despite this, she is making As and Bs. On the weekends, she goes to bed anytime between 11 PM and 3 AM and takes a long time to fall asleep despite a later bedtime. She wakes up anytime from 11 AM to 1 PM but often does not feel rested. She admits to staying in bed lounging for an extra hour. She needs coffee in the morning to get going on school days and has sweet tea every night with dinner. The patient denies leg discomfort, snoring, nasal congestion, or history of depression. Her only medication is occasional ibuprofen for aches. Her mother and grandmother both report similar difficulties falling asleep.

PHYSICAL EXAM

Vital signs: pulse 82, blood pressure 109/71; respiratory rate 12 breaths/min; afebrile, SpO_2 97%; weight 47.3 kg (40th percentile); height 1.62 m (50th percentile); and body mass index 18 (30th percentile).

Exam: head, eyes, ears, nose, and throat, normal; Mallampati 2; tonsils 1+. The remainder of the physical and neurologic exam was normal.

LABORATORY AND SLEEP FINDINGS

Modified Epworth Sleepiness Scale 11/24; sleep diary shown below (Fig. 27-1).

QUESTION

What is causing this patient's sleeping difficulties and what is the best way to help her?

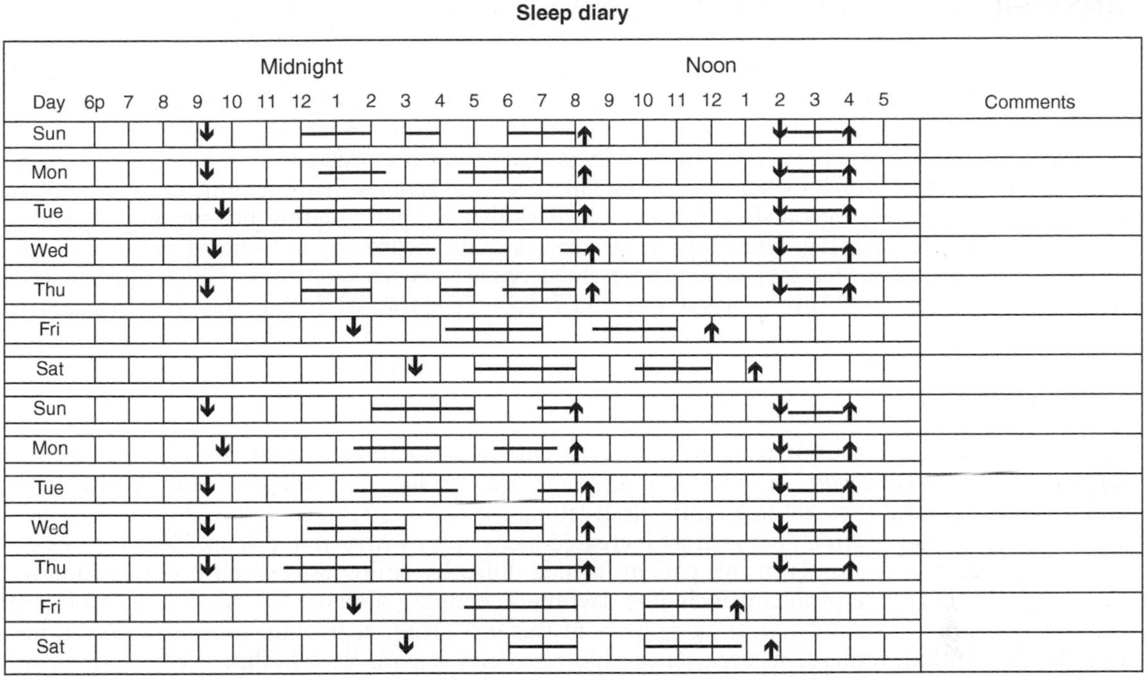

Sleep diary

FIGURE 27-1 ■ Sleep diary for 2 weeks, showing time in bed (↓) and time out of bed (↑), with time asleep indicated by *solid bars*. The diary shows in-bed time at 9 PM on school nights, with sleep onset at 12 to 2 AM and rise time of 8 AM. Sleep periods last 1 to 3 hours, with prolonged awakenings. It also shows napping from 2 to 4 PM on most weekdays. On weekend nights she gets into bed at 1 to 3 AM and takes a long time to fall asleep, awakening between 11 AM and 1 PM. She stays in bed on weekends for 1 hour after she awakens.

ANSWER

This patient has psychophysiological insomnia. Review of her sleep diary (Fig. 27-1) shows irregular sleep onset from 11:30 PM to 5 AM, with periods of sleep lasting from 1 to 3 hours, followed by prolonged awakenings. She has difficulty falling asleep on school and weekend nights and spends extended periods of time in bed not asleep. Her Epworth Sleepiness Scale score is consistent with mild daytime sleepiness. In addition, she worries when she cannot fall asleep and reports that it is difficult for her to calm her mind. She also has several sleep hygiene practices that are perpetuating her sleeping difficulties, including caffeine intake, daytime napping, electronics in the bedroom, and staying in bed for a prolonged period of time before sleep onset. When she sleeps in a new environment, she initially falls asleep more easily, but her sleep-onset issues return after 2 days as she tries to sleep in the new environment.

DISCUSSION

Psychophysiological insomnia is a subtype of the chronic insomnia disorder described in the third edition of the *International Classification of Sleep Disorders* as acquired sleep-preventing associations and increased arousal that results in difficulties falling asleep in the typical home sleep setting at the desired time.[1] Patients often demonstrate increased focus on or worry about sleep. Components consistent with chronic insomnia in this patient include difficulty falling asleep and dissatisfaction with sleep, as well as daytime problems including daytime sleepiness.[1] Further 9% to 13% of adolescents experience chronic insomnia, with up to 35% of this age group reporting insomnia many times a month.[2] In addition, adolescents experience a biologic delay in circadian rhythms, delaying their time of circadian sleepiness.[3]

Treatment approaches should include correcting her sleep hygiene practices to include no daytime napping and no caffeine intake, especially after 2 PM.[2,4] She should turn off her TV and cell phone an hour before bedtime and keep her room dimly lit. Bright light should be avoided in the evenings.

To improve her psychophysiological insomnia, approaches can include making a worry list before bed, using her bed only for sleep (no homework, TV, or texting in bed), and consideration for referral to a clinical psychologist for cognitive behavioral treatment of insomnia. These strategies have been well studied in adults, with fewer studies in adolescents and children.[2] She should be advised to get into bed closer to her sleep-onset time (12 AM) and arise at the same time each morning (8 AM) (sleep restriction). This should include the weekends. She should get out of bed after 15 to 20 minutes of trying to fall asleep if she is unable to sleep and engage in a relaxing and dimly lit activity (stimulus control).[2] She should also get out of bed on weekend mornings shortly after she awakens. Once she is falling asleep quickly at her bedtime, she can move her bedtime 15 minutes earlier and work toward a bedtime that will increase sleep on school nights. If she were age 16 years, she and her family should be advised not to allow driving with her inadequate sleep duration. A letter can be provided to the school to explain her sleep disorder, with suggestions to maximize her school performance, including testing at periods of maximum alertness and consideration of alternative ways to accomplish coursework such as online classes that could be completed in lieu of her early morning classes at school. She may need a caffeinated beverage to help her maintain alertness in the mornings initially, but caffeine should be avoided after 2 PM.

These suggestions were implemented, and at a 1-month follow-up visit, the patient reported being able to fall asleep at 12:30 AM and wake up more easily for school at 8 AM. She continues to work on moving her sleep onset earlier, with the goal of being able to fall asleep by 10:30 PM.

CLINICAL PEARLS

1. During development, many adolescents experience a biologic shift of their sleep phase, resulting in later circadian timing of sleepiness. A key feature on history in distinguishing psychophysiological insomnia from delayed sleep phase is sleep-onset insomnia persisting on weekends when the adolescent goes to bed later. The two conditions frequently coexist.
2. Appropriate sleep hygiene practices should be reviewed with adolescents with sleep issues, including avoidance of daytime napping, avoidance of caffeine, turning off electronics 1 hour before sleep time, setting sleep-onset and sleep-offset times to allow for adequate sleep, and establishing an appropriate sleep environment (dark, cool, and no electronics).
3. Cognitive behavioral therapy for insomnia should be considered for adolescents with psychophysiological insomnia not responsive to simple behavioral techniques.

REFERENCES

1. Chronic insomnia disorder. In: Sateia, M, ed. *International Classification of Sleep Disorders*. 3rd ed. Darien, IL: American Academy of Sleep Medicine; 2014:21–39.
2. Mindell JA, Owens JA. Insomnia. In: *A Clinical Guide to Pediatric Sleep-Diagnosis and Management of Sleep Problems*. 2nd ed. Philadelphia: Wolters Kluwer Lippincott Williams and Wilkins; 2010:153–160.
3. Crowley SJ, Tarokh L, Carskadon MA. Sleep during adolescence. In: Sheldon SH, Ferber R, Kryger MH, Gozal D, eds. *Principles and Practices of Pediatric Sleep Medicine*. 2nd ed. Philadelphia: Elsevier Saunders; 2014:45–49.
4. Owens JA, Mindell JA. Pediatric insomnia. *Pediatr Clin North Am*. 2011;58(3):555–569.

CASE 28

A 10-year-old boy with excessive sleepiness and new-onset parasomnia

Lourdes M. DelRosso

CASE PRESENTATION

A 10-year-old male presented with excessive daytime sleepiness for the last 6 months. The symptoms started without any apparent precipitating factor. The parents first noted that he was sleepy during the day and had started napping and dozing off in class. The parents also noticed that he had started having episodes of screaming or talking at night that occurred about 3 hours after falling asleep and lasted for about a minute. The patient did not have recollection of these events the next morning. His bedtime was 9 PM, and wake-up time was 6:30 AM. He took one daily nap for an hour, after which he woke up still feeling sleepy. The family denied snoring, sleepwalking, dream enactment, symptoms of restless legs, cataplexy, hypnagogic hallucinations, or sleep paralysis. There were no other past medical problems. His past surgical history was positive for tonsillectomy and adenoidectomy. His review of systems was negative for depression or anxiety.

PHYSICAL EXAM

Physical exam revealed vital signs within normal limits, and his weight was 38.4 kg (86th percentile) and height was 134.8 cm (35th percentile). He did not have an adenoid facies. His oropharynx was Mallampati class II, and tonsils were surgically absent. The remainder of the exam was normal.

LABORATORY AND SLEEP FINDINGS

A nocturnal polysomnogram (PSG) revealed total sleep time 516 minutes; total recording time 607 minutes; sleep efficiency 85%; sleep latency 3.5 minutes; and REM latency 14 minutes. The apnea–hypopnea index was 0.9/h. The leg movements per hour of sleep were 6.5/h. The periodic limb movements during sleep (PLMS) were not associated with arousals. Multiple Sleep Latency Test data are presented in Table 28-1.

QUESTIONS

What is the diagnosis in this child?

TABLE 28-1.	**Multiple sleep latency test results**				
	Nap 1 (min)	**Nap 2 (min)**	**Nap 3 (min)**	**Nap 4 (min)**	**Nap 5 (min)**
Sleep latency	1	2	3	1	2
REM latency	-	3	-	-	-

ANSWERS

The diagnosis is narcolepsy type 2.

DISCUSSION

The *International Classification of Sleep Disorders*, third edition (ICSD-3) diagnostic criteria for narcolepsy type 2 include daily symptoms of excessive sleepiness for 3 months with either cerebrospinal fluid hypocretin-1 levels not measured or levels >110 pg/mL or >1/3 normal values, absence of cataplexy, and positive MSLT. A positive MSLT includes a mean sleep onset <8 minutes and at least 2 sleep-onset REM periods (SOREMPs), one of which can be substituted by an REM onset within 15 minutes in the preceding nocturnal PSG, as in the case of this patient. The sleepiness or positive MSLT finding should not be better explained by insufficient sleep, obstructive sleep apnea, delayed sleep phase circadian disorder, effects of medications, or other medical problems.

The MSLT has been validated in children older than 6 years of age. Rarely, the onset of symptoms precedes the appearance of SOREMPs in the MSLT, and a repeat MSLT may be needed to confirm the diagnosis in patients with high clinical suspicion.[1] A PSG must be performed the night before the MSLT to assure adequate sleep and rule out sleep disorders. When possible, actigraphy and/or sleep diaries should be collected.[2]

Very little is known about the epidemiology and natural history of narcolepsy type 2. Unlike narcolepsy type 1, there are no biomarkers for narcolepsy type 2. There is current controversy as to whether narcolepsy type 2 is a pathophysiologically distinct diagnosis or part of the spectrum of manifestations of narcolepsy type 1, especially because a number of patients develop cataplexy later on and need to be rediagnosed as narcolepsy type 1. Hypnagogic or hypnopompic hallucinations occur in 28% of affected individuals.[3] Unlike adults, children with narcolepsy may present with sleep drunkenness lasting up to 30 minutes, a feature commonly seen in idiopathic hypersomnia. Other features of childhood onset narcolepsy may include precocious puberty, weight gain, and behavioral changes.[4]

Children with narcolepsy have a higher incidence of comorbid sleep disorders. Both REM and NREM parasomnias have been reported. REM sleep without atonia has been seen in up to 90% of affected patients, and up to 75% of patients have an increased periodic leg movement index. Other comorbidities include insomnia, sleep-disordered breathing, and bruxism. Sleep-related comorbidities appear to increase with age and may contribute to a delay in the diagnosis.[5,6]

CLINICAL PEARLS

1. The ICSD-3 diagnostic criteria for narcolepsy allow for substitution of a sleep-onset REM period during nocturnal PSG for one of the SOREMPs during MSLT.
2. Patients initially diagnosed with narcolepsy type 2 who later on develop cataplexy should be reclassified as narcolepsy type 1.
3. Children with narcolepsy are at increased risk for PLMS, NREM, and REM parasomnias, as well as insomnia and bruxism.
4. Unlike adults, children with narcolepsy may present with sleep drunkenness lasting up to 30 minutes, a feature commonly seen in idiopathic hypersomnia.

REFERENCES

1. Kubota H, Kanbayashi T, Tanabe Y, et al. Decreased cerebrospinal fluid hypocretin-1 levels near the onset of narcolepsy in 2 prepubertal children. *Sleep*. Aug 1 2003;26(5):555–557.
2. Littner MR, Kushida C, Wise M, et al. Practice parameters for clinical use of the multiple sleep latency test and the maintenance of wakefulness test. *Sleep*. Jan 2005;28(1):113–121.
3. Baumann CR, Mignot E, Lammers GJ, et al. Challenges in diagnosing narcolepsy without cataplexy: a consensus statement. *Sleep*. Jun 2014;37(6):1035–1042.
4. Nevsimalova S. The diagnosis and treatment of pediatric narcolepsy. *Curr Neurol Neurosci Rep*. Aug 2014;14(8):469.
5. Frauscher B, Ehrmann L, Mitterling T, et al. Delayed diagnosis, range of severity, and multiple sleep comorbidities: a clinical and polysomnographic analysis of 100 patients of the innsbruck narcolepsy cohort. *J Clin Sleep Med*. 2013;9(8):805–812.
6. Nevsimalova S, Pisko J, Buskova J, et al. Narcolepsy: clinical differences and association with other sleep disorders in different age groups. *J Neurol*. Mar 2013;260(3):767–775.

A 9-year-old girl with excessive daytime sleepiness and slurred speech

Lourdes M. DelRosso

CASE PRESENTATION

A 9-year-old girl presented with excessive daytime sleepiness that started 6 months earlier. Her mother stated that the child had always seemed to need more sleep compared with her peers, but recently, she had started taking naps during the day and fell asleep every time she sat down in a quiet environment. She went to bed at 8 PM and awoke at 6 AM, without nocturnal awakenings. She took 2 to 3 naps during the day. About once a week, the child reported seeing shadows in her room when she was falling asleep. The mother noted that when the child was excited, happy, or scared, her speech became slurred and her eyelids seemed droopy. On occasion she had fallen to the floor for a few seconds after laughing. Her mother did not notice any precipitating factors such as viral illness, head trauma, or a new stressful situation. She did not snore, and the mother denied symptoms of restless legs or episodes of sleep paralysis. There was no other past medical or surgical history. The patient did not take any medications. Review of systems was positive for weight gain and negative for depression or anxiety.

PHYSICAL EXAM

Physical exam revealed a sleepy girl in no distress. Her vital signs were within normal limits; her weight was 33.8 kg (76th percentile) and her height was 128.3 cm (20th percentile). Her oropharynx was Mallampati grade II. Her tonsils were size 2+. The remainder of the cardiovascular and neurologic exam was normal.

LABORATORY AND SLEEP FINDINGS

Polysomnography (PSG) revealed a total sleep time of 495 minutes; total recording time of 571 minutes; and sleep efficiency of 87%. The amount of REM sleep and the REM latency were normal for age. The apnea–hypopnea index was 0.8/h; SpO_2 nadir 97%; and periodic leg movement index 7/h. MSLT results are given in table 29-1.

QUESTION

What is the diagnosis in this child?

TABLE 29-1. **Multiple sleep latency test findings**

	Nap 1 (min)	Nap 2 (min)	Nap 3 (min)	Nap 4 (min)	Nap 5 (min)
Sleep latency	5	2	9.5	4.5	6
REM latency	2.5	3	—	1	—

ANSWER

Narcolepsy type 1.

DISCUSSION

Narcolepsy type 1 occurs in 0.02% to 0.18% of the US and Western European populations. First-degree relatives of affected patients are at slightly increased risk (1% to 2%). The pathophysiology of narcolepsy type 1 is attributed to loss of hypocretin-producing hypothalamic neurons. Hypocretin is an activating neuropeptide that regulates the sleep-wake cycle and REM sleep. The main manifestations of narcolepsy are rapid REM onset during sleep, sleep fragmentation, excessive daytime sleepiness, cataplexy, hypnagogic hallucinations, and sleep paralysis; the latter four are the classic "tetrad" of narcolepsy. Hypocretin also regulates the feeding cycle. Weight gain is another early manifestation of narcolepsy, with obesity occurring in at least 25% of affected children. In some patients, the onset of symptoms has been preceded by an inflammatory process, autoimmune condition, or stressful life event. It has also been associated with some specific types of influenza vaccines. About 50% of patients have onset of symptoms before 15 years of age, with up to 10% presenting before age 5.[1-3]

The *International Classification of Sleep Disorders*, third edition (ICSD-3) diagnostic criteria for narcolepsy type 1 include daily symptoms of excessive sleepiness for 3 months with either abnormal cerebrospinal fluid hypocretin-1 levels (<110 pg/mL or <1/3 normal values) or cataplexy with a positive Multiple Sleep Latency Test (MSLT). A positive MSLT includes a mean sleep onset ≤8 minutes and at least two sleep-onset REM periods (SOREMPs), one of which can be substituted by a SOREMP within 15 minutes in the preceding nocturnal PSG. The human leukocyte antigen (HLA) subtype DQB1*0602, present in 12% to 38% of the general population, is found in approximately 90% of patients with cataplexy.

Narcolepsy type 1 has a more severe course compared with that of narcolepsy type 2, with higher Epworth sleepiness scores and more sleep attacks per week. The onset of symptoms at a younger age has been correlated with the severity of symptoms. Patients with onset of symptoms at age younger than 15 years presented with shorter mean sleep onset on MSLT than older patients do; however, the number of SOREMPs does not differ.[4] Cataplexy may not occur at onset of symptoms. In children, cataplexy may present with facial weakness (such as a dropped jaw), tongue protrusion, and slurred speech. Hypnagogic or hypnopompic hallucinations and sleep paralysis occur in 20% to 60% of patients.[5] Note that young children may not be able to describe these symptoms. Of note, cataplexy is the only symptom that is specific for narcolepsy. However, it is often difficult to determine reliably if cataplexy is actually present.

Management of narcolepsy type 1 in children is aimed at consolidating sleep, improving alertness during the day, and controlling cataplexy. Nonpharmacologic recommendations include regular sleep-wake schedules and planned brief naps. Alerting medications include modafinil, armodafinil, atomoxetine, and methylphenidate. Pharmacologic options for control of cataplexy include venlafaxine, selective serotonin reuptake inhibitors, and tricyclic antidepressants. Sodium oxybate has been reported to treat all of the symptoms of narcolepsy: disrupted sleep, daytime sleepiness, cataplexy, sleep paralysis, and hypnagogic hallucinations. Treatment combinations are commonly used. Note that many of these medications are not approved by the US Food and Drug Administration for use in children but have been reported to be efficacious in the literature and are often prescribed off label.[2,6,7]

CLINICAL PEARLS

1. Of patients with narcolepsy type 1, 50% have onset of symptoms before 15 years of age.
2. Weight gain is a common symptom in children, with at least 25% of affected children being obese.
3. Of patients with narcolepsy type 1, 90% will test positive for HLA DQB1*0602.
4. Cataplexy in children may present with facial weakness (such as a dropped jaw), tongue protrusion, and slurred speech.

REFERENCES

1. Chen Q, de Lecea L, Hu Z, Gao D. The hypocretin/orexin system: an increasingly important role in neuropsychiatry. *Med Res Rev*. Jan 2015;35(1):152–197.
2. Aran A, Einen M, Lin L, Plazzi G, Nishino S, Mignot E. Clinical and therapeutic aspects of childhood narcolepsy-cataplexy: a retrospective study of 51 children. *Sleep*. Nov 2010;33(11):1457–1464.
3. Inocente CO, Lavault S, Lecendreux M, et al. Impact of obesity in children with narcolepsy. *CNS Neurosci Ther*. Jul 2013;19(7):521–528.
4. Nevsimalova S, Buskova J, Kemlink D, Sonka K, Skibova J. Does age at the onset of narcolepsy influence the course and severity of the disease? *Sleep Med*. Oct 2009;10(9):967–972.
5. Nevsimalova S. The diagnosis and treatment of pediatric narcolepsy. *Curr Neurol Neurosci Rep*. Aug 2014;14(8):469.
6. Peterson PC, Husain AM. Pediatric narcolepsy. *Brain Dev*. Nov 2008;30(10):609–623.
7. Lecendreux M, Bruni O, Franco P, et al. Clinical experience suggests that modafinil is an effective and safe treatment for paediatric narcolepsy. *J Sleep Res*. Aug 2012;21(4):481–483.

A 13-year-old boy with excessive sleepiness who falls asleep watching television

Lourdes M. DelRosso

CASE PRESENTATION

A 13-year-old boy presented with excessive daytime sleepiness. His mother first noticed that he had started napping during the day and dozing off during school a year before presentation. He also fell asleep during car rides. His bedtime was 10 PM. He slept in his own bed, in his own room. He usually watched television until falling asleep but he did not know at what time he fell asleep. Once he fell asleep, he did not have nocturnal awakenings. On weekdays, his mother woke him up at 6:30 AM to go to school; on weekends, he slept until noon. The family denied snoring, restless legs, cataplexy, sleep paralysis, hypnagogic hallucinations, or parasomnias. His modified Epworth sleepiness scale was 13/24. There were no other past surgical or medical problems. His review of systems was negative for depression or anxiety. He did not take any medications.

PHYSICAL EXAM

Physical exam revealed a cooperative boy in no distress. His vital signs were within normal limits, and his weight and height were at the 42nd percentile. The physical exam was normal.

LABORATORY AND SLEEP FINDINGS

Actigraphy results are presented in Figure 30-1.

QUESTION

What is the cause of this child's excessive daytime sleepiness?

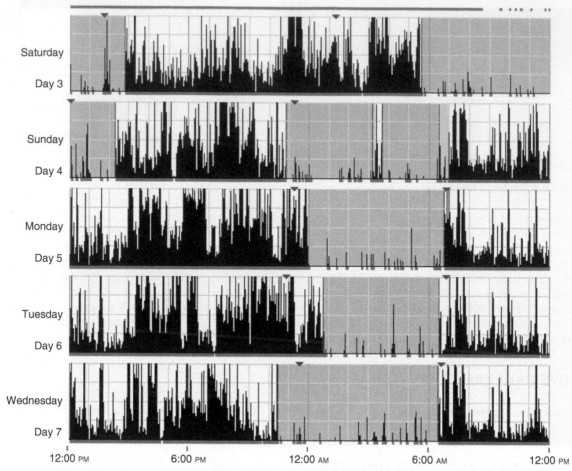

FIGURE 30-1 ■ **Five-day actigraphy results.**

ANSWER

The actigraphy shows that the patient is sleeping from 5 to 8 hours a night. On Saturday, he fell asleep at 5:30 AM and woke up on Sunday at 2 PM. From Sunday night until Wednesday, he went to sleep between 10:30 PM and 1 AM and woke up at 6:30 AM to go to school. The actigraphy reveals insufficient sleep.

DISCUSSION

Insufficient sleep syndrome is classified under central disorders of hypersomnolence. The *International Classification of Sleep Disorders*, third edition (ICSD-3) criteria for diagnosis include symptoms of excessive daytime sleepiness that are present for at least 3 months, longer periods of sleep when not awoken by an alarm or parental intervention, shorter than expected sleep time for age, resolution of symptoms when sleep time is extended, and symptoms not better explained by another disorder or medication effect.

The National Sleep Foundation Sleep for America poll revealed that 75% of twelfth graders self-reported sleeping <8 hours a night, whereas only 30% to 41% of younger adolescents reported sleeping 9 or more hours a night. The poll also reported that almost all adolescents used at least one electronic device at bedtime. The most common devices were music players (used by 90% of adolescents), followed by cell phones (64%) and television (57%). The use of electronic devices has been found to be associated with less nocturnal sleep and increased daytime sleepiness.[1]

Sleep insufficiency in adolescents has been demonstrated to affect executive functioning, attention, and modulation of emotion and drive. Adolescents with insufficient sleep demonstrate more apathy, less self-esteem, and increased self-reported likelihood of engaging in risky behaviors.[2] The causes of sleep insufficiency in adolescents are diverse. The most common cause is self-induced sleep restriction. Other contributors are homework, work after school hours in older adolescents, use of electronics, and comorbid sleep or medical disorders.

Actigraphy should be used to evaluate sleep patterns when sleep diaries or sleep history is not reliable.[3] Our patient could not accurately determine his bedtime because of falling asleep while watching TV, and actigraphy was necessary. Sleep extension was recommended for our patient. Excessive daytime sleepiness resolved with increased sleep.

CLINICAL PEARLS

1. Insufficient sleep syndrome is common in adolescents.
2. Actigraphy is a useful tool to evaluate sleep patterns in children.
3. Insufficient sleep has detrimental effects on behavior and cognition.

REFERENCES

1. Owens J. Insufficient sleep in adolescents and young adults: an update on causes and consequences. *Pediatrics*. Sep 2014;134(3):e921–e932.
2. Telzer EH, Fuligni AJ, Lieberman MD, Galvan A. The effects of poor quality sleep on brain function and risk taking in adolescence. *Neuroimage*. May 1 2013;71:275–283.
3. Morgenthaler T, Alessi C, Friedman L, et al. Practice parameters for the use of actigraphy in the assessment of sleep and sleep disorders: an update for 2007. *Sleep*. Apr 2007;30(4):519–529.

A 16-year-old boy who cannot stay up late on weekends

Lourdes M. DelRosso

CASE PRESENTATION

A 16-year-old male presented with episodes of excessive daytime sleepiness for the past 6 months. His parents did not notice any precipitating factors. He started going to bed at 7 PM and waking up drowsy at 7 AM. He dozed off in school. His grades dropped from A's and B's to D's. His parents sought medical advice from his primary care physician, but his laboratory workup was negative. The sleepiness resolved spontaneously after 4 to 5 weeks. However, 3 months later, he was noted to again sleep for prolonged periods. His parents noted that on the weekends, he rarely got up from bed except to use the bathroom and to eat. He missed a few school events on the weekends because he could not wake up, and the parents noted that he seemed drowsy and did not seem to be himself. The family visited the emergency department for further evaluation. Both a urine drug screen and magnetic resonance imaging (MRI) of the brain were normal. This second episode lasted 4 to 5 weeks and then resolved spontaneously. Between episodes, he went to bed at 10 PM and woke up at 6 AM. He did not take naps and he did not doze off in school. The family denied snoring, sleepwalking, dream enactment, symptoms of restless legs, cataplexy, hypnagogic hallucinations, or sleep paralysis. He had not traveled recently. There were no other past medical problems. His past surgical history was positive for tonsillectomy and adenoidectomy. His review of systems was positive for a 20-kg weight gain over the past 6 months and was negative for drug use, depression, anxiety, or increased irritability.

PHYSICAL EXAM

Physical exam revealed an alert and cooperative boy. His vital signs were within normal limits: his weight was at the 91st percentile, and height was at the 45th percentile; body mass index was at the 92nd percentile. His neurologic exam was normal.

LABORATORY AND SLEEP FINDINGS

Laboratory workup was within normal limits and included complete blood count, metabolic panel, and thyroid-stimulating hormone test and Lyme disease, cytomegalovirus, and Epstein-Barr virus serology. Urine drug screen was negative. MRI of the brain was normal.

QUESTION

What is the most likely diagnosis in this case?

ANSWER

Kleine-Levin syndrome (KLS), also known as recurrent hypersomnia or periodic hypersomnolence.

DISCUSSION

KLS is a hypersomnia syndrome characterized by recurrent periods of excessive sleepiness interspersed among periods of normal behavior, not attributed to a medical, neurologic, or psychiatric disorder or drug or medication use. The *International Classification of Sleep Disorders*, third edition (ICSD-3) criteria for KLS include at least two episodes of excessive sleepiness with prolonged sleep duration, lasting for 2 days to 5 weeks. These episodes must recur more than once a year or occur at least every 18 months. Cognitive dysfunction, altered perception, eating disorder, or disinhibited behavior must occur during the episode. The patient exhibits normal behavior between the episodes.

KLS is very rare, with a prevalence of one in a million individuals. The syndrome affects boys 4 times more than girls. The onset is during adolescence in 80% of patients, during childhood in 10%, and after adolescence in the remaining 10% of affected patients. The episodes of hypersomnolence decrease in frequency and severity with age, usually resolving by the third or fourth decade of life. An infection frequently precedes the onset of symptoms. Other triggering factors are alcohol or drug use, stress, sleep deprivation, history of recent travel, and head trauma. These events also trigger the recurrent episodes of hypersomnolence. The universal symptom is excessive sleepiness, present in 100% of patients. Other symptoms include altered perception or derealization (96%), increased or decreased appetite (95%), apathy (94%), hypersexuality (47%), and anxiety (72%).[1] Hypersexuality is seen more commonly in boys than in girls and is characterized by frequent masturbation and sexual comments or advances. Some have postulated a "triad" of hypersomnolence, hyperphagia, and hypersexuality to characterize KLS, but the three symptoms are concomitantly found in only 45% of affected patients. Apathy and anxiety can often be mistaken for a psychiatric diagnosis because patients often become withdrawn, with bursts of agitation or aggression. Cognitive dysfunction is transient and often includes memory, visuospatial, executive, and communication deficits.[2]

The pathophysiology of KLS is still unclear, but cerebral perfusion, examined by single photon emission computed tomography imaging studies, has been found to be decreased in the thalamus during the episodes. One study revealed that up to 56% of patients had persistence of hypoperfusion after remission of symptoms.[3]

There are no current diagnostic tests for KLS. Polysomnography helps to rule out other sleep disorders such as obstructive sleep apnea syndrome. The Multiple Sleep Latency Test is of limited utility and does not correlate with symptom onset or degree of sleepiness.[4] Routine cerebrospinal fluid (CSF) studies are normal in patients with KLS. One study revealed decreased CSF hypocretin levels during the hypersomnolence period, with normal levels during the recovery periods. MRI of the brain is typically normal.[2] Secondary KLS has been reported in cases of stroke, posttraumatic brain hematoma, hydrocephalus, paraneoplastic syndromes, and post neuroendoscopic surgery.[5]

There are no approved medications for the treatment of KLS. Lithium has been shown to decrease the duration of the episodes and relapses. Stimulants may improve alertness but are often ineffective.[6] Recent case reports have brought attention to the use of clarithromycin. In most cases, KLS resolves spontaneously.[7,8]

This patient and his family were educated on KLS. Weight loss was recommended through diet and exercise. The family was advised to contact the sleep center if another episode occurred.

CLINICAL PEARLS

1. KLS is a rare disorder of recurrent hypersomnolence.
2. KLS presents during adolescence and is more common in boys than in girls.
3. Typically, cognitive dysfunction, altered perception, eating disorder, or disinhibited behavior occur during the episode and resolve during the recovery period.
4. KLS resolves spontaneously in the majority of patients.

REFERENCES

1. Lavault S, Golmard JL, Groos E, et al. Kleine-Levin syndrome in 120 patients: differential diagnosis and long episodes. *Ann Neurol.* Mar 2015;77(3):529–540.
2. Miglis MG, Guilleminault C. Kleine-Levin syndrome: a review. *Nat Sci Sleep.* 2014;6:19–26.
3. Vigren P, Engstrom M, Landtblom AM. SPECT in the Kleine-Levin syndrome, a possible diagnostic and prognostic aid? *Front Neurol.* 2014;5:178.
4. Huang YS, Lin YH, Guilleminault C. Polysomnography in Kleine-Levin syndrome. *Neurology.* Mar 4 2008;70(10):795–801.
5. Nishikuni K, Oliveira MF, Takahashi LR, Rotta JM. Transient Kleine-Levin syndrome following a neuroendoscopic procedure. *J Neuropsychiatry Clin Neurosci.* 2014;26(3):E53–E55. Summer.
6. Arnulf I, Lin L, Gadoth N, et al. Kleine-Levin syndrome: a systematic study of 108 patients. *Ann Neurol.* Apr 2008;63(4):482–493.
7. Oliveira MM, Conti C, Prado GF. Pharmacological treatment for Kleine-Levin syndrome. *Cochrane Database Syst Rev.* 2013;8. CD006685.
8. Trotti LM, Bliwise DL, Rye DB. Further experience using clarithromycin in patients with Kleine-Levin syndrome. *J Clin Sleep Med.* Apr 15 2014;10(4):457–458.

A 4-year-old girl with septo-optic dysplasia and fragmented sleep

Lourdes M. DelRosso

CASE PRESENTATION

A 4-year-old girl with history of septo-optic dysplasia (SOD) with optic nerve hypoplasia and hypopituitarism (diabetes insipidus and adrenal insufficiency) presented to the clinic for evaluation of difficulty sleeping at night. She was diagnosed with SOD at 4 months of age after her parents noted that she did not follow objects or faces. A fundoscopic exam revealed optic disc hypoplasia.

The parents reported that the child has never been able to sleep at night. The parents brought a sleep diary, which revealed sleep cycles of 3 to 4 hours throughout the 24-hour period. Usually, the first cycle ranged from 4 AM until 8 AM. She napped from noon until 3 PM. Finally, she would sleep again from about 6 PM until 9 PM. The parents denied observing snoring, witnessed apneas, or parasomnias.

She was born full term without perinatal complications. Her medications included desmopressin (DDAVP) 0.1 mg twice a day and hydrocortisone 2.5 mg three times a day. Review of systems was positive for complete blindness, global developmental delay, and hypotonia (wheelchair bound).

PHYSICAL EXAM

The child was sitting in her wheelchair and appeared in no distress. Vital signs included weight 20.3 kg (86th percentile); height 100.3 cm (13th percentile); pulse 92; and blood pressure 105/74 mm Hg. Her pupils were reactive to light. She had wandering eye movements without nystagmus. On oral exam, Mallampati grade was III and tonsil size was 1+. Cardiovascular exam was normal.

LABORATORY AND SLEEP FINDINGS

Periodic leg movements index: total sleep time 300 minutes; total recording time 536 minutes; sleep efficiency 56% (because of multiple awakenings); arousal index 19/h; normal sleep stage distribution; obstructive apnea–hypopnea index (AHI) 1.3/h; central AHI 0/h; SpO_2 nadir 94%; no evidence of hypoventilation; leg movements per hour of sleep 1/h.

QUESTION

What is the sleep disorder in this patient?

ANSWER

The patient's history and sleep patterns are consistent with irregular sleep-wake circadian rhythm disorder. She meets all *International Classification of Sleep Disorders*, third edition (ICSD-3) criteria:

1. Irregular sleep and wake episodes throughout the 24-hour period, with symptoms of insomnia at the scheduled sleep time or excessive daytime sleepiness (napping) during the day.
2. Symptoms present for at least 3 months.
3. Sleep log or actigraphy shows at least three bouts of sleep without a major sleep period.
4. The disturbance is no better explained by another medical, mental, sleep disorder, medication, or substance abuse.

DISCUSSION

SOD is a congenital disorder that affects 1 in 10,000 children. The etiology is complex and it involves genetic, environmental, and degenerative factors. Smoking, alcohol, and cocaine use during pregnancy have been identified as potential contributors. Genetic abnormalities are identified in <1% of patients; the cause remains unknown in the majority of affected children.[1]

The diagnosis is made when two out of the three of following are present: optic nerve hypoplasia (found in up to 80% of patients), hypopituitarism, and midbrain defects (absent septum pellucidum, absent corpus callosum, and cerebellar hypoplasia); these constitute the "classic triad" of SOD (Fig. 32-1). The clinical picture is highly variable. Visual impairment, either unilateral or bilateral, is usually the presenting symptom. Pituitary insufficiency develops insidiously. Usually, the first hormonal abnormality found is an elevated prolactin level, followed by growth hormone insufficiency.[2] Other symptoms include obesity, developmental delay, seizure disorder, precocious puberty, and sleep disturbances.[3]

Actigraphy studies in children with SOD have shown decreased sleep efficiency because of frequent and prolonged nocturnal awakenings. Melatonin studies have been inconsistent. Two patients with SOD were found to produce no melatonin at all in a 24-hour cycle; however, children with normal 24-hour melatonin profiles would still exhibit significant sleep fragmentation.[4] Irregular sleep-wake cycle and sleep-wake inversion have also been reported.[5]

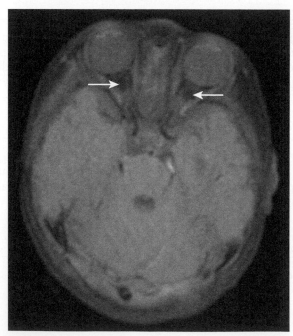

FIGURE 32-1 ■ Axial brain magnetic resonance imaging: bilateral optic nerve hypoplasia (*arrows*)

The most likely etiology of the sleep disturbances found in patients with SOD is disruption of the pathways involved in circadian entrainment. The circadian pacemaker, the suprachiasmatic nucleus (SCN), receives light signals from retinal photoreceptors. Melanopsin-containing retinal ganglion cells transmit these signals via the retinohypothalamic tract, which travels along the fibers of the optic nerve to the SCN.[6] Light signals travel to the superior cervical ganglia and the pineal gland, suppressing melatonin production (Fig. 32-2). Light and melatonin are the most powerful circadian entrainers (zeitgebers), but social cues such as feeding times are also important in circadian synchronization. The circadian pathway requires an intact optic nerve. Irregular sleep-wake cycle has been reported in a patient with bilaterally severed optic nerves and possible destruction of the SCN.[7]

Patients with SOD are at increased risk of circadian disorders, likely because of atrophy of the optic nerve affecting the integrity of the retinohypothalamic tract. However, other contributing factors must be considered, such as nocturnal seizures, hormonal imbalances, developmental delay, and obesity. A thorough sleep evaluation is recommended in these patients.

Treatment of patients with SOD is symptomatic and mainly consists of hormone replacement, management of comorbidities, and physical-occupational therapy. Sleep disturbances may be treated with exogenous melatonin and social zeitgebers. Our patient was successfully treated with melatonin 3 mg at 9 PM, a consistent bedtime and nap schedule, and planned activities during the day.

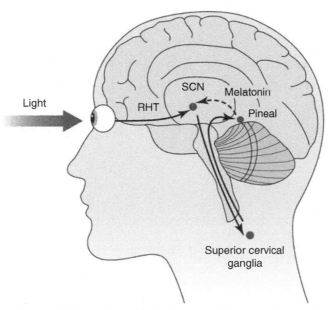

FIGURE 32-2 ■ **Circadian pathway.** *RHT,* Retinohypothalamic tract; *SCN,* suprachiasmatic nucleus. (From Berry RB. *Fundamentals of Sleep Medicine.* 1st ed. Philadelphia, PA: Elsevier; 2011 [Chapter 26, Table 26-1].)

CLINICAL PEARLS

1. Optic nerve hypoplasia is the most common finding in patients with SOD.
2. Circadian disorders are common in patients with SOD and may respond to treatment with melatonin and social zeitgebers.
3. Other contributors to sleep disruption in these patients may include nocturnal seizures, hormonal imbalances, developmental delay, and obesity.

REFERENCES

1. Webb EA, Dattani MT. Septo-optic dysplasia. *Eur J Hum Genet*. Apr 2010;18(4):393–397.
2. Saranac L, Gucev Z. New insights into septo-optic dysplasia. *Prilozi*. 2014;35(1):123–128.
3. Fard MA, Wu-Chen WY, Man BL, Miller NR. Septo-optic dysplasia. *Pediatr Endocrinol Rev*. Sep 2010;8(1):18–24.
4. Webb EA, O'Reilly MA, Orgill J, et al. Rest-activity disturbances in children with septo-optic dysplasia characterized by actigraphy and 24-hour plasma melatonin profiles. *J Clin Endocrinol Metab*. Oct 2010;95(10):E198–E203.
5. Rivkees SA. Arrhythmicity in a child with septo-optic dysplasia and establishment of sleep-wake cyclicity with melatonin. *J Pediatr*. Sep 2001;139(3):463–465.
6. LeGates TA, Fernandez DC, Hattar S. Light as a central modulator of circadian rhythms, sleep and affect. *Nat Rev Neurosci*. Jul 2014;15(7):443–454.
7. DelRosso LM, Hoque R, James S, Gonzalez-Toledo E, Chesson Jr AL. Sleep-wake pattern following gunshot suprachiasmatic damage. *J Clin Sleep Med*. Apr 15 2014;10(4):443–445.

A 13-year-old boy who falls asleep in school

Lourdes M. DelRosso

CASE PRESENTATION

A 13-year-old boy presented for evaluation of excessive daytime sleepiness. His parents have had difficulty waking him up in the mornings for the past 6 months. He has fallen asleep on the bus ride to school and during classes. His usual routine was to do homework until 10 PM and then read a book until midnight. He did not have a television in his bedroom or access to electronic devices after 9 PM. His bedtime was midnight, but most nights, he did not fall asleep until 1 to 2 AM. Rarely, he stayed up until 4 to 5 AM. Once he fell asleep, he did not have nocturnal awakenings. On weekdays his mother tried to wake him up at 6:30 AM to go to school. He had missed several days of school over the last few months because he was not able to wake up in the morning. On weekends he went to bed at 2 AM, fell asleep within 15 minutes, and woke up at 11 AM. He did not take naps. His modified Epworth sleepiness scale was 15/24. There were no past medical problems. His review of systems was negative. He did not take any medications.

PHYSICAL EXAM

Physical exam revealed a cooperative boy in no distress. His vital signs were within normal limits, and his weight and height were at the 50th percentile. The physical exam was normal.

LABORATORY AND SLEEP FINDINGS

Actigraphy results are presented in Figure 33-1.

QUESTIONS

What is the most likely cause of this boy's excessive daytime sleepiness on school days?

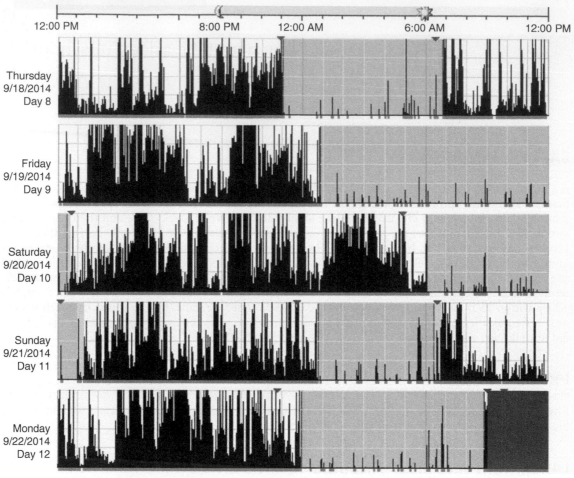

FIGURE 33-1 ■ **Five-day actigraphy results.** The actigraphy is consistent with the patient's history. The patient is falling asleep from midnight to 6 AM and waking up from 7 AM to noon.

ANSWERS

The most likely cause of his excessive daytime sleepiness on school days is insufficient sleep secondary to delayed sleep-wake phase disorder. On weekdays, the patient goes to bed at midnight but only falls asleep at 1 to 2 AM. His parents wake him up at 6:30 AM to go to school. This allows him only 4.5 to 5.5 hours of sleep. Sleepiness during the bus ride and during classes is likely secondary to insufficient sleep. On weekends his sleep latency is 15 minutes, and he sleeps about 9 hours and does not experience excessive sleepiness. This pattern of sleep, as confirmed by actigraphy, is consistent with delayed sleep-wake phase disorder.

DISCUSSION

To be diagnosed with delayed sleep-wake phase disorder, a patient must meet the *International Classification of Sleep Disorders*, third edition diagnostic criteria: delay in the phase of sleep with inability to fall asleep or wake up at a desired (or required) time for at least 3 months, sleep diaries or actigraphy demonstrating a delay in the sleep period, and improvement of daytime sleepiness when the patient is allowed to sleep on his or her own schedule. The sleep schedule disturbance cannot be secondary to a medication effect or medical or psychiatric condition. Delayed sleep-wake phase disorder is common in adolescents, with a prevalence of 3% to 8%.[1,2] Although the prevalence is higher in girls than in boys, the functional effect, measured by number of school absences, is higher in boys.[1]

Melatonin release from the pineal gland begins to increase in the evening and peaks in the early hours of the morning (about 2 hours before awakening).[3] Melatonin secretion is suppressed by daylight, and, therefore, melatonin production decreases after awakening. Melatonin can be measured in serum, saliva, or urine. The time of onset of endogenous melatonin secretion, called dim light melatonin onset (DLMO), is associated with sleep onset and wake-up time but not bedtime, making it a suitable marker of circadian phase.[3] DLMO measured in children and adolescents from 9 to 16 years of age has shown that DLMO starts to delay by 1 hour beginning at age 11 to 13 years, consistent with the physiologic delay in sleep-wake phase seen in adolescents.[4] The pattern of delayed sleep-wake disruption becomes pathologic when insomnia symptoms, excessive daytime sleepiness, distress, or impairment in any area of functioning (educational, occupational, social, mental, or physical) develops.

The major effect of delayed sleep-wake disorder in adolescents is increased school absences and poor school performance, likely secondary to insufficient sleep because of a mismatch between sleep phase and school hours, leading to less sleep than required for age.[5] Studies have shown that patients with delayed sleep-wake disorder are very difficult to wake up early in the morning, and some may not respond to an alarm clock.[6]

Delayed sleep-wake phase disorder can usually be diagnosed based on history and sleep diary alone. Treatment options include melatonin, light therapy, and cognitive behavioral therapy.[7] The response to melatonin is greater when given at times when endogenous melatonin levels are low (in the morning after awakening or in the evening before DLMO).[8] When given in the morning, melatonin produces a phase delay (shifts sleep to a later time), and when given in the evening, it produces a phase advance (shifts sleep to an earlier time). Bright light causes circadian phase shifts opposite to those of melatonin. Bright light in the evening causes phase delay, and bright light in the morning causes phase advance. In patients with delayed sleep-wake disorder, evening dim light in combination with morning bright light therapy is usually administered, with the goal to gradually advance the bedtime and rise time. Cognitive behavioral therapy includes stimulus control, education on sleep hygiene, and restructuring misconceptions about sleep.[7] Bright light in the morning and melatonin at bedtime were used successfully in our patient. Chronotherapy (having the patient progressively delay his or her bed time each day until he or she has "marched around the clock" and is going to bed at the desired time) is described in the literature but is seldom used because it tends to be impractical, and benefits are lost if the patient occasionally relapses and goes to bed late.[9]

CLINICAL PEARLS

1. Delayed sleep-wake phase disorder is common in adolescents.
2. When allowed to sleep and wake up at their endogenous circadian time, patients with delayed sleep-wake phase disorder usually fall asleep quicker, have adequate total sleep time for age, and experience resolution of symptoms.
3. Delayed sleep-wake phase disorder can affect school attendance and performance.
4. Treatment options for patients with delayed sleep-wake disorder include light therapy, melatonin, and cognitive behavioral therapy.

REFERENCES

1. Sivertsen B, Pallesen S, Stormark KM, Boe T, Lundervold AJ, Hysing M. Delayed sleep phase syndrome in adolescents: prevalence and correlates in a large population based study. *BMC Public Health*. 2013;13:1163.
2. Saxvig IW, Pallesen S, Wilhelmsen-Langeland A, Molde H, Bjorvatn B. Prevalence and correlates of delayed sleep phase in high school students. *Sleep Med*. Feb 2012;13(2):193–199.
3. Burgess HJ, Savic N, Sletten T, Roach G, Gilbert SS, Dawson D. The relationship between the dim light melatonin onset and sleep on a regular schedule in young healthy adults. *Behav Sleep Med*. 2003;1(2):102–114.
4. Crowley SJ, Van Reen E, LeBourgeois MK, et al. A longitudinal assessment of sleep timing, circadian phase, and phase angle of entrainment across human adolescence. *PLoS One*. 2014;9(11):e112199.
5. Sivertsen B, Glozier N, Harvey AG, Hysing M. Academic performance in adolescents with delayed sleep phase. *Sleep Med*. Sep 2015;16(9):1084–1090.
6. Solheim B, Langsrud K, Kallestad H, Olsen A, Bjorvatn B, Sand T. Difficult morning awakening from rapid eye movement sleep and impaired cognitive function in delayed sleep phase disorder patients. *Sleep Med*. Oct 2014;15(10):1264–1268.
7. Gradisar M, Dohnt H, Gardner G, et al. A randomized controlled trial of cognitive-behavior therapy plus bright light therapy for adolescent delayed sleep phase disorder. *Sleep*. Dec 2011;34(12):1671–1680.
8. Lewy A. Clinical implications of the melatonin phase response curve. *J Clin Endocrinol Metab*. Jul 2010;95(7):3158–3160.
9. Czeisler CA, Richardson GS, Coleman RM, et al. Chronotherapy: resetting the circadian clocks of patients with delayed sleep phase insomnia. *Sleep*. 1981;4(1):1–21.

A 1-month-old premature infant on an apnea monitor

Lourdes M. DelRosso

CASE PRESENTATION

A 1-month-old infant presented for evaluation of apnea of prematurity. The infant was born at 29 weeks postconceptional age via cesarean section delivery. His birth weight was 1450 g, his birth length was 42 cm, and his head circumference at birth measured 29 cm. The infant required supplemental oxygen for 2 days for hypoxemia. He was started on caffeine for observed apneas in the nursery and sent home with an apnea monitor.

The infant slept in a crib in his parent's room. The parents denied witnessing snoring, gasping, breathing pauses, or cyanosis. His mother reported breastfeeding every 4 to 5 hours. There was no choking or emesis. The parents reported hearing the apnea monitor alarm at least twice a day, usually during feeding periods. These episodes were not accompanied by cyanosis or witnessed apneas. The infant came to clinic for follow-up and evaluation of apnea monitor data. His medications included caffeine citrate 5 mg/kg/day.

PHYSICAL EXAM

Physical exam revealed a small infant in no distress. His vital signs were within normal limits. His weight was 1.28 kg, height was 43.5 cm, and head circumference was 31.8 cm. His lungs were clear to auscultation. His abdomen was not distended and without organomegaly or masses. The remainder of the exam was normal. Pulse oximetry while the infant was napping was 98%.

LABORATORY AND SLEEP FINDINGS

The apnea monitor recorded several events similar to the ones depicted in Figures 34-1 and 34-2.

QUESTION

What do Figures 34-1 and 34-2 from the apnea monitor show?

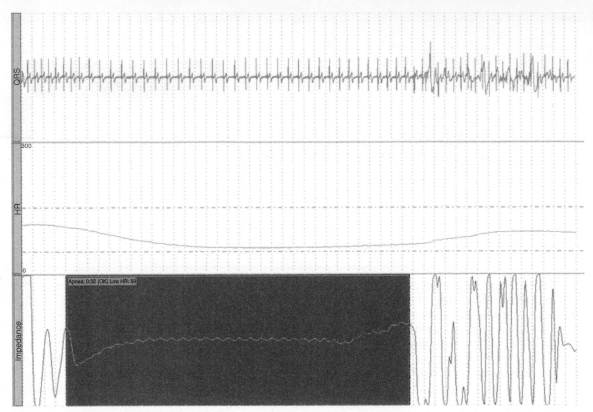

FIGURE 34-1 ■ Tracing from an apnea monitor is shown. The impedance tracing is from a belt around the abdomen. The ECG and heart rate are shown.

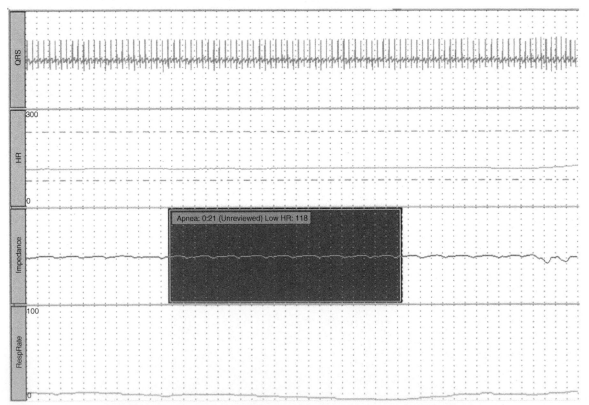

FIGURE 34-2 ■ Another tracing showing an event detected by the monitor.

ANSWER

Figure 34-1 shows a prolonged central apnea associated with bradycardia. Figure 34-2 shows a false-positive monitor-detected event because of chronic low-amplitude breathing signal.

DISCUSSION

Apnea monitors record breathing effort by detecting the difference in impedance between two electrodes placed on the infant's chest and secured with a belt. These electrodes also detect the heart rate. The standard monitor settings for home apnea monitoring include apnea delay of 20 seconds (the monitor records the previous 20 seconds after the alarm is triggered), low heart rate at 80 beats/min, and high heart rate at 210 beats/min. The monitors do not have a delay on the bradycardia alarm. Shallow breaths, loose electrodes, and/or inadequate placement or tightening of the impedance belt can also trigger the alarm. Figure 34-1 demonstrates a prolonged central apnea with bradycardia. Note that the small pulsations seen during the apnea are due to an electrocardiogram (ECG) artifact. In contrast, Figure 34-2 shows a prolonged period of low-amplitude artifact that was incorrectly identified as an apnea by the monitor software. Note that the amplitude on the respiratory channel is at a different frequency than that of the ECG, and there is no associated change in heart rate.

The *International Classification of Sleep Disorders*, third edition (ICSD-3) defines apnea of prematurity as observed apnea or cyanosis, or a detected central apnea, bradycardia, or desaturation on hospital cardiorespiratory monitoring, in an infant of postconceptional age <37 weeks at the time of presentation. A nocturnal polysomnogram (if performed) must show evidence of prolonged central apneas (more than 20 seconds duration) or periodic breathing (see Case 12 A 7 month-old infant with a series of central apneas) for more than 5% of the total sleep time. In many cases, the infant also has obstructive apneas and mixed apneas. Other medical, neurologic, or sleep disorders, as well as medication effects, must be ruled out. When the same diagnostic criteria are found in an infant born at 37 weeks conceptional age or later, but the diagnosis is changed to "apnea of infancy." The younger the conceptional age at birth, the greater the prevalence of apnea of prematurity.

The etiology of apnea of prematurity has been attributed to immaturity of the central nervous system. The central control of breathing, located in the brainstem, regulates ventilatory responses to CO_2. Studies have shown impaired hypercapnic responses in premature infants and increased ventilatory responses to CO_2 as the infant grows older. The peripheral carotid body receptors respond to hypoxia, hypercarbia, and acidosis, having a significant effect on ventilation. The chest wall compliance of a premature infant results in lower end-expiratory lung volume and distal airway closure. Bradycardia may result from stimulation of carotid chemoreceptors by hypoxia.[1,2]

Management of apnea of prematurity may include methylxanthine therapy, continuous positive airway pressure (if significant obstructive events are present), and home monitoring. Both theophylline and caffeine have been effective in increasing minute ventilation, improving CO_2 sensitivity, and decreasing periodic breathing. Apnea of prematurity generally resolves by 43 weeks postconceptional age.[3] If apnea persists past that time, the patient should be evaluated for other causes (e.g., gastroesophageal reflux or unsuspected hypoxemia from chronic lung disease).

The American Academy of Pediatrics recommends the use of home cardiorespiratory monitors for premature infants who are noted to have significant apnea, bradycardia, and/or hypoxemia in the newborn nursery or on the floor before discharge. Apnea monitors should be used up to 43 weeks postconceptional age or after the cessation of the cardiorespiratory episodes, whichever is later.[4] Caregivers must be instructed regarding appropriate responses to the monitors.

CLINICAL PEARLS

1. Apnea of prematurity is likely secondary to immaturity in the central control of breathing.
2. Management of apnea of prematurity may include methylxanthine therapy and home apnea monitoring.
3. Apnea monitors should be used in symptomatic infants up to 43 weeks postconceptional age or after the cessation of the cardiorespiratory episodes, whichever is later.
4. If apnea or bradycardia persists after 43 weeks, further investigation is warranted.
5. Many events labeled as apneas by monitor software automatic scoring are, in fact, artifacts.

REFERENCES

1. Martin RJ, Abu-Shaweesh JM. Control of breathing and neonatal apnea. *Biol Neonate.* 2005;87(4):288–295.
2. Di Fiore JM, Martin RJ, Gauda EB. Apnea of prematurity—perfect storm. *Respir Physiol Neurobiol.* Nov 1 2013;189(2):213–222.
3. Ramanathan R, Corwin MJ, Hunt CE, et al. Cardiorespiratory events recorded on home monitors: comparison of healthy infants with those at increased risk for SIDS. *JAMA.* 2001;285(17):2199–2207.
4. American Academy of Pediatrics. Apnea, sudden infant death syndrome, and home monitoring. *Pediatrics.* Apr 2003;111 (4 Pt 1):914–917.

A 2-month-old infant turns blue in front of his parents

Lourdes M. DelRosso

CASE PRESENTATION

A 2-month-old infant was brought to the emergency department for evaluation of cyanosis. The mother reported that the infant was asleep on his back in a bassinet when the parents noticed that he stopped breathing and his face turned blue. His mother picked him up from the crib and rubbed his back until he started breathing spontaneously. His skin color returned to normal within seconds. Further history revealed that the infant was born full term without complications and had been thriving since. His birth weight was at the 50th percentile. The parents denied any history of seizures, feeding difficulties, emesis, snoring, or gasping. The parents did not smoke.

PHYSICAL EXAM

The infant appeared well, interactive, and in no distress. He was afebrile, and his vital signs were within normal limits. His weight was at the 50th percentile; length at the 70th percentile; and head circumference at the 50th percentile. He did not appear syndromic or micrognathic. The fontanelle was open and flat. His oropharynx was normal. Cardiopulmonary, neurologic, and general exam were normal.

QUESTION

What is the diagnosis in this infant?

ANSWER

Apparent life-threatening event (ALTE).

DISCUSSION

ALTE is defined as "an episode that is frightening to the observer and that is characterized by some combination of apnea (central or occasionally obstructive), color change (usually cyanotic or pallid but occasionally erythematous or plethoric), marked change in muscle tone (usually marked limpness), choking, or gagging."[1] Note that this is a very broad description, given from the viewpoint of a layperson observer (typically a parent).

The incidence of ALTE is estimated at 0.6 per 1000 live births.[2] ALTEs were initially thought to be a precursor to the sudden infant death syndrome (SIDS), but this has been shown not to be the case. Only 7% of SIDS victims have ever had an ALTE.[1] Polysomnographic studies of infants who subsequently died of SIDS do not show pathologic central apneas.[3] The incidence of ALTE has not decreased with the "back-to-sleep" campaign as has the incidence of SIDS.[4]

The exact mechanism of ALTE is unclear, and ALTEs probably represent a response to a heterogeneous group of conditions, although a cause is often not found. Gastroesophageal reflux disease (GERD) is the most common diagnosis found in infants with ALTE (31% of cases with a diagnosis).[2] However, GERD is very common in young infants, and, therefore, causality is difficult to prove (see Clinical Pearls in Case 73: A 5-month-old baby who wakes up and spits up through the night). Other possible underlying diagnoses include seizures (10% of cases with a diagnosis),[2] respiratory infections (8% of cases with a diagnosis,[2] especially respiratory syncytial virus), hypoxemia (e.g., secondary to chronic lung disease of prematurity), sepsis, anemia, prolonged QT syndrome, inborn errors of metabolism, and child abuse.[2] A cause for the ALTE is not found in about 50% of cases,[4] and most infants do not have recurrent episodes.

The initial evaluation of infants with ALTE must include a careful history and physical exam. There is no evidence to recommend a specific battery of tests; as with other conditions in clinical medicine, further evaluation should be predicated by the results of the history and exam. A retrospective study of 150 cases evaluated in an emergency department found that only 2.5% of tests resulted in a diagnosis, and in all those cases, the diagnosis was suspected clinically.[5] A systematic review of the literature revealed that infants with a history of prematurity and those with recurrent ALTE are more likely to have an underlying condition[6] and, therefore, may warrant a more intensive evaluation. Other factors suggesting an underlying condition include severe ALTEs (infant requires intensive resuscitation), ALTEs that occur after fasting (suspect inborn errors of metabolism), or with a positive family history (suspect inborn errors of metabolism or child abuse, such as intentional smothering).[7] Potential selective tests based on the history and exam may include a complete blood count, electrolytes, serum glucose, pertussis, toxicology, electrocardiograph or Holter monitoring, electroencephalogram, and chest radiograph. Routine testing for GERD is not recommended in infants without GERD symptoms.[6] The American Academy of Sleep Medicine recommends polysomnography in the evaluation of infants with ALTE when there is clinical suspicion of obstructive sleep apnea (witnessed apnea, snoring, or gasping).[8]

The American Academy of Pediatrics emphasizes that home cardiorespiratory monitoring does not prevent SIDS but states that home cardiorespiratory monitoring may be used in infants with a history of ALTE to allow prompt parental response and recognition of central apnea or bradycardia.[9] The parents must be educated on the purpose, advantages, and limitations of the home cardiorespiratory monitors.

Our patient had a normal exam and noncontributory clinical history. He was discharged with a home cardiorespiratory monitor. The parents were educated on cardiopulmonary resuscitation, the use of the home monitor, and safe sleeping practices. The infant had no further events, and the monitor was subsequently discontinued.

CLINICAL PEARLS

1. ALTE is not associated with an increased risk of SIDS.
2. There is no consensus on the evaluation of ALTE. A careful history and physical exam must direct further testing as needed.
3. Recurrent ALTE and ALTE in premature infants may indicate an underlying condition.
4. Polysomnography is indicated if obstructive sleep apnea is suspected.
5. Home cardiopulmonary monitoring does not prevent SIDS, but it may be useful in recognition of central apnea or bradycardia.

REFERENCES

1. National Institutes of Health Consensus Development Conference on Infantile Apnea and Home Monitoring, Sept 29 to Oct 1, 1986. *Pediatrics*. Feb 1987;79(2):292–299.
2. McGovern MC, Smith MB. Causes of apparent life threatening events in infants: a systematic review. *Arch Dis Child*. Nov 2004;89(11):1043–1048.
3. Schechtman VL, Harper RM, Wilson AJ, Southall DP. Sleep apnea in infants who succumb to the sudden infant death syndrome. *Pediatrics*. Jun 1991;87(6):841–846.
4. Hall KL, Zalman B. Evaluation and management of apparent life-threatening events in children. *Am Fam Physician*. Jun 15 2005;71(12):2301–2308.
5. De Piero AD, Teach SJ, Chamberlain JM. ED evaluation of infants after an apparent life-threatening event. *Am J Emerg Med*. Mar 2004;22(2):83–86.
6. Tieder JS, Altman RL, Bonkowsky JL, et al. Management of apparent life-threatening events in infants: a systematic review. *J Pediatr*. Jul 2013;163(1):94–99. e91-96.
7. Southall DP, Plunkett MC, Banks MW, Falkov AF, Samuels MP. Covert video recordings of life-threatening child abuse: lessons for child protection. *Pediatrics*. Nov 1997;100(5):735–760.
8. Aurora RN, Zak RS, Karippot A, et al. Practice parameters for the respiratory indications for polysomnography in children. *Sleep*. Mar 2011;34(3):379–388.
9. American Academy of Pediatrics. Apnea, sudden infant death syndrome, and home monitoring. *Pediatrics*. Apr 2003;111 (4 Pt 1):914–917.

A 1-week-old infant with severely abnormal blood gases

Lourdes M. DelRosso

CASE PRESENTATION

The sleep medicine team was consulted on a 1-week-old infant with apneic events. The infant was born full term via cesarean section (because of premature rupture of membranes) to a 34-year-old G4P2 mother who received prenatal care and did not smoke or consume alcohol or drugs. His Apgar scores were 5 at 1 minute and 8 at 5 minutes. The nurses witnessed multiple central apneic events and desaturations and placed the infant on 0.25 L/min of supplemental oxygen by nasal cannula. Episodes continued, and the infant was intubated because of severely abnormal arterial blood gases (ABG; results below). A sepsis workup was performed, and a chest x-ray was obtained, which was unremarkable. Further, 3 hours after intubation, the ABG values normalized. The infant seemed vigorous and was therefore extubated. He continued having apneic episodes and desaturations during sleep. He received a bolus of caffeine without improvement and was reintubated.

PHYSICAL EXAM

Intubated infant. Vital signs were normal while awake. The physical exam was unremarkable.

LABORATORY AND SLEEP FINDINGS

Initial ABG showed pH 7.19, PCO_2 78 mm Hg, and PO_2 64 mm Hg. ABG after intubation showed pH 7.67, PCO_2 18 mm Hg, and PO_2 65 mm Hg. Chest x-ray: normal. Electroencephalogram: normal. Echocardiogram: normal. Diaphragm ultrasound: normal motion of both hemidiaphragms. Brain magnetic resonance imaging: normal

QUESTION

What diagnosis do you suspect in this infant? What test will confirm the diagnosis?

ANSWER

Congenital central hypoventilation syndrome (CCHS). Positive *PHOX2B* gene mutation testing will confirm the diagnosis.

DISCUSSION

CCHS is a rare genetic condition characterized by hypoventilation during sleep. The diagnosis is confirmed by a mutation on the *PHOX2B* gene. The *PHOX2B* gene is located on chromosome 4, and it encodes for a transcription factor that regulates neural crest cell migration, that is, autonomic nervous system neurons that control cardiovascular, digestive, and respiratory functions. Further, 90% of mutations consist of an expansion in the 20-residue polyalanine region. Patients with a higher number of polyalanine repeats (20/27-20/33) have a more severe presentation and may require ventilatory support during both wakefulness and sleep, whereas the typical patient with a lower number of polyalanine repeats (20/24-20/25) tends to have milder phenotypes and requires ventilatory support only during sleep.[1] Some patients with milder mutations have presented during adulthood, because of respiratory failure occurring with mild respiratory infections or emergence from general anesthesia.[2] The 10% of patients without expansion mutations are heterozygous for a nonpolyalanine repeat mutation in the *PHOX2B* gene or have a different mutation (e.g., nonsense or missense mutation) and are at higher risk of extensive gastrointestinal involvement (Hirshsprung disease), neural tumors, and the need for 24-hour ventilatory support.[3] The *PHOX2B* mutation is dominant but often occurs *de novo*.

CCHS is characterized by hypoxemia and hypercapnia during sleep, thought to be secondary to abnormal central integration of chemoreceptor signals. Central apneas may also be present. The degree of hypoventilation is more severe during NREM than REM sleep; however, hypoventilation is severe enough during REM sleep to warrant ventilatory support. The worsening of hypoventilation may be secondary to the tonic excitatory inputs to the respiratory centers that occur during both wakefulness and REM sleep.[4]

Positive pressure ventilation via tracheostomy is the treatment of choice during the first years of life, as noninvasive ventilation in infants is complicated by the paucity of well-fitting interfaces, poor triggering often seen with bi-level positive airway pressure devices (see Clinical Pearls Case 53 - d. A 3 year old girl with irregular breathing on BPAP), lack of a clear circadian rhythm, and the need for vigorous control of gas exchange to preserve cognitive potential. Noninvasive ventilation can be considered in older children who need ventilatory support only during sleep. Diaphragm pacing is a treatment option that is often reserved for patients requiring ventilation during wakefulness because it allows the child to be ambulatory. The implantable device converts radiofrequency signals into electric current that is then transmitted to the phrenic nerve, resulting in diaphragmatic contraction. In contrast to spontaneous breathing, diaphragmatic contraction is independent of vocal cord abduction; therefore, diaphragmatic pacing may result in obstructive apnea. Lengthening the inspiratory time or decreasing the inspiratory force may minimize obstructive apnea.[3]

Patients with CCHS will need lifelong support and do not "outgrow" their illness. However, if strict control of ventilation is maintained, patients are of normal cognition and can have an excellent quality of life.[5] Because of the dominant nature of the mutation, some patients with CCHS have had children with CCHS.

Our patient was too unstable extubated to have a polysomnogram. He underwent tracheostomy and required invasive positive pressure mechanical ventilation during sleep (Fig. 36-1).

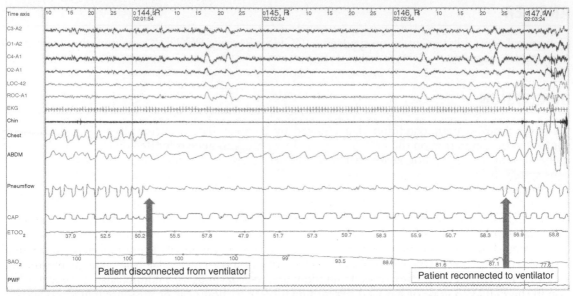

FIGURE 36-1 ■ Two-minute epoch from a different patient with CCHS who was transiently taken off his ventilator during sleep under controlled conditions for a research study. Note the rapid desaturation and hypercapnia. (Image used with permission from Cielo C, Marcus CL. Central hypoventilation syndromes. *Sleep Med Clin*. Mar 1 2014;9(1):105-118. doi:10.1016/j.jsmc.2013.10.005.[6])

CLINICAL PEARLS

1. CCHS is a rare genetic disorder that affects central control of breathing.
2. CCHS diagnosis requires a positive testing for a mutation in the *PHOX2B* gene.
3. The length of the polyalanine repeat expansion mutations correlates with disease severity.
4. Treatment options include invasive and noninvasive ventilation and diaphragmatic pacing.

REFERENCES

1. Healy F, Marcus CL. Congenital central hypoventilation syndrome in children. *Paediatr Respir Rev*. Dec 2011;12(4): 253–263.
2. Antic NA, Malow BA, Lange N, et al. PHOX2B mutation-confirmed congenital central hypoventilation syndrome: presentation in adulthood. *Am J Respir Crit Care Med*. Oct 15 2006;174(8):923–927.
3. Weese-Mayer DE, Berry-Kravis EM, Ceccherini I, Keens TG, Loghmanee DA, Trang H. An official ATS clinical policy statement: congenital central hypoventilation syndrome: genetic basis, diagnosis, and management. *Am J Respir Crit Care Med*. Mar 15 2010;181(6):626–644.
4. Huang J, Colrain IM, Panitch HB, et al. Effect of sleep stage on breathing in children with central hypoventilation. *J Appl Physiol (1985)*. Jul 2008;105(1):44–53.
5. Marcus CL, Jansen MT, Poulsen MK, et al. Medical and psychosocial outcome of children with congenital central hypoventilation syndrome. *J Pediatr*. Dec 1991;119(6):888–895.
6. Cielo C, Marcus CL. Central hypoventilation syndromes. *Sleep Med Clin*. Mar 1 2014;9(1):105–118.

A child with central sleep apnea treated with supplemental oxygen

Suzanne E. Beck

CASE PRESENTATION

A 3-year-old girl was referred for evaluation of suspected obstructive sleep apnea syndrome (OSAS). Her mother noticed restless sleep and frequent pauses in breathing during sleep but only occasional snoring. The child had mild developmental delay of unknown etiology but was slowly achieving developmental milestones. She had fine motor delay but was able to walk and talk. She had dysphagia and known aspiration of thin liquids but was able to tolerate thick liquids and solids. She had a gastrostomy tube for supplemental feedings. She did not choke or cough during sleep. She had difficulty handling secretions during colds and had a suction machine that was used along with chest physiotherapy and albuterol via nebulizer as needed. She was on no other medication. She was born full term. She had no history of rhinitis, asthma, pneumonia, or seizures. Genetic and neurologic evaluations had not identified a cause for her delay.

PHYSICAL EXAM

Vital signs: respiratory rate 24 breaths/min; pulse 120 beats/min; and blood pressure normal for age, SpO_2 96%. Weight was at the 5th percentile, height was at the 10th percentile, and head circumference was 5th percentile for age. Exam revealed a normal-appearing child with nondysmorphic facial features. She had a normal jaw, palate, and dentition. She had 1+ tonsils. Her neurologic exam was normal other than the developmental delays. The rest of her exam was otherwise unremarkable.

LABORATORY AND SLEEP FINDINGS

Chest radiograph: normal
Genetic evaluation: normal chromosomes
Brain magnetic resonance imaging (MRI): normal
   Polysomnography (PSG) revealed a total sleep time (TST) of 484 minutes; sleep efficiency of 86%; REM 22%; obstructive apnea–hypopnea index 0.9/h; central apnea index 4.1/h; arousal index 12.2/h; SpO_2 nadir 78%; time with SpO_2 ≤90% was 4% of TST; peak end-tidal CO_2 44 mm Hg. Periodic breathing occurred for 7% of TST. The longest central apnea was 19 seconds, with a mean duration of 14.5 seconds. Most central apneas occurred during REM sleep, but several occurred following arousals. Representative tracings of her events are shown in Figures 37-1 and 37-2.

QUESTIONS

1. What event is shown in Figure 37-1?
2. What event is shown in Figure 37-2?
3. What treatment would you offer this patient?

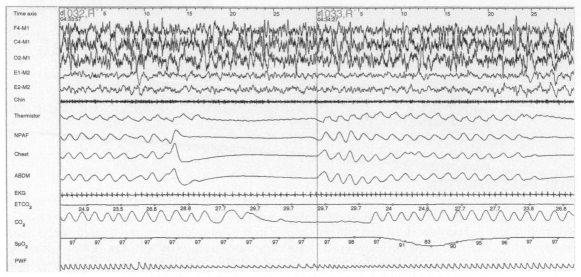

FIGURE 37-1 ■ A representative 60-second epoch of sleep.

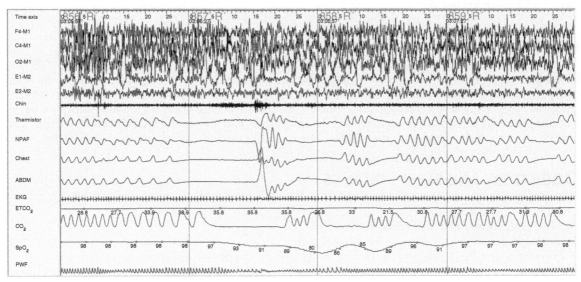

FIGURE 37-2 ■ A representative 120-second epoch of sleep.

ANSWERS

1. Figure 37-1 shows a 16-second central apnea followed by oxyhemoglobin desaturation to 83%, with quick recovery to baseline. The child's respiratory rate was 30 breaths/min, which is just above normal for a 3-year-old.[1]
2. Figure 37-2 shows a short run of periodic breathing with at least three central apneas ≥3 seconds duration, separated by no more than 20 seconds of normal breathing.[2] This run of periodic breathing was associated with oxyhemoglobin desaturation.
3. The patient was treated with supplemental oxygen during sleep.

DISCUSSION

Short central apneas in infants and children are common because of an active Hering-Breuer reflex, which is a compensatory central respiratory pause following the stimulation of pulmonary stretch receptors by a large breath, such as occurs with sighs or body movements. Central apneas in children are also very common during REM sleep[3,4] (see Clinical Pearls in Case 13: A 15-month-old with central apnea). However, brief central apneas associated with significant desaturation are less common and often indicate decreased pulmonary reserve. On the contrary, long or very frequent central apneas may indicate central nervous system (CNS) abnormalities or other pathology. Periodic breathing is common in preterm infants, but by 18 months of age, periodic breathing occurs for <2.5% of TST[5,6] (see Clinical Pearls in Case 12: A 7-month-old infant with a series of central apneas).

The cause of central apnea in children is not always known. In preterm infants, apnea of prematurity, because of developmental immaturity of respiratory control, is common. It is often treated with caffeine, monitoring, or nasal continuous positive airway pressure (CPAP) and usually resolves by term (see Clinical Pearls in Case 34: A 2-month-old premature infant on an apnea monitor). In neonates, increased central apnea and periodic breathing can be seen during metabolic stress, infections, or as a sign of CNS injury and may be nonspecific. In older infants and children, central apneas and periodic breathing are uncommon and are usually unresponsive to caffeine, as well as other drugs that have been tried in the past such as naloxone, progesterone, and theophylline.

Neurologic and metabolic diseases may cause central apnea. The brainstem is the primary site of the ventilatory pattern generator and the processing of respiratory afferent input from chemoreceptors and intrapulmonary receptors; therefore, any disease affecting this system can influence ventilation during sleep.[7] Pathologic central apnea may be seen in children with mitochondrial disease, Arnold Chiari malformations, and other CNS abnormalities such as tumor or hemorrhage, as well as chromosomal and developmental disorders such as with our patient.

Although primarily thought of as a cause of obstructive apnea, laryngochemoreceptor apnea can cause central apnea. Infants and children have prominent laryngeal chemoreceptors (irritant receptors in the mucosa of the epiglottic area innervated by unmyelinated C fibers of the superior laryngeal nerve) that are stimulated by noxious stimuli, particularly fluids with low chloride concentration. When this reflex is elicited, for example, during an aberrant swallow, the larynx closes, and swallowing occurs during a central apnea. If swallowing does not occur or fails to clear the liquid, the apneic portion of the response may be prolonged. After swallowing, if the airway remains closed, obstructive apnea can occur. This is a protective reflex against aspiration and is more prominent in the young. Given our patient's developmental delay and dysphagia, she may have an immature laryngochemoreceptor reflex. Infection with respiratory syncytial virus has been associated with a similar reflex and may present with central apneas in an acutely ill infant.[8]

Periodic breathing and/or isolated central apneas may be a normal phenomenon at sleep-wake transitions because of changes in the apneic threshold between wakefulness and sleep. The apneic threshold is the level of CO_2 that stimulates ventilation. During sleep, ventilation is driven by metabolic factors such as the PO_2 and PCO_2. During wakefulness, the cortical influence on breathing overrides the apneic threshold so that one breathes during wakefulness even if one's PCO_2 is low. Thus, an individual may have low CO_2 during wakefulness. When this individual transitions from wakefulness to N1 sleep, the PCO_2 is below the apneic threshold, and the PO_2 is normal, so there is no drive to breathe, and a central apnea ensues. The central apnea results in hypercapnia and hypoxemia, stimulating breathing to resume. In individuals with a high ventilatory drive, this may result in hyperpnea and overventilation, driving the PCO_2 below the apneic threshold and resulting in another central apnea. This ventilatory instability may lead to a few cycles of periodic breathing before ventilation stabilizes at a PCO_2 above the apneic threshold. This type of periodic breathing at sleep onset is considered normal. Any process that leads to increased arousals can result in increased central apneas. Gastroesophageal reflux, pain, pruritus, uncontrolled asthma, and OSAS (because of gasping) are conditions in children that may lead to an increase in arousals and subsequent central apnea. This pattern is also seen in children after crying.

Regardless of the cause of pathologic central apnea, there may be resultant significant desaturation. The degree of desaturation following a central apnea is related to the duration of the apnea, the lung volume at the time of the event, and the baseline SpO_2 before the event. Children and infants have smaller lungs and a more compliant chest wall than adults do, resulting in a lower functional residual capacity and a tendency for desaturation with brief central apneas. Desaturation is often more severe during REM sleep because of the negative effects of REM hypotonia on chest wall mechanics. Because young children spend a considerable amount of time in REM sleep, the desaturation may have important clinical consequences.

Our patient's PSG showed frequent central apneas and an increased percentage of periodic breathing for age. Her central apneas were not pathologic in duration but were associated with significant desaturation as shown in Figures 37-1 and 37-2. Because of the frequency of central apneas with desaturation, the amount of time that our patient spent with her SpO_2 <90% was clinically significant. The cause of her central apnea is most likely multifactorial as discussed above; the cerebral MRI ruled out any major CNS lesions that could be contributing to the central apnea. She was treated with ½ L/min supplemental oxygen via nasal cannula during sleep and her central apnea, saturations, and restless sleep improved. Because she had no hypoventilation or obstructive apnea, CPAP and bi-level positive airway pressure were not needed.

CLINICAL PEARLS

1. Central apneas syndrome in children is unusual.
2. Central apneas can be associated with significant oxyhemoglobin desaturation in infants and small children because of altered pulmonary mechanics and immature ventilatory reflexes.
3. Supplemental oxygen during sleep can be used to ameliorate the effects of central apnea with desaturation, if hypoventilation and/or OSAS are not also present.

REFERENCES

1. Rusconi F, Castagneto M, Gagliardi L, et al. Reference values for respiratory rate in the first 3 years of life. *Pediatrics*. 1994;94(3):350–355.
2. Berry RB, Gamaldo CE, Harding SM, Lloyd RM, Marcus CL, Vaughn BV. *The AASM Manual for the Scoring of Sleep and Associated Events: Rules, Terminology and Technical Specifications, Version 2.2*. Darien, IL: Academy of Sleep Medicine; 2015.
3. Stein IM, Fallon M, Merisalo RL, Kennedy Jr JL. The frequency of apnea and bradycardia in a population of healthy, normal infants. *Neuropediatrics*. 1983;14(2):73–75.
4. Montgomery-Downs HE, O'Brien LM, Gulliver TE, Gozal D. Polysomnographic characteristics in normal preschool and early school-aged children. *Pediatrics*. 2006;117(3):741–753.
5. Kelly DH, Riordan L, Smith MJ. Apnea and periodic breathing in healthy full-term infants, 12-18 months of age. *Pediatr Pulmonol*. 1992;13(3):169–171.
6. Oliveira AJ, Nunes ML, Fojo-Olmos A, Reis FM, da Costa JC. Clinical correlates of periodic breathing in neonatal polysomnography. *Clin Neurophysiol*. 2004;115(10):2247–2251.
7. Kryger MH, Roth T, Dement WC. *Principles and Practice of Sleep Medicine*. 4th ed. Philadelphia, PA: Elsevier Saunders; 2005:970–973.
8. Lindgren C, Grogaard J. Reflex apnoea response and inflammatory mediators in infants with respiratory tract infection. *Acta Paediatr*. 1996;85(7):798–803.

A toddler headed for tracheostomy decannulation

Suzanne E. Beck

CASE PRESENTATION

A 3½-year-old boy with a history of prematurity and a tracheostomy for subglottic stenosis was referred for evaluation before tracheostomy decannulation. He had occasional desaturations during sleep but no snoring or difficulty breathing. Past medical history revealed that he was born after a 27-week gestation and had pulmonary complications at birth, including respiratory distress syndrome, for which he was intubated and received mechanical ventilation for 2 weeks. He was subsequently extubated and required nasal continuous positive airway pressure (CPAP) but was not able to wean off this. He was diagnosed with subglottic stenosis and underwent tracheostomy at 6 months of age. Further, 6 months before evaluation, he underwent laryngotracheal reconstruction. He has been stable from a respiratory perspective since surgery, off CPAP and supplement oxygen. He has been growing and developing well with the exception of mild speech delay. He has well-controlled intermittent asthma. His only medication is albuterol as needed.

PHYSICAL EXAM

Physical exam revealed a well-developed toddler in no distress. His weight and height were at the 25th percentiles for age. Respiratory rate was 20 breaths/min, with pulse 90 beats/min and SpO_2 98%, while breathing spontaneously in room air. Oropharyngeal exam showed a normal palate and dentition. His tonsils extended to the pillars (2+). He had a 4.0 Bivona Flextend tracheostomy tube in place. He had a normal-shaped chest with clear breath sounds and normal heart sounds. There was no clubbing. The rest of his exam was normal.

LABORATORY AND SLEEP FINDINGS

Polysomnography (PSG) was performed with a downsized tracheotomy tube (3.0 Bivona), which was capped for the first part of the study. Total sleep time (TST) was 238 minutes; sleep efficiency 61%; REM sleep was decreased at 39 minutes (17% of TST); arousal index 53.4/h; obstructive apnea–hypopnea index (AHI) 144/h (trach capped) and 0/h (trach uncapped); SpO_2 nadir 90%; peak end-tidal CO_2 49 mm Hg (Fig. 38-1).

QUESTIONS

1. What are the findings on the PSG hypnogram in Figure 38-1 and the tracing in Figure 38-2?
2. Based on the information presented in Figures 38-1 through 38-3, would you recommend tracheostomy decannulation at this point?

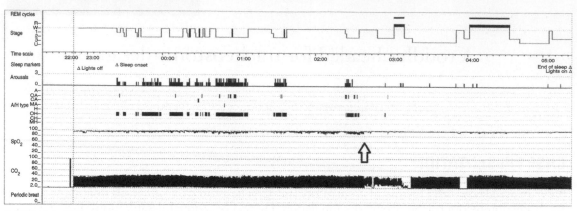

FIGURE 38-1 ■ Hypnogram indicating the timing of tracheostomy uncapping (*arrow*) and relationship to sleep architecture and respiratory events.

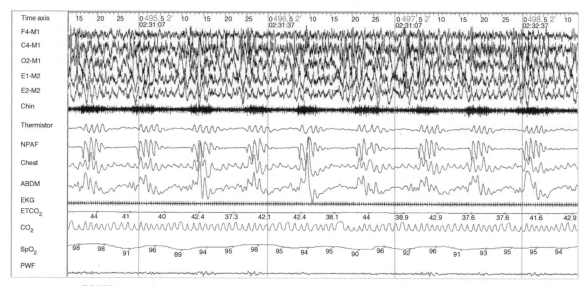

FIGURE 38-2 ■ Representative 120-second epoch of sleep with tracheostomy capped.

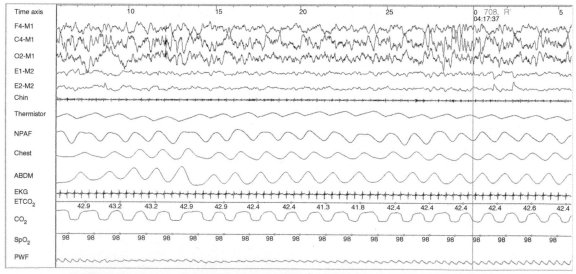

FIGURE 38-3 ■ Representative 30-second epoch of sleep after tracheostomy uncapping.

ANSWERS

1. There are frequent obstructive events associated with arousals, episodic oxyhemoglobin desaturation, and sleep fragmentation with the tracheostomy capped.
2. Figure 38-3 shows improvement in airflow, arousals, and oxyhemoglobin saturation, as well as consolidated sleep when the tracheostomy was uncapped. The patient needs further medical or surgical management before decannulation.

DISCUSSION

The majority of tracheostomies in pediatric patients are performed to treat upper-airway obstruction, most commonly caused by craniofacial syndromes or subglottic stenosis, or for long-term mechanical ventilation requirements for underlying neuromuscular or respiratory problems.[1] Many children with tracheostomies will undergo eventual decannulation.

Subglottic stenosis is a narrowing of the airway below the vocal cords involving the cricoid ring, the only complete cartilaginous ring of the airway. Subglottic stenosis is graded on a scale of 1 to 4, based on the degree of narrowing (grade 1, <50% obstruction; grade 2, 51% to 70% obstruction; grade 3, 71% to 99% obstruction; and grade 4, no detectable lumen).[2] Subglottic stenosis can be either congenital or acquired, and it is often a complication of prolonged intubation. Treatment varies and depends on the degree of narrowing and symptoms. Most cases of severe subglottic stenosis require tracheostomy until endoscopic laryngoplasty or surgical cricotracheal or laryngo-tracheal reconstruction can be performed.[3] Following healing, the tracheostomy can be removed in most patients.

Because the indications for tracheostomy and associated comorbidities vary widely in children, the approach to decannulation readiness also varies and should be tailored to the patient. Most agree that direct visualization of the airway with microlaryngoscopy and bronchoscopy is indicated before decannulation to examine and remove obstructing lesions such as granulomas. PSG can be useful in planning for tracheostomy decannulation in pediatric patients,[4] especially those with complex airway issues or underlying sleep-disordered breathing.[5] This is because patients may breathe adequately during wakefulness with the tracheotomy tube capped but during sleep may have upper-airway muscle hypotonia or additional issues such as adenotonsillar hypertrophy, leading to upper-airway obstruction. Based on small retrospective studies, several centers[6-8] have published multistep protocols for decannulation following long-term tracheostomy in children, similar to the following: (1) assess for clinical readiness; (2) perform flexible laryngoscopy; (3) downsize the tracheotomy tube over several weeks and start daytime capping of the tube; (4) perform bronchoscopy to remove suspected granulomas; (5) perform PSG with a capped, down-sized tracheotomy tube; and (6) decannulate in the intensive care unit and observe for 24 hours if the PSG is reassuring. In a recent retrospective study of 59 patients in a tertiary care center, favorable PSG parameters (obstructive AHI ≤5/h and absence of hypoventilation with end-tidal CO_2 >50 mm Hg for <25% of TST) along with favorable airway endoscopy predicted successful decannulation.[8] These authors point out that clinical concerns drove the decision against decannulation in one third of patients despite having favorable PSG and airway endoscopy findings. This finding highlights the complexity and variability of the population.

Our patient seemed to be doing clinically well following surgical correction of his subglottic stenosis. As part of readiness for decannulation, he underwent airway endoscopy, which showed 2+ tonsils, non-obstructing adenoids, and no other obstructing tissue. PSG showed significant obstructive sleep apnea syndrome with a small capped tracheostomy in place (Figs. 38-1 and 38-2). The discrepancy in these findings may be due to the tracheostomy itself acting to obstruct the airway or may be due to patient-related anatomic or dynamic causes of obstruction. This discrepancy underscores that endoscopy evaluates anatomic abnormalities and PSG assesses physiologic function and dynamics during sleep. Our patient underwent adenotonsillectomy. Subsequent PSG with a downsized capped tracheostomy was normal. He was observed overnight in the intensive care unit while the tracheostomy was capped and then underwent successful decannulation.

CLINICAL PEARLS

1. PSG is useful in planning for tracheotomy decannulation in pediatric patients, especially those with complex airway issues or underlying sleep-disordered breathing.
2. Upper-airway obstruction may occur during sleep because of upper-airway hypotonia or additional issues such as adenotonsillar hypertrophy, even if the primary indication for the tracheotomy has been resolved.
3. A capped tracheostomy tube may itself obstruct the airway. Repeat PSG with a downsized capped tracheostomy tube could be considered.

REFERENCES

1. Yaneza MM, James HP, Davies P, et al. Changing indications for paediatric tracheostomy and the role of a multidisciplinary tracheostomy clinic. *J Laryngol Otol*. 2015;129(9):882–886.
2. Myer 3rd CM, O'Connor DM, Cotton RT. Proposed grading system for subglottic stenosis based on endotracheal tube sizes. *Ann Otol Rhinol Laryngol*. 1994;103(4 Pt 1):319–323.
3. Triglia JM, Nicollas R, Roman S. Management of subglottic stenosis in infancy and childhood. *Eur Arch Otorhinolaryngol*. 2000;257(7):382–385.
4. Wise MS, Nichols CD, Grigg-Damberger MM, et al. Executive summary of respiratory indications for polysomnography in children: an evidence-based review. *Sleep*. 2011;34(3):389–398.
5. Aurora RN, Zak RS, Karippot A, et al. Practice parameters for the respiratory indications for polysomnography in children. *Sleep*. 2011;34(3):379–388.
6. Robison JG, Thottam PJ, Greenberg LL, Maguire RC, Simons JP, Mehta DK. Role of polysomnography in the development of an algorithm for planning tracheostomy decannulation. *Otolaryngol Head Neck Surg*. 2015;152(1):180–184.
7. Tunkel DE, McColley SA, Baroody FM, Marcus CL, Carroll JL, Loughlin GM. Polysomnography in the evaluation of readiness for decannulation in children. *Arch Otolaryngol Head Neck Surg*. 1996;122(7):721–724.
8. Gurbani N, Promyothin U, Rutter M, Fenchel MC, Szczesniak RD, Simakajornboon N. Using polysomnography and airway evaluation to predict successful decannulation in children. *Otolaryngol Head Neck Surg*. 2015;153(4):649–655.

A school-aged child with snoring

Suzanne E. Beck

CASE PRESENTATION

A 6-year-old girl was seen for evaluation of snoring. The snoring occurred on most nights and was worse with upper-respiratory infections. Her parents also noticed that she was very restless during sleep, breathed primarily through her mouth, and sometimes had deep pauses in breathing. She slept from 8:30 PM to 7:30 AM. Her weekend schedule was similar. She was doing well in school. She was typically developing. She had no medical problems and was on no medications. Her mother smoked inside the house. Family history was unremarkable. The parents were concerned that her snoring was a sign of sleep apnea and requested further evaluation.

PHYSICAL EXAM

Physical exam revealed a well-developed, well-nourished girl with normal vital signs for age. Her growth parameters were at the 40th percentiles. She had nondysmorphic features, a normal palate, and normal dentition. Her tonsils extended beyond the pillars (3+). Her nares were patent and nasal mucosa was normal. The rest of her exam was normal.

LABORATORY AND SLEEP FINDINGS

Polysomnography (PSG) revealed a total sleep time (TST) of 420 minutes; sleep efficiency 92%; normal sleep architecture with 138 minutes REM sleep (33% of TST); arousal index 9.2/h; obstructive apnea–hypopnea index (AHI) 0.8/h; SpO_2 nadir 93%; 5% of TST with end-tidal CO_2 >50 mm Hg.

QUESTIONS

1. What are the findings on the 60-second epoch in Figure 39-1?
2. Based on the sleep history and the PSG results, what is the sleep diagnosis?

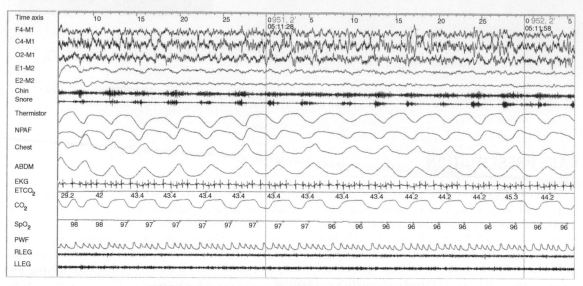

FIGURE 39-1 ■ Representative 60-second epoch of sleep.

ANSWERS

1. Figure 39-1 shows rhythmic snoring in the chin and snore leads. There is heart-rate variability in synchrony with respiration in which the R-R interval on the electrocardiogram (EKG) is shorter during inspiration and longer during expiration, consistent with respiratory sinus arrhythmia, which is a normal finding. There are no respiratory events that meet scoring criteria.
2. The results of the PSG, showing snoring with otherwise normal breathing during sleep, together with the clinical presentation of normal growth and development, are consistent with the diagnosis of primary snoring.

DISCUSSION

Snoring is often concerning to caregivers and clinicians alike because it is a hallmark feature of obstructive sleep apnea syndrome (OSAS). However, not all children who snore have OSAS. OSAS has a prevalence of 2% to 5.7% in the general pediatric population and has well-recognized neurobehavioral, neurocognitive, cardiovascular, and growth sequelae if left untreated.[1] Primary snoring, on the contrary, is much more common than OSAS, with an estimated overall population prevalence of approximately 10% in children.[2] *Primary snoring* is defined as snoring without associated apneas, hypopneas, hypoxemia, hypercapnia, or sleep fragmentation,[3] and its sequelae are not well understood. Whether primary snoring, that is, snoring in the absence of frank obstructive events and gas-exchange abnormalities, has the same neurobehavioral sequelae as OSAS is of much interest. The American Academy of Pediatrics recommends that all children be screened for snoring and that further evaluation is warranted to determine whether the snoring is part of OSAS.[3] The guidelines recommend a thorough history and physical exam as the first step; PSG is not indicated in every child with snoring alone.

Habitual snoring is very common in preschool and school-aged children. A longitudinal study of more than 12,000 children followed from birth to age almost 7 years found that parent-reported habitual snoring ranged from 9.6% to 21% and peaked at age 3.5 years.[4] Risk factors for snoring at all ages included maternal smoking, lower maternal education, and wheezing, while race and gender effects were significant only at age 1.5 years (increased snoring in non-white and male children).[4] In another large British study, parent-reported habitual snoring in 1- to 4-year-olds was found in 7.9% of the study group and was positively associated with socioeconomic deprivation, but when adjusted for wheeze and other atopic disorders, respiratory symptoms, body mass index, and exposure to pollutants, socioeconomic status was no longer significant.[5] Other studies have shown that prematurity and black race are associated with increased risk of symptoms of sleep-disordered breathing among 8- to 11-year-old children.[6]

Snoring and OSAS have always been presented as opposite ends of the continuum of the sleep-disordered breathing spectrum; however, it is not fully understood whether snoring in the absence of frank obstruction and gas-exchange abnormalities is a benign condition in children or how the two syndromes overlap. Snoring is due to vibration of upper-airway tissues during sleep secondary to upper-airway narrowing and sleep-induced pharyngeal hypotonia and results from increased upper-airway resistance. The consequence is airflow limitation, which may result in a variety of physiologic consequences, including sleep fragmentation and autonomic dysfunction. Small, observational studies have shown impaired vigilance, social problems, anxiety, and depressive symptoms in snoring children without OSAS.[7,8] Another small, nonrandomized study showed that children with snoring have worse behavior problems and hyperactivity compared with controls, which improves after adenotonsillectomy, similar to children with OSAS.[9] However, many of these studies have shown that children with primary snoring differ from non-snoring controls but are still within the normal range. Further, studies have also been nonrandomized and have not controlled for important factors such as socioeconomic status. Therefore, whether PSG-proven snoring in the absence of frank obstructive breathing is associated with neurobehavioral consequences similar to OSAS, and whether surgical treatment is effective at reversal of those consequences, is still unclear. Further study of the neurobehavioral and neurocognitive outcomes of primary snoring in preschool and school-aged children is indicated.

Determining whether a child has primary snoring versus OSAS is difficult without a PSG. Most questionnaires have shown insufficient predictive accuracy.[10] The Pediatric Sleep Questionnaire had a sensitivity of 0.85 and specificity of 0.87 in one study and may be as predictive as the AHI for neurocognitive impairment associated with OSAS.[11] However, the sensitivity and specificity are low for clinical purposes. Clinical history and exam are not sufficient to discern primary snoring from OSAS, but they are helpful in determining which children need further evaluation. For example, if the snoring is only intermittent with upper-respiratory-tract infections, and is not associated with observed apneas, daytime symptoms, or a worrisome exam, further evaluation may not be necessary. If OSAS is suspected based on clinical manifestations of sleep-disordered breathing, the American Academy of Pediatrics recommends overnight, attended, in-laboratory PSG as the gold standard tool for the diagnosis of OSAS in children (see Clinical Pearls in Case 1: Pediatric sleep history: a 4 year old with snoring, gasping, and witnessed apnea).[3]

Nocturnal pulse oximetry has been proposed as a low-cost and easy-to-use diagnostic alternative to identify OSAS when PSG is not available.[12] In this scenario, oxygen desaturation indices can be used as a surrogate for AHI as detailed in a recent review.[12] However, the sensitivity and specificity of overnight pulse oximetry to identify OSAS with an obstructive AHI >5/h are low: 67% and 60%, respectively.[13] Oximetry algorithms tend to overestimate the AHI at low levels and underestimate it at high levels, and it is not sufficient to diagnose OSAS,[1] but it might be used as a screening tool. Because only a small proportion of children who are subjected to adenotonsillectomy for sleep-disordered breathing in the United States undergo preoperative PSG,[14] alternative diagnostic tools that are less costly and more available are warranted.

Our patient's PSG showed snoring with no evidence of OSAS, gas-exchange abnormalities, or sleep fragmentation. Our patient was diagnosed with primary snoring. The parents were reassured that the findings on the PSG were normal. Because our patient was growing well and functioning well in school with no problems with attention, behavior, or performance, it was recommended that she reduce risk factors such as exposure to secondhand tobacco smoke and that she continue to follow with her pediatrician, who, along with her parents, will keep a vigilant watch on her symptoms.

CLINICAL PEARLS

1. The prevalence of habitual snoring in the pediatric population is common; much more common compared with OSAS.
2. The American Academy of Pediatrics recommends that all children be screened for snoring and that further evaluation is warranted to determine whether the snoring is part of OSAS.[3] The guidelines recommend a thorough history and physical exam as the first step; PSG is not indicated in every child with snoring alone.
3. Overnight, attended, in-laboratory PSG is the gold standard tool to determine whether a child has OSAS.
4. Overnight oximetry and sleep questionnaires are not sufficient to differentiate primary snoring from OSAS.
5. Tobacco smoke exposure is a modifiable risk factor for snoring.

REFERENCES

1. Marcus CL, Brooks LJ, Draper KA, et al. Diagnosis and management of childhood obstructive sleep apnea syndrome. *Pediatrics*. 2012;130(3):e714–e755.
2. Goodwin JL, Babar SI, Kaemingk KL, et al. Symptoms related to sleep-disordered breathing in white and Hispanic children: the Tucson Children's Assessment of Sleep Apnea Study. *Chest*. 2003;124(1):196–203.
3. Clinical practice guideline: diagnosis and management of childhood obstructive sleep apnea syndrome. *Pediatrics*. 2002;109(4):704–712.
4. Bonuck KA, Chervin RD, Cole TJ, et al. Prevalence and persistence of sleep disordered breathing symptoms in young children: a 6-year population-based cohort study. *Sleep*. 2011;34(7):875–884.
5. Kuehni CE, Strippoli MP, Chauliac ES, Silverman M. Snoring in preschool children: prevalence, severity and risk factors. *Eur Respir J*. 2008;31(2):326–333.
6. Rosen CL, Larkin EK, Kirchner HL, et al. Prevalence and risk factors for sleep-disordered breathing in 8- to 11-year-old children: association with race and prematurity. *J Pediatr*. 2003;142(4):383–389.
7. O'Brien LM, Mervis CB, Holbrook CR, et al. Neurobehavioral implications of habitual snoring in children. *Pediatrics*. 2004;114(1):44–49.
8. Blunden S, Lushington K, Kennedy D, Martin J, Dawson D. Behavior and neurocognitive performance in children aged 5-10 years who snore compared to controls. *J Clin Exp Neuropsychol*. 2000;22(5):554–568.
9. Chervin RD, Ruzicka DL, Giordani BJ, et al. Sleep-disordered breathing, behavior, and cognition in children before and after adenotonsillectomy. *Pediatrics*. 2006;117(4):e769–e778.
10. Brockmann PE, Schlaud M, Poets CF, Urschitz MS. Predicting poor school performance in children suspected for sleep-disordered breathing. *Sleep Med*. 2015;16(9):1077–1083.
11. Chervin RD, Weatherly RA, Garetz SL, et al. Pediatric sleep questionnaire: prediction of sleep apnea and outcomes. *Arch Otolaryngol Head Neck Surg*. 2007;133(3):216–222.
12. Kaditis A, Kheirandish-Gozal L, Gozal D. Pediatric OSAS: oximetry can provide answers when polysomnography is not available. *Sleep Med Rev*. 2015;27:96–105.
13. Kirk VG, Bohn SG, Flemons WW, Remmers JE. Comparison of home oximetry monitoring with laboratory polysomnography in children. *Chest*. 2003;124(5):1702–1708.
14. Friedman NR, Perkins JN, McNair B, Mitchell RB. Current practice patterns for sleep-disordered breathing in children. *Laryngoscope*. 2013;123(4):1055–1058.

Double trouble: Tween siblings with obesity, daytime somnolence, and snoring

Suzanne E. Beck

CASE PRESENTATION

An 11-year-old boy was evaluated for snoring and daytime somnolence at the suggestion of his school counselor. His parent reported that the child was struggling with his grades, and he often fell asleep in class despite getting adequate nocturnal sleep. His bedtime was at 9 PM and wake time was 7 AM. He often took a 2-hour nap after school. He had snoring on most nights for the past several years. He had been overweight since the age of 2 years and developed dyslipidemia, vitamin D deficiency, and intermittently elevated blood pressure at the age of 10 years. There was a family history of obesity, type 2 diabetes, hypertension, and heart disease in his parents. He took vitamin D supplements but was on no other medications.

His sister, a 12-year-old girl, was evaluated on the same day, at the request of the parent because of concerns over similar symptoms of snoring, daytime somnolence, and poor grades in school. Her sleep schedule and napping pattern were similar. She had been obese since the age of 3 years. She was recently diagnosed with dyslipidemia, vitamin D deficiency, and diabetes. Her medications included metformin and vitamin D.

PHYSICAL EXAM (11-YEAR-OLD BOY)

Vital signs: pulse 76 beats/min; blood pressure (BP) 137/70 mm Hg; respiratory rate 20 breaths/min; SpO_2 98%; weight 101.6 kg (>99th percentile); height 161.1 cm (99th percentile); and body mass index (BMI) 39.2 kg/m^2 (>99th percentile).

He was a severely obese male with nondysmorphic features. His oropharynx was narrow, with a Mallampati score of II, and 2+ tonsils. Lungs were clear to auscultation. Cardiac exam was normal. There was no cyanosis, clubbing, or edema. Muscle strength was normal. Development was normal.

PHYSICAL EXAM (12-YEAR-OLD GIRL)

Vital signs: pulse 100 beats/min; BP 128/67; respiratory rate 20 breaths/min; SpO_2 99%; weight 113.8 kg (>99th percentile); height 162.7 cm (95th percentile); and BMI 43.0 kg/m^2 (>99th percentile).

She was a severely obese female with nondysmorphic features. Her oropharynx was narrow, with a Mallampati score of III, and 2+ tonsils. Lungs were clear to auscultation. Cardiac exam was normal. Acanthosis nigricans was present on the neck and axillae. There was no cyanosis, clubbing, or edema. Muscle strength was normal. Development was normal.

LABORATORY AND SLEEP FINDINGS

The boy's polysomnography (PSG) revealed a total sleep time (TST) of 442 min; SE 72%; REM sleep 59 min (18.5% of TST); arousal index 4.7/h; obstructive apnea–hypopnea index (AHI) 13.8/h; central apnea index 0/h; SpO_2 nadir 85%; and peak end-tidal CO_2 was 54 mm Hg, and end-tidal CO_2 was >50 mm Hg for 0.2 % of TST.

The girl's PSG revealed a TST of 442 min; SE 82%; REM sleep 46 min (13% of TST); arousal index 8.4/h; obstructive AHI 11.6/h; central apnea index 0/h; SpO_2 nadir 85%; and peak end-tidal CO_2 54 mm Hg, and end-tidal CO_2 was >50 mm Hg for 4.7% of TST.

QUESTIONS

1. What are the risk factors for obstructive sleep apnea in our patients?
2. What are the next steps in treatment for our patients?

ANSWERS

1. Risk factors for obstructive sleep apnea syndrome (OSAS) in both patients include tonsillar hypertrophy and obesity.
2. The first step in treatment is referral to otolaryngology for evaluation for adenotonsillectomy. Treatment with continuous positive airway pressure (CPAP) during sleep is indicated if the patient is not a surgical candidate or OSAS persists after surgery.

DISCUSSION

The prevalence of obesity in the pediatric population is high. More than one third of children and adolescents in the United States are overweight or obese.[1] Globally, the number of overweight or obese infants and young children has increased from 32 million in 1990 to 42 million in 2013[2] and is clearly a public health concern. Being obese as a child increases the likelihood of being obese as an adult, and obesity in adulthood is strongly associated with comorbities that contribute to cardiovascular disease and diabetes.[3] Obese children with OSAS may also be at risk for metabolic syndrome.[4] In addition to metabolic and cardiovascular sequelae, obese adolescents with OSAS show impairment in neurobehavioral function, which may be an etiologic factor in attention, behavior, mood, and school problems.[5]

With the rise of obesity in children, the epidemiology of pediatric OSAS has broadened from the classic picture of failure to thrive and adenotonsillar hypertrophy in a preschool-aged child to include obese school-aged children and adolescents with daytime somnolence or school problems. The estimated prevalence of OSAS in adolescents is 2%[6] and much higher in selected obese adolescent cohorts, ranging from 14% to 78%, as detailed in a recent review.[7]

The mechanisms of increased OSAS in obese children are not well understood. Adipose tissue is deposited around the upper airway (i.e., the "double chin"), as well as within the airway, invading intrinsic muscles of the upper airway such as the tongue,[8] and resulting in airway narrowing. However, parapharyngeal fat pads are not increased in adolescents or adults with OSAS.[9,10] Many obese children, especially if prepubertal, have adenotonsillar hypertrophy that results in further airway narrowing.[11] Although children have a greater ventilatory drive than adults do, the obese sleeping child may have impaired ventilation because of a mechanical load on the chest wall and abdomen imposed by central adiposity, resulting in decreased chest wall compliance and reduced diaphragmatic excursion. The impaired respiratory mechanics can lead to worsening of gas exchange during sleep or when lying down.

The first line of treatment for children and adolescents with OSAS is tonsillectomy and adenoidectomy (T&A) if patients have enlarged tonsils and adenoids.[12] However, after T&A, residual OSAS or symptoms persist in about one third of obese prepubertal children, compared with about 15% of nonobese children.[13] Further, it has also been shown that obese patients who undergo T&A may gain weight following surgery.[14] CPAP is indicated for residual OSAS following surgery, in patients who do not have adenotonsillar hypertrophy or who are not surgical candidates. However, surgery is generally recommended as the first-line treatment because it is curative in many patients and because adherence is a major obstacle to CPAP treatment.[12] Weight loss and exercise are also recommended for overweight patients. Although bariatric surgery has been successful in achieving weight loss and improving symptoms of OSAS in extremely obese children and adolescents,[15] this procedure is not commonly performed in children.

Our patient and his sibling were both at risk for OSAS, given their obesity and tonsillar hypertrophy, and both had cardiovascular disease (elevated blood pressure and dyslipidemia), metabolic dysfunction (glucose intolerance and vitamin D deficiency), and neurobehavioral problems (sleepiness and poor school performance). Both children had moderate OSAS on PSG. In both cases, the severity of the findings was felt to be underestimated because of decreased REM sleep (Figs. 40-1 and 40-2). Our patients and their parent were counseled on the association of untreated OSAS with cardiovascular, metabolic, and neurobehavioral consequences. Both children underwent adenotonsillectomy but ultimately required CPAP for residual OSAS following T&A. During the office visit at the Sleep Center each child underwent fitting for the appropriate-sized mask, and education on the use of the CPAP device. Also during the visit, to optimize adherence, both children and their parent underwent counseling and were given guidance by a sleep psychologist on desensitization strategies including sleep hygiene and cognitive behavioral therapy. Close phone surveillance and follow-up were arranged. CPAP titration PSGs were ordered. The children were also referred to a weight-management program.

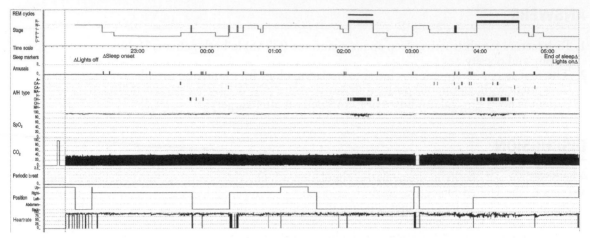

FIGURE 40-1 ■ Hypnogram of 11-year-old boy's overnight PSG.

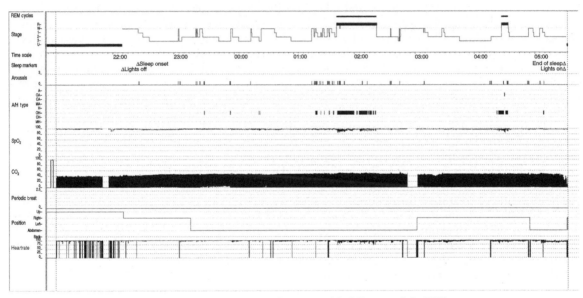

FIGURE 40-2 ■ Hypnogram of 12-year-old girl's overnight PSG.

CLINICAL PEARLS

1. The prevalence of OSAS in obese children and adolescents is high; therefore, obese children should be screened for symptoms of OSAS.
2. Obese children and adolescents with OSAS are at risk for cardiovascular sequelae and neurobehavioral impairment including poor attention and school performance, sleepiness, and behavioral and mood problems, which may be a factor in their ability to cope with treatment.
3. T&A is often effective in improving or resolving OSAS, even in obese pediatric patients. However, a repeat polysomnogram should be performed after surgery to evaluate for residual OSAS requiring further treatment.
4. CPAP is indicated for residual OSAS following surgery, in patients who do not have adenotonsillar hypertrophy, and in those who are not surgical candidates.
5. Treatment strategies should be comprehensive and include medical and surgical evaluation, weight loss and exercise, supportive care, and follow-up.

REFERENCES

1. Ogden CL, Carroll MD, Kit BK, Flegal KM. Prevalence of childhood and adult obesity in the United States, 2011-2012. *JAMA*. Feb 26 2014;311(8):806–814.
2. Obesity and Overweight. http://www.who.int/mediacentre/factsheets/fs311/en/: updated January 2015, Accessed 20.07.2015.
3. Litwin SE. Childhood obesity and adulthood cardiovascular disease: quantifying the lifetime cumulative burden of cardiovascular risk factors. *J Am Coll Cardiol*. Oct 14 2014;64(15):1588–1590.
4. Gozal D, Capdevila OS, Kheirandish-Gozal L. Metabolic alterations and systemic inflammation in obstructive sleep apnea among nonobese and obese prepubertal children. *Am J Respir Crit Care Med*. May 15 2008;177(10):1142–1149.
5. Xanthopoulos MS, Gallagher PR, Berkowitz RI, Radcliffe J, Bradford R, Marcus CL. Neurobehavioral functioning in adolescents with and without obesity and obstructive sleep apnea. *Sleep*. Mar 2015;38(3):401–410.
6. Sanchez-Armengol A, Fuentes-Pradera MA, Capote-Gil F, et al. Sleep-related breathing disorders in adolescents aged 12 to 16 years: clinical and polygraphic findings. *Chest*. May 2001;119(5):1393–1400.
7. Mathew JL, Narang I. Sleeping too close together: obesity and obstructive sleep apnea in childhood and adolescence. *Paediatr Respir Rev*. Sep 2014;15(3):211–218.
8. Kim AM, Keenan BT, Jackson N, et al. Tongue fat and its relationship to obstructive sleep apnea. *Sleep*. Oct 2014;37(10):1639–1648.
9. Schwab RJ, Gupta KB, Gefter WB, Metzger LJ, Hoffman EA, Pack AI. Upper airway and soft tissue anatomy in normal subjects and patients with sleep-disordered breathing. Significance of the lateral pharyngeal walls. *Am J Respir Crit Care Med*. Nov 1995;152(5 Pt 1):1673–1689.
10. Schwab RJ, Kim C, Bagchi S, et al. Understanding the anatomic basis for obstructive sleep apnea syndrome in adolescents. *Am J Respir Crit Care Med*. Jun 1 2015;191(11):1295–1309.
11. Wing YK, Hui SH, Pak WM, et al. A controlled study of sleep related disordered breathing in obese children. *Arch Dis Child*. Dec 2003;88(12):1043–1047.
12. Marcus CL, Brooks LJ, Draper KA, et al. Diagnosis and management of childhood obstructive sleep apnea syndrome. *Pediatrics*. Sep 2012;130(3):e714–e755.
13. Marcus CL, Moore RH, Rosen CL, et al. A randomized trial of adenotonsillectomy for childhood sleep apnea. *N Engl J Med*. Jun 20 2013;368(25):2366–2376.
14. Katz ES, Moore RH, Rosen CL, et al. Growth after adenotonsillectomy for obstructive sleep apnea: an RCT. *Pediatrics*. Aug 2014;134(2):282–289.
15. Alqahtani AR, Antonisamy B, Alamri H, Elahmedi M, Zimmerman VA. Laparoscopic sleeve gastrectomy in 108 obese children and adolescents aged 5 to 21 years. *Ann Surg*. Aug 2012;256(2):266–273.

An infant with respiratory muscle weakness and lethargy

Suzanne E. Beck

CASE PRESENTATION

A 12-month-old boy with spinal muscular atrophy (SMA) was evaluated for increasing fatigue. He had generalized weakness and hypotonia. He recently developed a mild respiratory infection with mild hypoxemia and was treated with ½ L/min supplemental oxygen. Despite the supplemental oxygen use and resolution of the cold symptoms, he became less energetic and was eating less.

Past medical history: He was born full term. He was diagnosed with SMA type II at 10 months of age. He had normal development in the first 6 months of life but, thereafter, showed delay of physical developmental milestones. He sat with support by 11 months of age but never learned to crawl or pull to stand. He required nasogastric feeds to supplement his oral feeding. He had a weak cough regularly, no snoring, and no symptoms of gastroesophageal reflux. He was on no medications.

PHYSICAL EXAM

Physical exam revealed an alert infant in no apparent distress. His weight and height were at the 25th percentiles for age. Respiratory rate was 28 breaths/min; pulse 120 beats/min; blood pressure normal for age; and SpO_2 95% in room air. His head had a flattened occiput. Oropharyngeal exam showed a high-arched palate, tongue fasciculations, and decreased facial expression. His tonsils were visible behind the pillars (1+). He had a small bell-shaped chest, mild pectus excavatum, mild scoliosis, and thoracoabdominal asynchrony at rest. Lungs were clear to auscultation with good air exchange, and heart sounds were normal. The abdomen was protuberant, but soft and without organomegaly. Muscle tone was decreased, and he had poor head control. Patellar reflexes were absent. The infant was able to reach for an object against gravity and transfer from hand to hand but was not able to roll over or lift his chest off the examination table when he was in the prone position. He could sit with support.

LABORATORY AND SLEEP FINDINGS

Previous genetic analysis showed a homozygous deletion of exon 7 of the telomeric survival motor neuron gene (SMN1).

Polysomnography (PSG) revealed a total sleep time (TST) of 440 minutes; sleep efficiency 81%; normal sleep architecture, with 90 minutes REM sleep (25% of TST); arousal index 18.4/h; obstructive apnea–hypopnea index 3.4/h; SpO_2 nadir 68%; SpO_2 <90% for 60% of TST; peak end-tidal CO_2 74 mm Hg; end-tidal CO_2 >50 mm Hg for 78% of TST; mean transcutaneous CO_2 68 mm Hg.

QUESTIONS

1. What are the findings on the PSG tracing in Figure 41-1?
2. What is the diagnosis?
3. Based on the information presented in Figure 41-2, was the intervention effective?

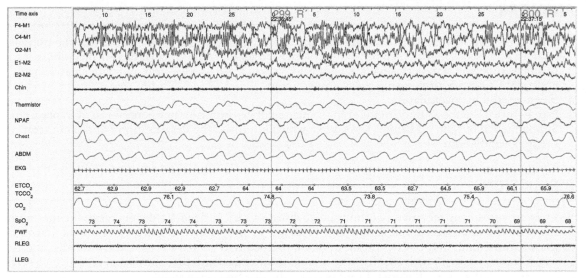

FIGURE 41-1 ■ Representative 60-second epoch of sleep.

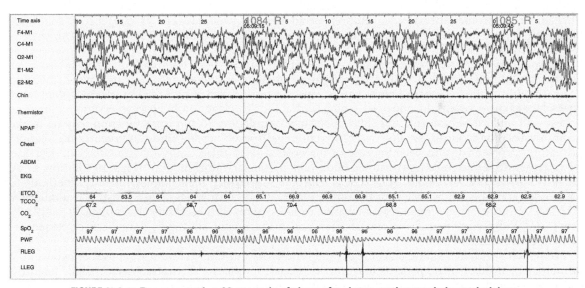

FIGURE 41-2 ■ Representative 60 seconds of sleep after intervention made by technician.

ANSWERS

1. Figure 41-1 shows persistent desaturation and hypercapnia without apneas (note that the transcutaneous CO_2 reads higher than the end-tidal CO_2 because of a number of factors including sensor response time and skin perfusion; see Clinical Pearls in Case 6: A 14-year-old with an abnormal end-tidal CO_2 waveform during polysomnography).
2. Sleep-related hypoventilation.
3. No. Figure 41-2 shows improvement in oxyhemoglobin saturation but persistence of hypercapnia. Supplemental oxygen (½ L/min) was added, which improved the desaturation but did not treat the hypoventilation.

DISCUSSION

SMA is an autosomal recessive neuromuscular disease characterized by degeneration of the motor neurons of the spinal cord and brainstem, resulting in progressive muscle weakness and atrophy of the proximal limb and bulbar muscles. The incidence is 1/6000 to 1/10,000 live births, and the carrier frequency is 1/40 to 1/60.[1] It is the second most common lethal autosomal recessive disorder in Caucasians (after cystic fibrosis). In most cases, the disease is caused by homozygous mutations of the survival motor neuron 1 (SMN1) gene, which is on chromosome 5q13.[2] The phenotype is variable, and patients have been classified as SMA types I-IV based on age of onset and functional level achieved. Type I SMA or infantile SMA, also called Werdnig-Hoffmann disease, usually presents in the first 6 months of life with hypotonia and progressive respiratory insufficiency and is rapidly fatal unless ventilatory support is instituted. Type II or intermediate SMA is usually recognized between 6 and 18 months of age, and it progresses gradually over the life span. Type III, known as Kugelberg-Welander syndrome, affects older children or adolescents, whereas type IV presents in adulthood; these are milder forms. Pulmonary disease is the major cause of morbidity and mortality in children with SMA types I and II.[3]

Respiratory compromise in children with SMA is caused by a combination of inspiratory and expiratory muscle weakness with relative sparing of the diaphragm, resulting in a weak, mechanically disadvantaged bell-shaped chest with sternal depression and paradoxical breathing.[3] Ventilatory muscle weakness results in impaired cough and ability to clear lower airway secretions, lung and chest wall underdevelopment, and subsequent hypoventilation. Respiratory function may be further compromised by scoliosis, swallowing dysfunction, gastroesophageal reflux, and recurrent infections. Breathing worsens during sleep because of the normal sleep-related physiologic effects of decreased ventilatory drive and respiratory muscle inhibition, particularly during REM sleep. In addition, OSAS may occur because of bulbar dysfunction. Chronic respiratory management includes methods for airway clearance, such as mechanical insufflation-exsufflation, manual cough assist, and noninvasive (bi-level positive airway pressure) or invasive (tracheostomy and mechanical ventilation) ventilatory support.[3] Pulmonary manifestations of SMA and management strategies have been discussed in a recent consensus statement.[3]

In patients with neuromuscular disease and ventilatory muscle weakness, the onset of hypoventilation may be insidious, and patients may initially be asymptomatic.[4] Symptoms may include nocturnal awakenings and restless sleep, daytime sleepiness, and morning headache. Fatigue, swallowing difficulties, weakened cough, weight loss, and frequent respiratory infections may suggest worsening of nocturnal ventilation. Initially, hypoventilation may occur only during sleep (particularly REM sleep), but as deterioration progresses, daytime respiratory function becomes impaired. Overnight oximetry can be useful to detect hypoxemia, but it fails to detect hypoventilation. PSG with end-tidal and transcutaneous CO_2 measurements should be performed to assess sleep-related hypoventilation and sleep-disordered breathing. Hypoventilation is diagnosed when the end-tidal CO_2 is >50 mm Hg for >25% of sleep time. Patients with nocturnal hypoventilation secondary to neuromuscular disease (regardless of the underlying condition) are at risk of developing daytime respiratory failure, which is likely to ensue within the following 12 to 24 months if the nocturnal hypoventilation is not treated.[5]

Noninvasive positive pressure ventilation has a favorable long-term effect on nocturnal and diurnal gas exchange and sleep in patients with neuromuscular disorders, although the decision to institute ventilatory support needs to be made together with the patient and family in view of the overall prognosis, family goals, and quality of life. A 5-year prospective study of children with muscular dystrophy treated with nocturnal noninvasive positive pressure ventilation showed an improved respiratory disturbance index, decreased arousals from sleep, improved sleep architecture, and decreased nocturnal heart rate.[6] A randomized controlled trial in patients with neuromuscular disease with nocturnal hypoventilation and daytime normocapnia showed that noninvasive ventilation significantly improved nocturnal blood gas tensions.[5] Noninvasive ventilation may improve gas exchange by increasing tidal ventilation, unloading respiratory muscles, and, possibly, by resetting respiratory central chemosensitivity.[7] Importantly, nocturnal noninvasive ventilation also reduces symptoms of sleep disturbance and morning headaches and improves appetite, concentration, and quality of life in children with neuromuscular disorders and sleep-disordered breathing.[8]

Noninvasive ventilation with bi-level positive pressure support is the most effective strategy for improving ventilation in children with ventilatory muscle weakness and hypoventilation. The expiratory positive airway pressure is adjusted to maintain upper airway patency, whereas the pressure support, that is, the difference between the inspiratory and expiratory pressures, is adjusted to augment tidal volume. Infants and children with neuromuscular disease are usually too weak to trigger the machine; therefore, a backup rate in the pressure control mode is usually used. Continuous positive airway pressure is not indicated because it does not reduce the ventilatory load. Oxygen therapy alone in neuromuscular patients is usually contraindicated in view of the risk of exacerbating hypercapnia.[5]

Our patient had respiratory muscle weakness because of SMA type II and was diagnosed with sleep-related hypoventilation because of a medical condition. To meet diagnostic criteria, sleep-related hypoventilation must be present as indicated by elevated arterial, transcutaneous, or end-tidal CO_2, as was the case for our patient, who had end-tidal CO_2 >50 mm Hg for 78% of TST. Sustained oxygen desaturation during sleep that is unexplained by discrete apnea-hypopnea is common but is not sufficient to establish the diagnosis of sleep-related hypoventilation.[9] Obstructive or central apneas may be present but must not be believed to be the primary cause of the hypoventilation. Hypoventilation may also be present during wakefulness but is not required for the diagnosis.

As demonstrated in Figure 41-2, supplemental oxygen alone does not treat the underlying hypoventilation. Our patient was treated with nocturnal bi-level positive airway pressure. A daily regimen of airway clearance regimen with insufflation-exsufflation therapy was also instituted. His fatigue improved, and a titration polysomnogram showed resolution of nocturnal hypoventilation on bi-level positive airway pressure without supplemental oxygen.

CLINICAL PEARLS

1. Children with neuromuscular disease are susceptible to both upper airway obstruction and hypoventilation during sleep because of impaired ventilatory muscle function. The onset of nocturnal hypoventilation may be insidious.
2. CO_2 should be monitored during PSG to assess for sleep-related hypoventilation.
3. Noninvasive ventilation with bi-level positive pressure support is an effective strategy for improving ventilation in children with ventilatory muscle weakness and hypoventilation.
4. Oxygen therapy alone in neuromuscular patients with hypoventilation is usually contraindicated in view of the risk of exacerbating hypercapnia.

REFERENCES

1. Pearn JH. The gene frequency of acute Werdnig-Hoffmann disease (SMA type 1). A total population survey in North-East England. *J Med Genet*. 1973;10(3):260–265.
2. Brzustowicz LM, Lehner T, Castilla LH, et al. Genetic mapping of chronic childhood-onset spinal muscular atrophy to chromosome 5q11.2-13.3. *Nature*. 1990;344(6266):540–541.
3. Wang CH, Finkel RS, Bertini ES, et al. Consensus statement for standard of care in spinal muscular atrophy. *J Child Neurol*. 2007;22(8):1027–1049.
4. Ragette R, Mellies U, Schwake C, Voit T, Teschler H. Patterns and predictors of sleep disordered breathing in primary myopathies. *Thorax*. 2002;57(8):724–728.
5. Ward S, Chatwin M, Heather S, Simonds AK. Randomised controlled trial of non-invasive ventilation (NIV) for nocturnal hypoventilation in neuromuscular and chest wall disease patients with daytime normocapnia. *Thorax*. 2005;60(12):1019–1024.
6. Mellies U, Ragette R, Dohna Schwake C, Boehm H, Voit T, Teschler H. Long-term noninvasive ventilation in children and adolescents with neuromuscular disorders. *Eur Respir J*. 2003;22(4):631–636.
7. Piper AJ, Sullivan CE. Effects of long-term nocturnal nasal ventilation on spontaneous breathing during sleep in neuromuscular and chest wall disorders. *Eur Respir J*. 1996;9(7):1515–1522.
8. Mellies U, Dohna-Schwake C, Stehling F, Voit T. Sleep disordered breathing in spinal muscular atrophy. *Neuromuscul Disord*. 2004;14(12):797–803.
9. American Academy of Sleep Medicine. *International Classification of Sleep Disorders*. 3rd ed. Darien, IL: American Academy of Sleep Medicine; 2014.

A 7-year-old boy with snoring, restless sleep, and obstructive sleep apnea

Suzanne E. Beck

CASE PRESENTATION

A 7-year-old boy was referred for evaluation and treatment of recently diagnosed obstructive sleep apnea. His pediatrician ordered a polysomnogram (PSG) because of loud snoring and restless sleep. The snoring had occurred every night for the past few years, was associated with occasional gasping, and seemed to be getting worse. He had labored breathing during sleep. He slept for 11 hours per night without nighttime awakenings and did not seem sleepy during the day. He did well in school and got along with friends. He had occasional rhinitis in the spring and fall but did not take any medications. He did not have a cough or asthma. He was born full term and had no other medical problems. Family history was unremarkable. His parents requested an expert opinion on treatment of obstructive sleep apnea and wished to avoid surgery.

PHYSICAL EXAM

Physical exam revealed a healthy-appearing Caucasian boy with normal vital signs. His weight, height, and body mass index were at the 50th percentiles for age. He had non-dysmorphic features, a normal jaw, and a slight adenoid facies. Nares were patent without polyps. Nasal mucosa showed mild edema with mild erythema and clear rhinitis. Examination of the oropharynx revealed symmetric tonsils that protruded beyond the anterior pillars (3+), a slightly crowded oropharynx (Mallampati III) with a normal palate, and normal dentition. Chest wall was normal. Lungs were clear to auscultation. Cardiac exam was normal. Skin was normal. There was no cyanosis, clubbing, or edema. Muscle strength was normal for age, as was development.

LABORATORY AND SLEEP FINDINGS

PSG revealed a total sleep time (TST) of 566 minutes; sleep efficiency 93%; REM 20% of TST; arousal index 11.2/h; obstructive apnea–hypopnea index (AHI) 9.3/h; peak end-tidal CO_2 51 mm Hg; and SpO_2 nadir 87%. In Figure 42-1 a 120-second epoch of sleep is shown. There is an obstructive hypopnea (*A*) with a >3% arterial oxygen desaturation, as well an obstructive apnea (*B*), as shown in Figure 42-2.

QUESTIONS

1. What is the recommended treatment for uncomplicated pediatric obstructive sleep apnea syndrome (OSAS)?
2. What advice would you give this family regarding OSAS treatment for this patient?

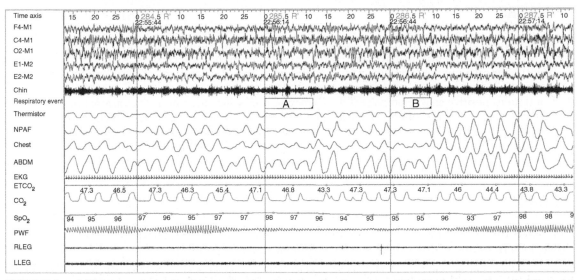

FIGURE 42-1 ■ A 120-second epoch of sleep showing 1 obstructive hypopnea (**A**) with desaturation of >3% and 1 obstructive apnea (**B**).

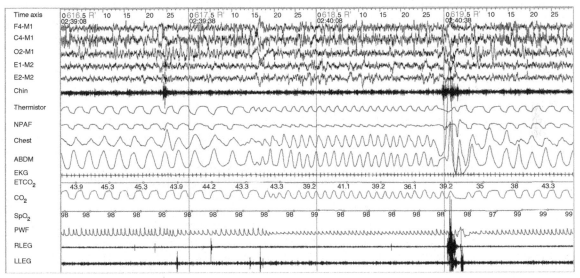

FIGURE 42-2 ■ A 120-second epoch of sleep showing a long obstructive hypopnea followed by an arousal. Note the shift from in-phase breathing to thoraco-abdominal asynchrony on the chest and abdominal leads during the hypopnea.

ANSWERS

1. Adenotonsillectomy is considered the first line of treatment for uncomplicated OSAS in pediatric patients with adenotonsillar hypertrophy, according to the American Academy of Pediatrics (AAP) Clinical Practice Guidelines on the Diagnosis and Management of Childhood Obstructive Sleep Apnea Syndrome.[1]
2. Continuous positive airway pressure (CPAP) may be used when adenotonsillectomy is not indicated or performed. In mild cases of OSAS, intranasal corticosteroids can be considered. Weight loss is recommended if a child is overweight, but other modalities should be used until weight loss is sufficient. In some cases of mild OSAS where adenotonsillectomy or CPAP is not preferred, recent research indicates that a period of watchful waiting with supportive care may be a reasonable approach.[2]

DISCUSSION

Childhood OSAS may be associated with neurocognitive impairment, behavioral problems, failure to thrive, hypertension, cardiac dysfunction, and systemic inflammation. Even though early treatment and diagnosis of pediatric OSAS is recommended,[3] there are no universally accepted guidelines as to when to treat OSAS in children. The American Academy of Sleep Medicine (AASM) considers an obstructive AHI >1/h to be statistically abnormal.[4] However, there are no clear-cut data as to the level of AHI that merits clinical treatment. The decision to treat is individualized and is not predicated solely by the AHI but also by clinical features and additional PSG abnormalities, and risks and benefits must be weighed.

Adenotonsillectomy is the first line of treatment for an otherwise healthy child diagnosed with uncomplicated OSAS and adenotonsillar hypertrophy.[1] Most children with uncomplicated OSAS show a marked improvement in the number and severity of obstructive events on PSG following adenotonsillectomy, even if they are obese.[2,3] For a discussion of resolution rates and postoperative complications after adenotonsillectomy, see Clinical Pearls in Case 43: 2-year-old girl with snoring, restless sleep, and severe obstructive sleep apnea.

Nasal CPAP is effective in treating OSAS in children, but adherence can be a limiting factor to effective use.[3] A multicenter trial of PAP demonstrated significant improvement in sleepiness, snoring, AHI, and oxyhemoglobin saturation while using PAP.[5] However, a third of the participants dropped out of the study.[5] Another study showed that bi-level positive airway pressure (BPAP) or CPAP was effective but both were associated with limited adherence.[6] Further, CPAP needs to be used long term (possibly lifelong), whereas adenotonsillectomy is a one-time only procedure. Therefore, CPAP is not recommended as a first-line option for treating children with OSAS and adenotonsillar hypertrophy.[1,3] CPAP may be considered for patients or families who prefer alternative treatments to surgery or who are at very high risk for surgery. CPAP is also used in children with significant residual OSAS after surgery and in children with conditions other than adenotonsillar hypertrophy leading to OSAS, such as children with craniofacial anomalies or neuromuscular disease. When CPAP is prescribed, it should be managed by a clinician with expertise in caring for children using CPAP.[1] CPAP pressures should be objectively evaluated in the sleep lab and periodically titrated because pressure needs may change over time in a growing child.[3] In addition, objective assessments of use (i.e., equipment downloads) should be performed, as adherence is often overestimated and children may not be able to communicate changes in treatment effects. The family should be taught how to use the equipment and be provided with behavioral modification to support proper use and adherence.[7] Note that CPAP is not approved by the US Food and Drug Administration for children younger than 7 years of age, or weighing <40 lb, but is often used off label.

The AAP guidelines indicate that intranasal corticosteroids may be considered for children with mild OSAS in whom adenotonsillectomy is contraindicated or who have residual mild OSAS following surgery.[1] This recommendation is based on several small studies that show topical steroids may ameliorate mild OSAS steroids but should not be used as the primary treatment for moderate or severe OSAS.[1,3] Because long-term side effects of these medications in children and their effects on OSAS are not known, follow-up and further research are essential.

Orthodontic intervention, such as rapid maxillary expansion, is another approach in selected children with high-arched palates and irregular dentition (cross bite) (see Clinical Pearls in Case 50: A 5-year-old boy with obstructive sleep apnea not tolerating continuous positive airway pressure). However, it has not been studied thoroughly. One small study in 31 children with OSAS showed a reduction in AHI from 12 to 1/h 4 months after rapid maxillary expansion.[8]

Environmental factors such as allergens, tobacco smoke, and other pollutants should be controlled when possible, but this should not delay definitive treatment.

Recently, a large, multicenter, randomized controlled trial of early adenotonsillectomy versus watchful waiting with supportive care for childhood OSAS without prolonged oxyhemoglobin desaturation (called the "Childhood Adenotonsillectomy" or "CHAT" trial) was undertaken to determine whether adenotonsillectomy would, in fact, result in improved outcomes.[2] This study showed that early surgery resulted in improved behavior and quality of life. At 6 months, the PSG normalized in 79% of patients in the surgical group compared to 46% of those in the watchful waiting group.[2] Although this study failed to show an association between OSAS and cognitive outcomes, children assigned to adenotonsillectomy showed greater improvements in behavior, daytime sleepiness, and sleep symptoms and larger improvements on the Connor's Rating Scale measuring restlessness, impulsivity, and emotional liability compared with the watchful-waiting group,[2] supporting the AAP clinical practice guidelines that adenotonsillectomy is beneficial and is the recommended first-line treatment for uncomplicated pediatric OSAS. Note that this study was limited to 5- to 9-year-olds without prolonged desaturation, and study findings may not apply to younger or more severely affected patients.

The CHAT study also found normalization of PSG findings in nearly half of the children (46%) assigned to the watchful-waiting group. The reasons for spontaneous resolution are unclear but may include growth of the airway or regression of lymphoid tissue over the 6 months.[2] Therefore, watchful waiting with supportive care and close follow-up has become an acceptable approach in appropriate patients (otherwise healthy school-aged children without prolonged desaturation and without major symptoms or sequelae of OSAS).

Our patient had adenotonsillar hypertrophy and OSAS in the moderate range with an obstructive AHI of 9.3/h; a normal arousal index; normocapnia during sleep; and mild, episodic desaturation. Most pediatric sleep physicians would agree that this needs further treatment. The child was referred to otolaryngology to discuss the surgical risks of adenotonsillectomy. The parents were reluctant to have surgery despite being reassured that complications were typically minimal and that adenotonsillectomy was successful in the majority of cases. Sequelae of untreated OSAS in children and alternative treatments were discussed further, including CPAP and medical management. Their rationale to forgo surgery and treatment with CPAP was that they did not perceive behavioral or learning problems in their child, and they preferred a period of watchful waiting with medical treatment. Given the results of the CHAT study showing normalization of AHI in nearly half of the subjects over a 6-month period and that our patient had no significant underlying medical or behavioral problems and his PSG did not show severe OSAS or gas-exchange abnormalities, the sleep physician agreed to conservative therapy. Intranasal corticosteroids were prescribed. At the 6-month follow-up, our patient continued to have nightly snoring but had good grades and behavior. His exam showed slightly smaller tonsils and resolved rhinitis. A follow-up PSG showed improvement in the obstructive AHI to 1.8/h. The patient was scheduled for follow-up in 6 months and instructed to return sooner if snoring worsened or daytime symptoms developed.

CLINICAL PEARLS

1. Adenotonsillectomy is the recommended first line of treatment for uncomplicated OSAS in children.
2. CPAP is used for the treatment of OSAS in children when OSAS persists after surgery, there is no adenotonsillar hypertrophy, or adenotonsillectomy is contraindicated. The clinician should be aware that optimal adherence may require family education and behavioral modification and that the growing pediatric patient's CPAP needs may change, requiring frequent CPAP titration studies.
3. Nasal steroids may be considered for treatment of OSAS in mild cases.
4. Weight loss is recommended if a child is overweight, but other treatment should be instituted until weight loss is sufficient.
5. Orthodontic procedures may be considered in selected patients with specific orthodontic abnormalities.
6. A period of watchful waiting and medical management with close follow-up is a reasonable approach for school-aged children with uncomplicated mild-to-moderate OSAS.
7. Treatment for OSAS should not be based on AHI alone but should be determined in the context of all variables measured on a sleep study, as well as the child's daytime functional impairment.

REFERENCES

1. Marcus CL, Brooks LJ, Draper KA, et al. Diagnosis and management of childhood obstructive sleep apnea syndrome. *Pediatrics*. Sep 2012;130(3):576–584.
2. Marcus CL, Moore RH, Rosen CL, et al. A randomized trial of adenotonsillectomy for childhood sleep apnea. *N Engl J Med*. Jun 20 2013;368(25):2366–2376.
3. Marcus CL, Brooks LJ, Draper KA, et al. Diagnosis and management of childhood obstructive sleep apnea syndrome. *Pediatrics*. Sep 2012;130(3):e714–e755.
4. American Academy of Sleep Medicine *International Classification of Sleep Disorders*. Darien, IL: American Academy of Sleep Medicine; 2014.
5. Marcus CL, Rosen G, Ward SL, et al. Adherence to and effectiveness of positive airway pressure therapy in children with obstructive sleep apnea. *Pediatrics*. Mar 2006;117(3):e442–e451.
6. Marcus CL, Beck SE, Traylor J, et al. Randomized, double-blind clinical trial of two different modes of positive airway pressure therapy on adherence and efficacy in children. *J Clin Sleep Med*. Feb 15 2012;8(1):37–42.
7. King MS, Xanthopoulos MS, Marcus CL. Improving positive airway pressure adherence in children. *Sleep Med Clin*. Jun 1 2014;9(2):219–234.
8. Pirelli P, Saponara M, Guilleminault C. Rapid maxillary expansion in children with obstructive sleep apnea syndrome. *Sleep*. Jun 15 2004;27(4):761–766.

A 2½-year-old girl with snoring, restless sleep, and severe obstructive sleep apnea

Suzanne E. Beck

CASE PRESENTATION

A 2½-year-old girl was referred for evaluation of suspected obstructive sleep apnea syndrome (OSAS). She had loud snoring and labored breathing during sleep over the past year. Snoring occurred on most nights and was worse when she had a cold. She had frequent upper respiratory infections and recurrent ear infections but had not had a recent infection. She had some behavioral problems at day care in the form of temper tantrums but had not been diagnosed with a behavioral disorder. She had mild speech delay but was otherwise typically developing. She was difficult to settle at bedtime but slept through the night for 12 hours and took two short naps per day. She tended to fall asleep during car rides. She was born after a 35-week gestation and had no known medical problems. She did not take any medications. Family history was negative.

PHYSICAL EXAM

Physical exam revealed an interactive, healthy-appearing female child with normal vital signs. Her weight was 10.6 kg (<5th percentiles for age), height 87.5 cm (20th percentile for age), and body mass index 14.1 kg/m^2 (3rd percentile for age). She had nondysmorphic features, 4+ cryptic tonsils that protruded beyond the anterior pillar on the right and to the midline on the left occupying >75% of the oropharyngeal width (Fig. 43-1), a normal palate, and normal dentition. She breathed with her mouth

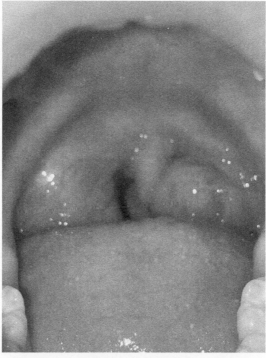

FIGURE 43-1 ■ Enlarged tonsils extending beyond the anterior tonsillar pillars on the patient's right and to the midline on the left, occupying >75% of the pharyngeal width (4+).

open. Nares were patent with mild edema and clear rhinorrhea. The chest wall was symmetric. Lungs were clear to auscultation. Cardiac exam was normal. There was no cyanosis, clubbing, or edema. Muscle tone and strength were normal for age.

LABORATORY AND SLEEP FINDINGS

Polysomnography (PSG) (Figs. 43-2 and 43-3): total sleep time (TST) was 426.5 minutes; sleep efficiency 80%; N1 5.5% of TST; N2 18.4%; N3 41.7%; rapid eye movement (REM) 34%; arousal index 16.3/h; obstructive apnea–hypopnea index (AHI) 30.1/h; peak end-tidal CO_2 66 mm Hg, with CO_2 >50 mm Hg for 35% of TST; SpO_2 nadir 67%, with SpO_2 <90% for 10.9% of TST.

QUESTIONS

1. What is the recommended treatment for OSAS in this patient?
2. What are the predictors of perioperative complications related to adenotonsillectomy in children?

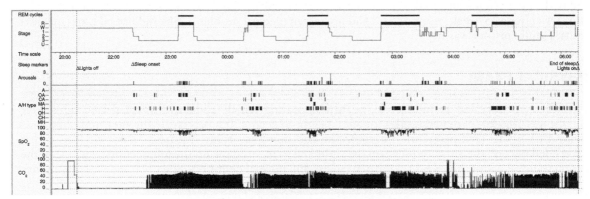

FIGURE 43-2 ■ Hypnogram from overnight PSG showing REM-related severe OSAS with hypoxemia and hypercapnia.

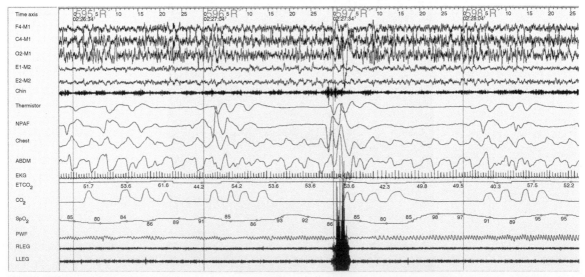

FIGURE 43-3 ■ Representative 120-second epoch of REM sleep showing repetitive obstructive apneas and obstructive hypopneas with oxyhemoglobin desaturation with poor recovery and hypercapnia.

ANSWERS

1. Adenotonsillectomy is the first line of treatment for uncomplicated OSAS in otherwise healthy pediatric patients with adenotonsillar hypertrophy.[1]
2. Predictors of perioperative complications include age <3 years, severe OSAS or gas exchange abnormalities on PSG, cardiac complications of OSAS, failure to thrive, obesity, craniofacial anomalies, neuromuscular disorders, and current respiratory infection.[1]

DISCUSSION

Adenotonsillar hypertrophy is the most common cause of OSAS in children.[1] Other risk factors include obesity, craniofacial anomalies, and neuromuscular disorders. When an otherwise healthy child is diagnosed with uncomplicated OSAS and has adenotonsillar hypertrophy, the clinician should recommend adenotonsillectomy as the first line of treatment, according to the American Academy of Pediatrics Clinical Practice Guidelines on the Diagnosis and Management of Childhood Obstructive Sleep Apnea Syndrome.[1]

Most patients with uncomplicated OSAS show a marked improvement in the number and severity of obstructive events on PSG following adenotonsillectomy.[1,2,3] In uncomplicated cases, the operation may result in complete elimination of OSAS symptoms in 70% to 90% of patients; however, full resolution of OSAS symptoms may not occur for 6 to 8 weeks owing to postoperative swelling. Previous literature has suggested widely varying rates of persistent postoperative OSAS, but a randomized controlled trial of 460 children showed resolution of OSAS (to an AHI <2/h) in 79% of otherwise healthy 5- to 9-year-olds, including some with moderate obesity.[2] Risk factors for residual OSAS following adenotonsillectomy include obesity, a higher degree of severity on baseline PSG, African American race, young children with complicated medical or craniofacial anomalies, and children >7 years of age.[3] Clinical follow-up is important after treatment, and postoperative PSG should be considered, depending on the child's symptoms, severity of OSAS, and underlying risk factors.

Adenotonsillectomy is usually well tolerated in most children, with only minor complications such as pain and decreased oral intake related to postoperative nausea or vomiting. More significant complications include hemorrhage (~3% of patients), velopharyngeal incompetence, nasopharyngeal stenosis, respiratory decompensation, anesthetic complications, and death.[1] Perioperative complications were found to be very low in school-aged children with uncomplicated OSAS without severe oxyhemoglobin desaturation.[2] Polysomnographic parameters, in particular oxyhemoglobin saturation nadir <80% and peak end-tidal CO_2 >60 mm Hg, young age (<3 years), the presence of failure to thrive, and black race are associated with increased postoperative respiratory complications.[4] Because of the increased risk, the American Academy of Pediatrics recommends that children <3 years of age, those with severe OSAS, and those with underlying high risk medical conditions should be monitored as inpatients following surgery.[1] High-risk patients should undergo surgery in a center capable of treating complex pediatric patients.[1] Having a concurrent respiratory infection at the time of surgery is a risk factor for perioperative respiratory decompensation, and surgery is usually rescheduled unless the OSAS is very severe.

Our patient had failure to thrive (height and weight <5th percentile). Poor growth is a sequela of obstructive sleep apnea, and in the past, it was a common presenting sign.[5] The mechanism is not clear, but it is thought to be due to increased energy expenditure related to increased work of breathing during sleep[6] or effects of OSAS on growth factors.[7] Failure to thrive is a risk factor for perioperative complications.[1,4]

Our patient had severe OSAS with an obstructive AHI of 30.1/h (normal in a child being <1.5/h) with prolonged oxyhemoglobin desaturation and hypoventilation. Pediatric OSAS is predominately a REM phenomenon, highlighting the importance of monitoring sleep architecture and ensuring adequate REM sleep duration so that OSAS is not underestimated.[8] Regardless of the severity of OSAS, sleep architecture is usually preserved, unlike with adults.[8]

Because of the severe findings and high risk for complications before surgery, our patient was admitted to the hospital for adenotonsillectomy and was monitored as an inpatient after surgery. On her first postoperative night, she required supportive care with supplemental oxygen and frequent suctioning, although she did not need continuous positive airway pressure, but, by the second night, she was stable and was discharged home the next day. Clinical follow-up revealed her snoring had improved immediately and appetite and weight improved in 1 month. Follow-up PSG at 3 months showed improvement in obstructive AHI to 1.8/h, SpO_2 nadir 94%, and peak end-tidal CO_2 52 mm Hg.

CLINICAL PEARLS

1. Adenotonsillectomy is the recommended first-line treatment of uncomplicated OSAS in children, and most children improve following surgery.
2. Risk factors for postoperative complications include age <3 years, severe OSAS or gas exchange abnormalities on PSG, cardiac complications of OSAS, failure to thrive, obesity, craniofacial anomalies, neuromuscular disorders, or current respiratory infection. These children should be admitted postoperatively.
3. Because of the high rate of residual OSAS after treatment, all patients should be clinically reassessed for residual symptoms to determine if further treatment is necessary, and high-risk patients should be objectively assessed with PSG.
4. Obstructive sleep apnea in children is usually a REM phenomenon, and it tends to worsen over the night; sleep architecture is usually preserved regardless of the severity.

REFERENCES

1. Marcus CL, Brooks LJ, Draper KA, et al. Diagnosis and management of childhood obstructive sleep apnea syndrome. *Pediatrics*. Sep 2012;130(3):576–584.
2. Marcus CL, Moore RH, Rosen CL, et al. A randomized trial of adenotonsillectomy for childhood sleep apnea. *N Engl J Med*. Jun 20 2013;368(25):2366–2376.
3. Bhattacharjee R, Kheirandish-Gozal L, Spruyt K, et al. Adenotonsillectomy outcomes in treatment of obstructive sleep apnea in children: a multicenter retrospective study. *Am J Respir Crit Care Med*. Sep 1 2010;182(5):676–683.
4. Thongyam A, Marcus CL, Lockman JL, et al. Predictors of perioperative complications in higher risk children after adenotonsillectomy for obstructive sleep apnea: a prospective study. *Otolaryngol Head Neck Surg*. Dec 2014;151(6):1046–1054.
5. Guilleminault C, Korobkin R, Winkle R. A review of 50 children with obstructive sleep apnea syndrome. *Lung*. 1981;159(5):275–287.
6. Marcus CL, Carroll JL, Koerner CB, Hamer A, Lutz J, Loughlin GM. Determinants of growth in children with the obstructive sleep apnea syndrome. *J Pediatr*. Oct 1994;125(4):556–562.
7. Tatlipinar A, Atalay S, Esen E, Yilmaz G, Koksal S, Gokceer T. The effect of adenotonsillectomy on serum insulin like growth factors and the adenoid/nasopharynx ratio in pediatric patients: a blind, prospective clinical study. *Int J Pediatr Otorhinolaryngol*. Feb 2012;76(2):248–252.
8. Goh DY, Galster P, Marcus CL. Sleep architecture and respiratory disturbances in children with obstructive sleep apnea. *Am J Respir Crit Care Med*. Aug 2000;162(2 Pt 1):682–686.

A school-aged boy with snoring and attention-deficit hyperactivity disorder

Suzanne E. Beck

CASE PRESENTATION

A 12-year-old boy was seen for evaluation of snoring, hyperactivity, and poor school performance. Snoring had been present since infancy and was worse with upper respiratory infections. He was always a restless sleeper and a "mouth breather." His parents noticed occasional gasping and apnea but never cyanosis. He slept from 9:00 PM to 7:00 AM and was difficult to wake in the morning. He slept 2 hours later on weekends despite the same bedtime but never took naps or fell asleep during the day. He had always been hyperactive and had difficulty completing homework, but this year he was also doing poorly in school. He was evaluated by a developmental specialist and diagnosed with attention-deficit hyperactivity disorder (ADHD). He was otherwise developing typically and growing normally. He had allergic rhinitis, which was treated with nasal steroids as needed. Family history was positive for obstructive sleep apnea syndrome (OSAS) in his father. The parents were concerned that the child's hyperactivity and poor school performance might be related to his snoring and requested an expert opinion before starting medication for ADHD.

PHYSICAL EXAM

Physical exam revealed an alert boy with normal vital signs for age. His weight was at the 25th percentile, and height was at the 50th percentile for age. He had an adenoid facies, a slightly high-arched palate, and normal dentition. His tonsils were visible just at the pillars (2+). Nares were patent, and the nasal mucosa was mildly inflamed. The rest of his exam was normal.

LABORATORY AND SLEEP FINDINGS

Polysomnography (PSG) revealed a total sleep time (TST) of 450 minutes; sleep efficiency 88%; normal sleep architecture with 94 minutes REM sleep (21% of TST); arousal index 17.2/h; obstructive apnea–hypopnea index (AHI) 4.4/h; SpO_2 nadir 89%; periodic limb movement index 4.3/h.

QUESTION

Based on the history and the PSG results, what advice would you give this family?

ANSWER

Figure 44-1 shows a 9.5-second obstructive hypopnea followed by an arousal. This event meets pediatric scoring criteria for an obstructive hypopnea and is representative of the obstructive events this child had during sleep. The results of the PSG are consistent with mild obstructive sleep apnea. The child's symptoms of hyperactivity and poor school performance may be a manifestation of obstructive sleep apnea syndrome (OSAS). The child may benefit from treatment for OSAS, such as adenotonsillectomy.

DISCUSSION

Habitual snoring may be abnormal in otherwise healthy children. Snoring can be a sign of a respiratory infection or allergies; other times it may be a symptom of OSAS. *OSAS*, defined as a "disorder of breathing during sleep characterized by prolonged partial upper airway obstruction and/or intermittent complete obstruction (obstructive apnea) that disrupts normal ventilation during sleep and normal sleep patterns,"[1] may be associated with impairments in growth, neurocognitive, neurobehavioral, and cardiovascular abnormalities if left untreated. In 2002, the American Academy of Pediatrics recommended that all children be screened for snoring and that an affirmative answer be followed by a detailed history and examination to determine whether further evaluation for OSAS is needed.[2]

Habitual snoring in children may be associated with poor school performance or behavioral problems. Studies have shown that young children who habitually snore are at greater risk for poor academic performance in later years, well after snoring has resolved.[3] In a large, population-based longitudinal study of more than 11,000 children from infancy through 7 years, it was found that symptoms of sleep-disordered breathing early in life (snoring, witnessed apnea, and mouth breathing) had strong, persistent effects on subsequent behavior in childhood, in particular hyperactivity.[4] Children in the symptomatic groups were 20% to 60% more likely to exhibit behavioral difficulties such as hyperactivity at 4 years of age and 40% to 100% more likely by 7 years of age.[4] These findings, from the largest pediatric cohort study of sleep-disordered breathing and neurobehavioral morbidity to date, provide epidemiologic evidence that the effects of sleep-disordered breathing in early childhood may be linked to behavioral problems in later childhood.[4] However, this study did not make the distinction between symptoms of OSAS and actual PSG-confirmed OSAS.

The association between OSAS and ADHD is evolving. OSAS may contribute to ADHD symptomatology in some patients with ADHD.[5,6] A cross-sectional, community-based survey of 5- to 7-year-old children found that the prevalence of snoring and OSAS in children with severe ADHD (per the Conner's Parent Rating Scale) was not more common than in the general population (5%);

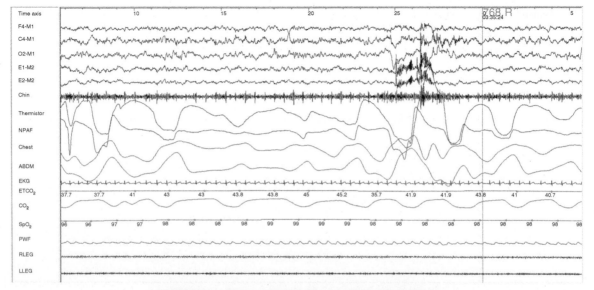

FIGURE 44-1 ■ **Representative 30-second epoch of sleep.**

however, the prevalence of OSAS was 5 times more common in children with mild ADHD compared with the general population (26%).[7] These authors suggested that mild ADHD-like behaviors may be manifestations of sleep-disordered breathing and can be potentially misperceived, misdiagnosed, and mistreated.[7]

Treatment of OSAS has been shown to have favorable effects on ADHD symptoms.[5] A prospective, nonrandomized, open trial was performed to determine the best treatment for children with ADHD plus OSAS (adenotonsillectomy vs. ADHD medication [methylphenidate] vs. no treatment). Of 125 children (aged 6 to 12 years) with suspected ADHD referred to a university-based child psychiatry clinic in Taiwan, 66 children (55.2%) had PSG-proven mild OSAS (AHI >1<5) and met the ADHD entry criteria (*Diagnostic and Statistical Manual of Mental Disorders*, 4th edition [DSM-IV] diagnosis of ADHD). At 6-month follow-up, ADHD symptoms had significantly improved in both the methylphenidate and adenotonsillectomy groups as compared with the no-treatment group, emphasizing the nonspecific positive neurocognitive effects of stimulants. However, the adenotonsillectomy group showed significant improvement in inattention (and PSG parameters) compared with the methylphenidate group, and these children no longer met DSM-IV ADHD criteria at the 6-month follow-up.[8] Thus, recognition and surgical treatment of underlying mild OSAS in children with ADHD may prevent unnecessary long-term stimulant usage and potential side effects associated therewith.[8]

More recently, the childhood adenotonsillectomy study found that children with OSAS had improved parent- and teacher-rated behavior and attention following surgical treatment for OSAS, despite normal results on neurocognitive tests,[9] giving insight that poor school performance (because of behavior and attention problems) may be a more sensitive "real-world" marker of neurocognitive impairment in young children.[10] Although more randomized, controlled, interventional trials are needed to better understand the relationship between OSAS and ADHD, OSAS should be considered when evaluating a child with symptoms of ADHD, as the clinical presentations of these two disorders may overlap. Treating OSAS, even mild OSAS, should be considered before a medication trial for ADHD in children.

Our patient had symptoms and signs of OSAS (chronic habitual snoring, mouth breathing, neurobehavioral problems, nasal congestion, adenotonsillar hypertrophy, and adenoid facies). An obstructive AHI of 4.4/h on his PSG confirmed the diagnosis of mild OSAS. He underwent adenotonsillectomy, following which his snoring and restless sleep improved. His hyperactivity and ability to complete homework assignments also improved. It is important for the sleep physician to know that it is usually not standard or routine practice to rule out OSAS (or insufficient sleep and other sleep disorders for that matter) before diagnosing or treating ADHD in children. In fact, the DSM-IV for ADHD does not have exclusion criteria for ruling out sleep disorders.

CLINICAL PEARLS

1. Obstructive events may be <10 seconds duration in children because children have a shorter respiratory cycle compared with adults. The American Academy of Sleep Medicine pediatric scoring guidelines recommend scoring obstructive apneas >2 breaths duration.[11]
2. OSAS may contribute to ADHD symptomatology in some patients with ADHD.
3. Treatment of OSAS (even mild OSAS) often has favorable effects on ADHD symptoms.

REFERENCES

1. Standards and indications for cardiopulmonary sleep studies in children. American Thoracic Society. *Am J Respir Crit Care Med*. Feb 1996;153(2):866–878.
2. Marcus CL, Brooks LJ, Draper KA, et al. Diagnosis and management of childhood obstructive sleep apnea syndrome. *Pediatrics*. Sep 2012;130(3):576–584.
3. O'Brien LM, Gozal D. Behavioural and neurocognitive implications of snoring and obstructive sleep apnoea in children: facts and theory. *Paediatr Respir Rev*. Mar 2002;3(1):3–9.
4. Freeman K, Bonuck K. Snoring, mouth-breathing, and apnea trajectories in a population-based cohort followed from infancy to 81 months: a cluster analysis. *Int J Pediatr Otorhinolaryngol*. Jan 2012;76(1):122–130.
5. Youssef NA, Ege M, Angly SS, Strauss JL, Marx CE. Is obstructive sleep apnea associated with ADHD? *Ann Clin Psychiatry*. Aug 2011;23(3):213–224.
6. Chervin RD, Archbold KH, Dillon JE, et al. Inattention, hyperactivity, and symptoms of sleep-disordered breathing. *Pediatrics*. Mar 2002;109(3):449–456.
7. O'Brien LM, Holbrook CR, Mervis CB, et al. Sleep and neurobehavioral characteristics of 5- to 7-year-old children with parentally reported symptoms of attention-deficit/hyperactivity disorder. *Pediatrics*. Mar 2003;111(3):554–563.
8. Huang YS, Guilleminault C, Li HY, Yang CM, Wu YY, Chen NH. Attention-deficit/hyperactivity disorder with obstructive sleep apnea: a treatment outcome study. *Sleep Med*. Jan 2007;8(1):18–30.

9. Marcus CL, Moore RH, Rosen CL, et al. A randomized trial of adenotonsillectomy for childhood sleep apnea. *N Engl J Med.* Jun 20 2013;368(25):2366–2376.

10. Brockmann PE, Schlaud M, Poets CF, Urschitz MS. Predicting poor school performance in children suspected for sleep-disordered breathing. *Sleep Med.* Sep 2015;16(9):1077–1083.

11. Berry RB, Brooks R, Gamaldo CE, et al. *The AASM Manual for the Scoring of Sleep and Associated Events: Rules, Terminology and Technical Specifications, Version 2.2.* Darien, IL: American Academy of Sleep Medicine; 2015. <www.aasmnet.org>.

A 7-year-old boy with obesity and persistent hypoventilation

Suzanne E. Beck

CASE PRESENTATION

A 7-year-old boy with obesity was evaluated for persistent hypoventilation after an episode of pneumonia. The child developed a low-grade fever and cough for 2 days, without shortness of breath. On the third day of illness, the parents noticed that the child's lips and fingers turned blue while he was taking a bath and attributed this to his being cold. Later that evening the child developed cyanosis of the face and trunk, prompting medical attention. He was initially treated with antibiotics and supplemental oxygen but developed hypercapnic hypoxemic respiratory failure requiring noninvasive ventilation. Following resolution of his pneumonia and hypoxemia, the hypoventilation persisted. He was referred to the inpatient pulmonary service for further evaluation.

Past medical history revealed that he was born full term with no medical problems or illnesses with the exception of obesity, which developed rapidly over the past year. His parents noted that he was growing along the 50th percentiles before he suddenly gained 45 pounds over the past 12 months. Efforts to curb his weight gain had failed. He had an insatiable appetite and food-seeking behavior. He was doing well in school and was otherwise developing typically; however, recently, he had become fatigued and disinterested in sports. He recently developed secondary enuresis. He slept for 10 hours at night and recently began snoring. Family history was negative for obesity and obstructive sleep apnea syndrome.

PHYSICAL EXAM

Physical exam revealed an obese boy in no obvious distress but with cyanotic lips. Respiratory rate was 16 breaths/min, pulse 110 beats/min, and blood pressure 105/76 mm Hg. SpO_2 on room air was 86%. Weight was 45 kg (greater than 97th percentile for age), height was 130 cm (90th percentile for age), and body mass index was 26.6 kg/m^2 (greater than 95th percentile for age). He had a normal jaw, dentition, and palate. Tonsils were visible behind the pillars (1+). His thyroid was not enlarged. Chest exam revealed no retractions, symmetric thoracic excursion, and crackles in the right lower lobe. Heart sounds were normal. The abdomen was obese without palpable organomegaly. Neurologic exam was normal. His genitalia and pubic hair were Tanner 4 (late puberty). He had acne on his forehead. The rest of his exam was normal.

LABORATORY AND SLEEP FINDINGS

Initial chest radiograph: Infiltrate right lower lobe. Follow-up chest radiograph 4 weeks following acute illness: normal.

Arterial blood gas at acute presentation: pH 7.27, PCO_2 91 mm Hg, PO_2 46 mm Hg, bicarbonate 41 mmol/L.

Venous blood gas after resolution of acute processes: pH 7.34, PCO_2 68 mm Hg, bicarbonate 36 mmol/L.

Venous blood gas after initiation of nighttime bi-level positive pressure noninvasive ventilation: pH 7.39, PCO_2 48 mm Hg, bicarbonate 28 mmol/L.

Na: 150 mmol/L (normal 134 to 144 mmol/L).

Prolactin: 36.5 ng/mL (normal 2 to 11 ng/mL).

Thyroid studies: normal with the exception of a low free thyroxine (T_4) of 0.8 ng/dL (normal 1.0 to 1.8 ng/dL) in combination with thyroid-stimulating hormone (TSH) 1.75 μIU/mL (normal 0.5 to 3.8 μIU/mL) (inappropriately normal TSH).

Testosterone: 34 ng/dL (reference range, 6 months to 9 years, <7 to 20 ng/dL; by Tanner stage I (prepubertal), <7 to 20 ng/dL; II, 8 to 66 ng/dL; III, 26 to 800 ng/dL; IV, 85 to 1200 ng/dL; V (young adult), 300 to 950 ng/dL).

Luteinizing hormone: 0.853 mIU/mL (reference range, prepubertal males 0.3 to 6 mIU/mL; adult males 1.8 to 12.0 mIU/mL).

Insulin-like growth factor-I: 201 ng/mL (normal 42 to 311 ng/mL).

Cardiac evaluation: normal electrocardiogram and echocardiogram.

Magnetic resonance imaging (MRI) head, chest, abdomen: normal.

Ultrasound of diaphragm: normal diaphragmatic excursion.

Genetic testing: negative for Prader-Willi syndrome and paired-like homeobox 2b (*PHOX2B*) mutations.

Polysomnography (PSG) performed 4 weeks following the acute illness revealed a total sleep time (TST) of 485 minutes, sleep efficiency 92%, normal sleep architecture, arousal index 6.2/h, obstructive apnea–hypopnea index 0.8/h, central apnea index 0.8/h, SpO_2 nadir 79% with 45% of TST having SpO_2 <90%, peak end-tidal CO_2 68 mm Hg with 85% of TST having end-tidal CO_2 >50 mm Hg. Respiratory rate was 20 to 22 breaths/min during sleep, there were no paradoxical respiratory efforts, and snoring was not present.

QUESTIONS

1. What are the findings shown in Figure 45-1?
2. What abnormalities are demonstrated on the PSG tracing in Figure 45-2?
3. What is our patient's diagnosis?

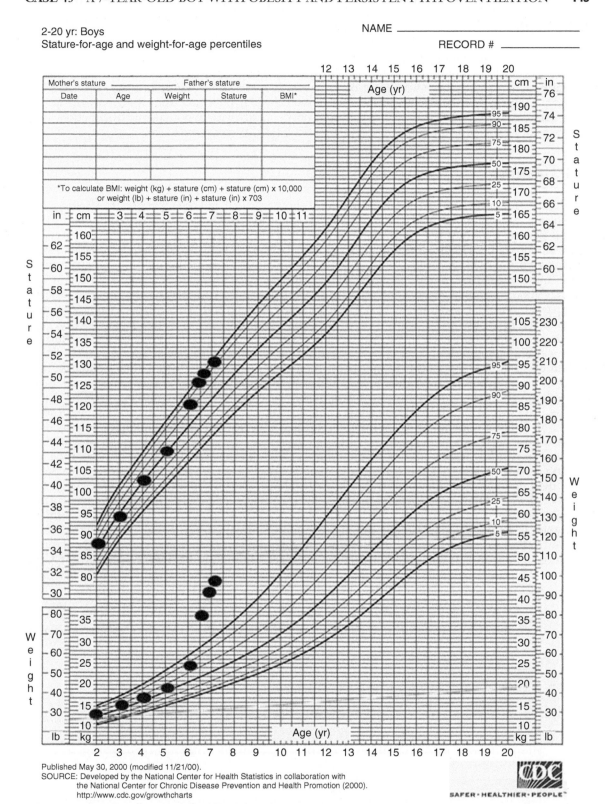

2-20 yr: Boys
Stature-for-age and weight-for-age percentiles

NAME _____

RECORD # _____

Mother's stature _____ Father's stature _____

Date	Age	Weight	Stature	BMI*

*To calculate BMI: weight (kg) + stature (cm) + stature (cm) x 10,000
or weight (lb) + stature (in) + stature (in) x 703

Published May 30, 2000 (modified 11/21/00).
SOURCE: Developed by the National Center for Health Statistics in collaboration with
the National Center for Chronic Disease Prevention and Health Promotion (2000).
http://www.cdc.gov/growthcharts

SAFER · HEALTHIER · PEOPLE

FIGURE 45-1 ■ Growth curve for our patient.

ANSWERS

1. Figure 45-1 shows rapid onset of obesity.
2. Figure 45-2 shows nonobstructive hypoventilation with desaturation.
3. Our patient was diagnosed with rapid-onset obesity, hypothalamic dysfunction, hypoventilation, and autonomic dysregulation, known as late-onset central hypoventilation with hypothalamic dysfunction (LO-CHS/HD) (ICD-3) or rapid-onset obesity with hypothalamic dysfunction, hypoventilation, and autonomic dysregulation (ROHHAD) syndrome.

DISCUSSION

LO-CHS/HD was recognized as a distinct clinical entity in 2000[1] and the term *ROHHAD* was coined in 2007, to distinguish patients with LO-CHS/HD from the genetically distinct clinical entity congenital central hypoventilation syndrome (CCHS).[2] Both syndromes are associated with central hypoventilation. CCHS usually presents in the newborn period with alveolar hypoventilation (in the absence of primary lung, cardiac, or neurologic abnormalities that can account for the hypoventilation)[3] and is caused by mutations in the PHOX2B gene[4] (see Case 36: A 1-week-old infant with severely abnormal blood gases). Children with ROHHAD, on the contrary, have a remarkable period of apparently normal development and growth in their first several years. Hypothalamic obesity is typically the first sign, and it tends to have a sudden onset, typically with insatiable appetite, rapid weight gain, and obesity early in life. Autonomic dysregulation, hypothalamic endocrine dysfunction, and hypoventilation develop later. The hypoventilation is worse during sleep but may persist during wakefulness as well. If hypoventilation is not recognized or adequately treated, then significant morbidity or mortality ensues, as evidenced by the high incidence of cardiorespiratory arrest in this group of children.[2] ROHHAD is not associated with mutations in the PHOX2B *gene*.[2,5]

The diagnosis of ROHHAD is based on clinical criteria, and disorders with overlapping features should be ruled out, including CCHS, Prader-Willi syndrome, and cardiopulmonary, neuromuscular, or central nervous system disorders. Although there is a wide variation in the onset of symptoms, weight gain typically begins after 18 months of age and within the first 10 years of life (median age of 3 years), with later onset of alveolar hypoventilation (median age of 6.2 years).[2,6] Evidence of hypothalamic dysfunction may include obesity, hyperprolactinemia, central hypothyroidism (increased TSH), disordered water balance with hyponatremia or hypernatremia, decreased growth hormone, corticotrophin deficiency, or precocious or delayed puberty.[2,6] Features of autonomic nervous system dysregulation in ROHHAD are variable and may include abnormal pupillary responses to light, altered thermoregulation, gastrointestinal dysmotility, and altered pain perception.[2] Tumors of neural crest origin (ganglioneuromas and ganglioneuroblastomas) are common in ROHHAD, similar to CCHS,

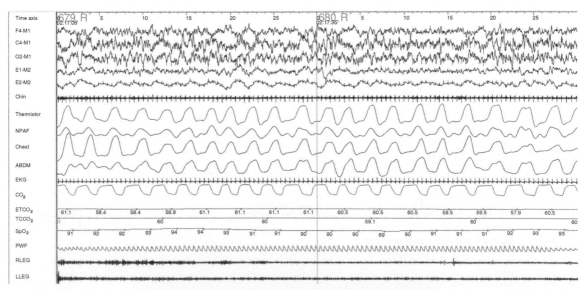

FIGURE 45-2 ■ Representative 60-second epoch of sleep.

occurring in 30% to 40% of cases; thus, appropriate imaging is recommended.[3,5] Severe behavioral abnormalities, autism, and developmental delay occur in some patients, whereas others have normal behavior and cognition. It is important to recognize that ROHHAD is a heterogeneous condition, with patients having various combinations of abnormalities. Thus, one patient may have hypothyroidism and hypernatremia, whereas another may have growth-hormone deficiency and autism. However, the current level of knowledge of this syndrome is that all patients have obesity, hypoventilation severe enough to warrant nocturnal ventilatory support, and at least one endocrine abnormality.

Patients with ROHHAD have blunted ventilatory responses to hypoxia and hypercapnia. The etiology of ROHHAD is not known. Epigenetic, paraneoplastic, and autoimmune etiologies have been considered.[6] Recently, oligoclonal bands were reported in the cerebrospinal fluid in two children with ROHHAD, indicating a possible underlying aberrant immune response,[7] but this is nonspecific evidence.

Our patient was diagnosed with ROHHAD syndrome. He had rapid-onset obesity, as shown in Figure 45-1. He had hypothalamic dysfunction, as evidenced by central hypothyroidism, hyperprolactinemia, precocious puberty, and hypernatremia. He had acute on chronic respiratory failure at presentation. Notably, the patient appeared comfortable despite being hypoxemic, as is typical of patients with central hypoventilation. Following resolution of his pneumonia and treatment of hypothyroidism, his hypoventilation persisted, as evidenced on his follow-up blood gas showing chronic respiratory acidosis with metabolic compensation. Subsequent PSG confirmed nonobstructive hypoventilation and desaturation during sleep in the absence of obstructive sleep apnea, paradoxical respiratory efforts, or snoring (see Fig. 45-2). Obesity hypoventilation syndrome was considered; however, given the rapid onset of weight gain and hypothalamic dysfunction, ROHHAD was diagnosed. Cardiopulmonary and neuromuscular disorders were ruled out clinically or by testing as described previously. Genetic testing was negative for Prader-Willi syndrome and CCHS. He had no neural crest tumors on MRI.

ROHHAD is a complex disorder. There is no cure. Treatment is supportive but must include ventilatory support during sleep and monitoring for additional complications, because failure to do so may have devastating consequences. Symptoms may evolve over time, so vigilant follow-up and evaluation are paramount. Our patient was treated with bi-level positive pressure ventilation during sleep, which resulted in improved gas exchange during sleep and wakefulness. He undergoes frequent pulmonary-sleep, endocrine, and cardiology evaluation, with re-evaluation of his ventilatory support requirements, management of his endocrine abnormalities and sodium-water balance, and imaging for tumors.

CLINICAL PEARLS

1. ROHHAD can be diagnosed in children older than 18 months based on development of rapid weight gain, endocrine abnormalities, and central hypoventilation with additional associated features of hypothalamic dysfunction.
2. Repeated evaluations may be necessary in children as the syndrome evolves. Rapid onset of weight gain occurs first; however, hypoventilation, hypothalamic dysfunction, or tumors may bring the patient to medical attention.
3. Treatment is supportive and includes ventilatory support during sleep.
4. Unrecognized or inadequately treated hypoventilation may have devastating consequences including death.

REFERENCES

1. Katz ES, McGrath S, Marcus CL. Late-onset central hypoventilation with hypothalamic dysfunction: a distinct clinical syndrome. *Pediatr Pulmonol*. Jan 2000;29(1):62–68.
2. Ize-Ludlow D, Gray JA, Sperling MA, et al. Rapid-onset obesity with hypothalamic dysfunction, hypoventilation, and autonomic dysregulation presenting in childhood. *Pediatrics*. Jul 2007;120(1):e179–e188.
3. Weese-Mayer DE, Berry-Kravis EM, Ceccherini I, Keens TG, Loghmanee DA, Trang H. An official ATS clinical policy statement: congenital central hypoventilation syndrome: genetic basis, diagnosis, and management. *Am J Respir Crit Care Med*. Mar 15 2010;181(6):626–644.
4. Weese-Mayer DE, Berry-Kravis EM, Zhou L, et al. Idiopathic congenital central hypoventilation syndrome: analysis of genes pertinent to early autonomic nervous system embryologic development and identification of mutations in PHOX2b. *Am J Med Genet A*. Dec 15 2003;123A(3):267–278.
5. De Pontual L, Trochet D, Caillat-Zucman S, et al. Delineation of late onset hypoventilation associated with hypothalamic dysfunction syndrome. *Pediatr Res*. Dec 2008;64(6):689–694.
6. Patwari PP, Wolfe LF. Rapid-onset obesity with hypothalamic dysfunction, hypoventilation, and autonomic dysregulation: review and update. *Curr Opin Pediatr*. Aug 2014;26(4):487–492.
7. Sartori S, Priante E, Pettenazzo A, et al. Intrathecal synthesis of oligoclonal bands in rapid-onset obesity with hypothalamic dysfunction, hypoventilation, and autonomic dysregulation syndrome: new evidence supporting immunological pathogenesis. *J Child Neurol*. Mar 2014;29(3):421–425.

A 6-month-old with laryngomalacia and stridor in sleep

Suzanne E. Beck

CASE PRESENTATION

A 6-month-old baby was seen for evaluation of stridor, snoring, and difficulty breathing during sleep. He was born full term with no complications. The stridor began in the first few weeks after birth and had become progressively louder. It was worse with agitation but was also present during quiet times and sleep. It was less pronounced when the infant was prone compared with supine. There were occasional episodes of perioral cyanosis. None of the episodes was prolonged or associated with loss of consciousness or change in muscle tone. He was noisy when feeding, but there was no cough or chest congestion. He was being treated empirically with lansoprazole for gastroesophageal reflux with minimal improvement. Weight had dropped from the 40th percentile to the 5th percentile. Development was normal.

PHYSICAL EXAM

Physical exam revealed a thin infant who was alert and not dysmorphic. Respiratory rate was 30 breaths/min, and heart rate 120 beats/min. Weight was at the 5th percentile, and length was at the 25th percentile. He had audible high-pitched stridor. His voice was normal. He had nondysmorphic features and a normal jaw. Nares were patent. The oropharynx was of a normal diameter, with tonsils visible behind the tonsillar pillars (1+). The chest wall was symmetrical but with suprasternal and subcostal retractions. Lungs were clear to auscultation. Cardiac exam was normal. Muscle tone was normal.

A chest radiograph and barium swallow were normal, and a videofluoroscopic swallow study did not show aspiration.

Airway endoscopy findings are shown in Figures 46-1 and 2.

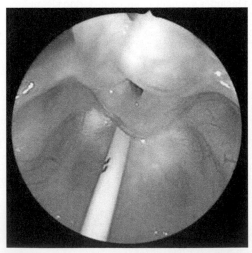

FIGURE 46-1 ■ **Direct microlaryngoscopy of the patient's larynx during inspiration.** (Courtesy of Steven Sobol, MD [from the Department of Otolaryngology, Children's Hospital of Philadelphia].)

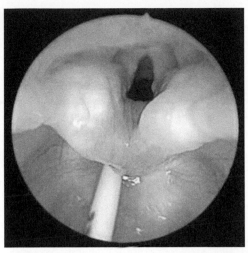

FIGURE 46-2 ■ **Direct microlaryngoscopy of the same child during expiration is shown for comparison.** (Courtesy of Steven Sobol, MD [from the Department of Otolaryngology, Children's Hospital of Philadelphia].)

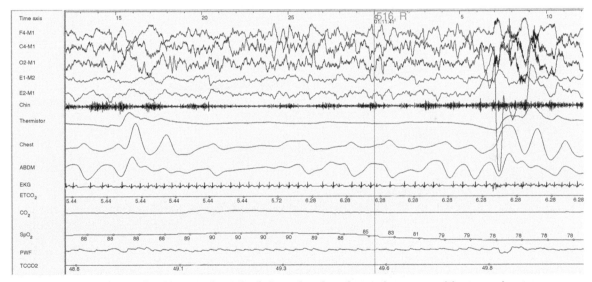

FIGURE 46-3 ■ **Representative 30-second epoch of sleep showing obstructive apnea with severe desaturation.** Note: nasal pressure airflow (NPAF) is not shown because of artifact.

LABORATORY AND SLEEP FINDINGS

Polysomnography (PSG) revealed total sleep time (TST) of 509 minutes; sleep efficiency 93%; REM sleep: 35% of TST; obstructive apnea–hypopnea index 114/h; central apnea index 0.1/h; SpO_2 nadir 78% with SpO_2 <90% for 3.5% TST; peak end-tidal CO_2 58 mm Hg; time with end-tidal CO_2 >50 mm Hg 1% TST (Figs. 46-3 and 46-4).

QUESTIONS

1. What abnormality is shown in Figure 46-1?
2. What type of event is shown in Figure 46-4? Does it meet the scoring criteria?

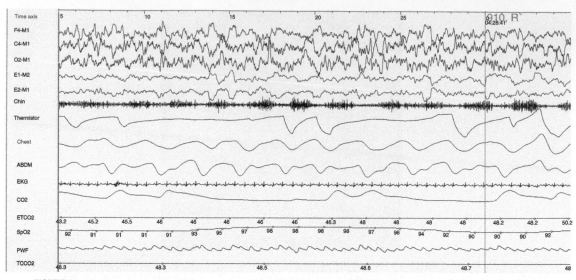

FIGURE 46-4 ■ **Representative 30-second epoch of sleep.** Note: NPAF is not shown because of artifact.

ANSWERS

1. Figure 46-1 shows collapse of the epiglottis and arytenoid cartilages during inspiration, consistent with laryngomalacia (compare with the patent (non-collapsed) airway during exhalation. Fig. 46-2).
2. Figure 46-4 shows two short obstructive apneas. In children, obstructive apneas and hypopneas are scored if they are at least two breaths in duration; hypopneas also require an arousal or a 3% desaturation.[1] In children, shorter obstructive events are of significance because children have a shorter respiratory cycle.

DISCUSSION

Laryngomalacia refers to collapse of the supraglottic airway structures during inspiration, as shown in Figure 46-1. Laryngomalacia is the most common congenital anomaly of the larynx and is the most common cause of stridor in infants.[2] Stridor results from rapid, turbulent air flow through a narrowed airway during inspiration. It is often worse during crying, feeding, agitation, and upper respiratory tract infections and is better during sleep. Stridor may be worse in the supine position and improve when prone.[3] Symptoms usually begin within the first few weeks after birth, peak between 4 and 8 months of age, and often resolve by 12 to 24 months of age, although subclinical findings may persist. In a series of 88 children with confirmed laryngomalacia, most patients presented with stridor alone, but atypical presentations of snoring or obstructive sleep apnea syndrome (OSAS) occurred in 25%, and swallowing dysfunction occurred in 11%.[4] Laryngomalacia has also been recognized as a cause of OSAS in older children and may occur alone or in concert with additional dynamic or fixed lesions to cause OSAS.[5] Acquired laryngomalacia has been reported in a few cases following adenotonsillectomy.[6]

Proposed mechanisms of laryngomalacia include delayed maturation or hypotonia of the supporting cartilaginous structures of the larynx, redundant soft tissue in the supraglottis, a foreshortened or tight aryepiglottic fold, underlying neuromuscular disorders, and supraglottic edema (possibly related to gastroesophageal reflux).[3,7,8] In the majority of cases, the natural history of laryngomalacia is benign, and patients recover spontaneously. However, in about 10% to 15% of patients, like our patient, laryngomalacia results in severe upper airway obstruction with cyanosis, increased work of breathing, feeding difficulties, and failure to thrive, and it requires surgical intervention.[9] Children with underlying neurologic disorders such as cerebral palsy may present with a clinical picture similar to laryngomalacia, but because of pharyngeal neuromotor hypotonia and collapse rather than cartilaginous abnormalities.[10] This type of dynamic collapse is less amenable to surgery. In these patients, endoscopy may be a useful tool to determine the site and type of collapse as a guide for therapy.[11]

PSG should be performed when severe laryngomalacia is suspected. In patients with severe laryngomalacia, surgical management with supraglottoplasty is indicated. Epiglottoplasty (also referred to as supraglottoplasty) is the procedure of choice, and it involves excision of redundant mucosa over the lateral edges of the epiglottis, aryepiglottic folds, arytenoids, and other structures of the supraglottis performed endoscopically.[9] Continuous positive airway pressure can be used in some cases but is difficult to use in very young infants because of limited availability of appropriate interfaces, frequent napping, etc., and will not help with airway obstruction during wakefulness or feeding difficulties. Tracheotomy may be needed in very severe cases.

Our patient with stridor and failure to thrive had severe OSAS because of congenital laryngomalacia. PSG showed severe obstructive apnea in the prone and supine positions manifested as frequent short obstructive events associated with episodic hypoxemia and mild hypercapnia. Airway endoscopy identified collapse of the supraglottic structures during inspiration as the primary cause of obstruction, without pharyngeal collapse or adenotonsillar hypertrophy (see Fig. 46-1). Despite medical management, our patient had persistent symptoms of sleep-disordered breathing and was failing to thrive. PSG was useful to diagnose the severity of the OSAS and guide further intervention. Our patient underwent successful supraglottoplasty at the age of 7 months. At his follow-up visit, stridor had markedly improved, and he had gained weight. PSG 4 months after the procedure showed resolution of his OSAS.

CLINICAL PEARLS

1. Laryngomalacia is the most common cause of stridor in infancy, and it is usually benign.
2. A small subset of infants with laryngomalacia may present with severe upper airway obstruction necessitating surgical intervention.
3. PSG is a useful tool to help guide medical and/or surgical management.
4. Obstructive apneic events in infants and children are often shorter than 10 seconds duration, because of their faster respiratory cycle.

REFERENCES

1. Berry RB, Gamaldo CE, Harding SM, Marcus CL, Vaughn BV. *The AASM Manual for the Scoring of Sleep and Associated Events: Rules, Terminology and Technical Specifications. Version 2.0.* Darien, IL: American Academy of Sleep Medicine; 2012.
2. Jones KL. Dysmorphology approach and classification. In: Jones KL, Jones MC, Del Campo Casanelles M, eds. *Smith's Recognizable Patterns of Human Malformation.* 6th ed. Philadelphia, PA: Elsevier Saunders; 2006:1.
3. Cotton RT, Richardson MA. Congenital laryngeal anomalies. *Otolaryngol Clin North Am.* Feb 1981;14(1):203–218.
4. Cooper T, Benoit M, Erickson B, El-Hakim H. Primary presentations of laryngomalacia. *JAMA Otolaryngol Head Neck Surg.* Jun 2014;140(6):521–526.
5. Revell SM, Clark WD. Late-onset laryngomalacia: a cause of pediatric obstructive sleep apnea. *Int J Pediatr Otorhinolaryngol.* Feb 2011;75(2):231–238.
6. Cunningham MJ, Anonsen CK, Kinane B. Acquired laryngomalacia secondary to obstructive adenotonsillar hypertrophy. *Am J Otolaryngol.* Mar-Apr 1993;14(2):132–136.
7. Richter GT, Thompson DM. The surgical management of laryngomalacia. *Otolaryngol Clin North Am.* Oct 2008;41(5):837–864. vii.
8. Thompson DM. Abnormal sensorimotor integrative function of the larynx in congenital laryngomalacia: a new theory of etiology. *Laryngoscope.* Jun 2007;117(6 Pt 2 Suppl 114):1–33.
9. Zalzal GH, Anon JB, Cotton RT. Epiglottoplasty for the treatment of laryngomalacia. *Ann Otol Rhinol Laryngol.* Jan-Feb 1987;96(1 Pt 1):72–76.
10. Seddon PC, Khan Y. Respiratory problems in children with neurological impairment. *Arch Dis Child.* Jan 2003;88(1):75–78.
11. Truong MT, Woo VG, Koltai PJ. Sleep endoscopy as a diagnostic tool in pediatric obstructive sleep apnea. *Int J Pediatr Otorhinolaryngol.* May 2012;76(5):722–727.

Disturbed sleep in a patient with Duchenne muscular dystrophy*,†

Mary H. Wagner and Richard B. Berry

CASE PRESENTATION

A 17-year-old white male with Duchenne muscular dystrophy (DMD) presented to the pediatric pulmonary clinic for a follow-up evaluation after being hospitalized for pneumonia. During the hospital stay, he was noted to have nocturnal desaturation intermittently during sleep. The patient has been wheelchair bound since age 12 years. His father's two current concerns include the patient's difficulty in both swallowing and breathing during sleep.

PHYSICAL EXAM

The patient is a thin young man sitting in a wheelchair. He has decreased breath sounds at his lung bases and exhibits a weak cough. Auscultation of his heart reveals a regular rate and rhythm with a rapid rate and an S3 gallop. No pedal edema is present.

Pulmonary Function Testing

He is unable to perform testing.

Chest Radiograph

Scoliosis and elevation of both hemidiaphragms with no focal infiltrates or atelectasis are revealed by chest radiograph.

Polysomnography (PSG) was requested because of the history of nocturnal desaturation and difficulty breathing during sleep.

PSG findings:

Total sleep time	380 min
Sleep efficiency	71%
Sleep latency	70 min
Sleep stages as (%TST)	
Stage W	32%
Stage N1 + N2	51%
Stage N3	13%
Stage R	4%
AHI (#/h)	9.6
REM AHI	22.7
Events	30 obstructive apneas and 31 hypopneas

*This entire chapter is taken from Wagner MH, Berry RB. Disturbed sleep in a patient with Duchenne muscular dystrophy. *J Clin Sleep Med*. 2008;4(2):173-175.
†This study was not industry supported. Dr. Berry has received research support from Itamar Medical.

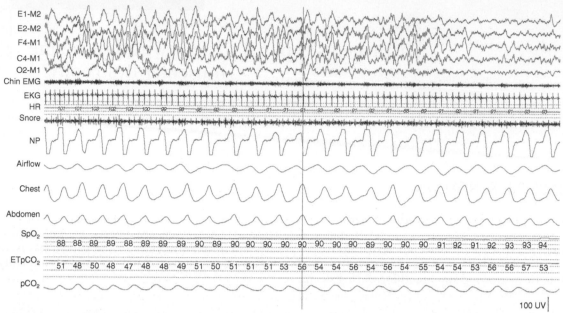

FIGURE 47-1 ■ A tracing from NREM sleep while the patient breathed room air. These epochs show continued respiratory effort with decreased oxygen saturation to 88% to 94% and increased $ETCO_2$ to 47 to 57 torr. The CO_2 tracings do not show a clear plateau; therefore, the end-tidal CO_2 value underestimates the true alveolar-arterial PCO_2. The depicted derivations include left and right electro-oculographic tracings; frontal, central, and occipital electroencephalogram (EEG) tracings; chin electromyogram (EMG) tracing; electrocardiogram (EKG); heart rate derived from the oximeter; snore, nasal pressure, and nasal-oral airflow by a thermal device; chest and abdomen by piezoelectric belts; pulse oximetry; end-tidal CO_2; and a CO_2 tracing.

Min SpO_2	83%
Awake Baseline SpO_2	97%-98%
Awake $ETCO_2$	45-47 torr

A representative 60-second tracing of the patient's sleep is shown in Figure 47-1.

QUESTION

What is the appropriate therapy for this young man's gas exchange abnormalities during sleep?

ANSWER

Nocturnal positive pressure ventilation, not oxygen therapy alone.

DMD is an X-linked trait occurring in 1:3000 male births.[1] The disease results from a mutation of the dystrophin gene and leads to progressive decrease in muscle strength. This results in loss of ambulation and respiratory muscle weakness. Progressive deterioration in respiratory muscle strength results in hypoventilation. Death is due to respiratory failure in greater than 80% of cases.[2] The earliest signs of respiratory insufficiency are seen in sleep, as shown by Suresh et al.[3] They examined 34 patients with DMD, ranging in age from 1 to 15 years. They found that almost two thirds had sleep symptoms. On PSG, one third had hypoventilation and one third had obstructive sleep apnea. Others have reported an increased risk of sleep-related breathing disorders, including hypoventilation, central apnea, and obstructive apnea and hypopnea.[1]

The American Thoracic Society consensus statement on the respiratory care of patients with DMD recommends a regular review of the sleep history with a focus on symptoms of sleep-related breathing disorders at every visit.[1] Patients should have an annual evaluation of their sleep when they become wheelchair bound or sooner as clinically indicated. Most develop problems with scoliosis when they become wheelchair bound.[4] The preferred method for evaluation of sleep in DMD patients is PSG with continuous CO_2 monitoring.[1] Other methods, though less optimal, include oximetry with CO_2 monitoring or capillary blood gas upon arising in the morning. Simple oximetry alone will provide a direct measure of nocturnal arterial oxygen saturation but only indirect information on the adequacy of nocturnal ventilation or the presence of obstructive apnea and hypopnea.

Nocturnal arterial PCO_2 can be estimated by the value of the end-tidal CO_2 obtained by measuring exhaled CO_2. During a sleep study, the exhaled CO_2 is typically measured by the side-stream method with a device that continually samples (suctions) air from a nasal cannula worn by the patient. With each breath, the CO_2 tracing rises and then exhibits a plateau (the end-tidal CO_2 value). The actual arterial PCO_2 exceeds the end-tidal CO_2 (except in rare circumstances). The difference between the arterial and end-tidal CO_2 values depends on the physiology of the patient's lung and the CO_2 monitoring device. Ideally, both the end-tidal value and a CO_2 versus time tracing should be recorded. If the CO_2 versus time tracing does not show a plateau (see Fig. 47-1), the actual end-tidal CO_2 is higher than the measured value. Lack of a plateau can occur with rapid or shallow breaths. One can monitor exhaled CO_2 during nocturnal ventilation either using a connection to the mask or via a small nasal cannula worn under the mask. In either case, the measured value may not reflect the true end-tidal CO_2. In this circumstance, measurement of transcutaneous CO_2 can be useful.

The treatment of choice for obstructive sleep apnea (OSA) and hypoventilation in DMD patients is positive pressure ventilation, which can be delivered using a nasal mask noninvasively (non invasive positive pressure ventilation or NIPPV) or with a mechanical ventilator through a tracheotomy. Benefits of treatment with NIPPV include improved sleep quality, quality of life, and daytime gas exchange, as well as decreased daytime sleepiness and a slower decline in the pulmonary function.[1,3] The level of therapeutic support needs should be determined in the sleep laboratory. Oxygen saturation and carbon dioxide status should be monitored in addition to patient tolerance of the mask and pressure. Pressure levels should be adjusted to maintain oxygen saturation above 94% with attention to carbon dioxide status as well. Carbon dioxide can be monitored using $ETCO_2$; however, this can be difficult to interpret with nasal ventilation if a nasal $ETCO_2$ cannula is used. In this case, transcutaneous carbon dioxide monitoring can be useful. The carbon dioxide level that can be achieved will depend on the starting CO_2 and effectiveness of the positive pressure. Using bi-level pressure with an inspiratory to expiratory pressure difference of greater than 6 cm is often effective. A backup rate can also be helpful to stabilize the ventilatory pattern, provide respiratory muscle rest, and improve ventilation. Blood gas determination during the study will help correlate arterial or venous CO_2 levels with $ETCO_2$ or $TcPCO_2$. Serial evaluation should be performed to evaluate changing needs with disease progression or other changes in clinical status.

Complications of positive pressure have included gastric distention and issues related to the continuous positive airway pressure (CPAP) mask. There is one case report of a pneumothorax in a patient with DMD and subpleral blebs.[5] DMD patients treated with NIPPV may need an oximeter with an alarm at home to monitor their status at night because displacement of the positive pressure mask may result in severe hypoxemia and hypercarbia. Another consideration for treatment of hypoxemia

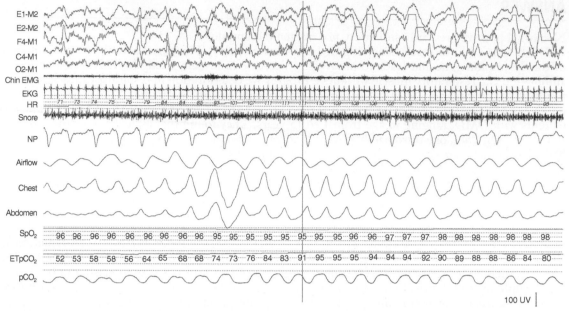

FIGURE 47-2 ■ A tracing from NREM sleep while the patient breathed supplemental oxygen at 0.5 L/min. He has continued respiratory effort during these epochs with no discrete respiratory events. Gas exchange parameters show increased arterial oxygen saturation to 95% to 98% with a concomitant significant rise in the $ETCO_2$ to 83 to 95 torr. The depicted derivations include left and right electro-oculographic tracings; frontal, central, and occipital EEG tracings; chin EMG tracing; EKG; heart rate derived from the oximeter; snore, nasal pressure, and nasal-oral airflow by a thermal device; chest and abdomen by piezoelectric belts; pulse oximetry; end-tidal CO_2; and a CO_2 tracing.

because of hypoventilation is tracheotomy with volume ventilation. Treatment with oxygen alone should be avoided without ventilatory support because these patients may develop worsening of their hypoventilation and hypercarbia.

In the current patient after sleep onset, the SpO_2 fell to 88% to 91% without events, with $ETCO_2$ 47 to 57 torr (see Fig. 47-1). With respiratory events, $ETCO_2$ increased to a high of 69 torr, with oxygen desaturation as low as 83%. He would not tolerate placement of a mask for CPAP, and his father requested a trial of oxygen therapy. On oxygen at 0.5 L/min, his baseline saturation increased to 95% to 98%, but $ETCO_2$ increased as high as 95 torr (Fig. 47-2). His oxygen flow rate was decreased using a pediatric flow meter that can deliver oxygen in increments of 0.1 to 0.2 L/min. At this flow rate, his saturation ranged from 88% to 91% with $ETCO_2$ 50 to 60 torr. Arterial blood gas in the morning on 0.2 L/min showed pH 7.34, $PaCO_2$ 75.6, PaO_2 77, and HCO_3 40.8. The patient underwent a program of mask desensitization at home and eventually had a positive airway pressure titration in the sleep laboratory.

CLINICAL PEARLS

1. Patients with DMD are at risk for sleep-related breathing disorders including OSA and alveolar hypoventilation.
2. Nocturnal oximetry will detect arterial oxygen desaturation (hypoxemia) but will not reflect the degree of hypoventilation. PSG with monitoring of end-tidal CO_2 or transcutaneous CO_2 is more informative.
3. The earliest signs of respiratory failure in DMD patients are generally detectable during sleep.
4. Yearly evaluation for sleep-related breathing disorders should be performed in patients with DMD starting when they are confined to a wheelchair or sooner for clinical symptoms. The test of choice is PSG with CO_2 monitoring.
5. Sleep-related hypoventilation and/or OSA should be treated with ventilatory assistance by NIPPV. Another option is tracheotomy and volume ventilation.
6. Oxygen alone should not be used to treat nocturnal hypoxemia because it is usually due to hypoventilation. Oxygen may worsen nocturnal hypoventilation and lead to significant hypercarbia.

REFERENCES

1. Finder JD, Birnkrant D, Carl J, et al. Respiratory care of the patient with Duchenne muscular dystrophy. ATS consensus statement. *Am J Respir Crit Care Med*. 2004;170:456–465.
2. Nagi T. Prognostic evaluation of congestive heart failure in patients with Duchenne muscular dystrophy–Retrospective study using non-invasive cardiac function tests. *Jpn Circ J*. 1989;53:406–415.
3. Suresh S, Wales P, Dakin C, et al. Sleep-related breathing disorder in Duchenne muscular dystrophy: disease spectrum in the paediatric population. *J Paediatr Child Health*. 2005;41:500–503.
4. Karol LA. Scoliosis in patients with Duchenne muscular dystrophy. *J Bone Joint Surg*. 2007;89:155–162.
5. Choo-Kang LR, Ogunlesi FO, McGrath-Morrow SA, et al. Recurrent pneumothoraces associated with nocturnal noninvasive ventilation in a patient with muscular dystrophy. *Pediatr Pulmonol*. 2002;34:73–78.

A 17-year-old with morning headaches

Mary H. Wagner

CASE PRESENTATION

A 17-year-old boy was referred to the sleep clinic for evaluation of nocturnal hypoxemia noted in an outside emergency department after receiving pain medication for treatment of an orthopedic injury. The patient moved to this area recently and had been followed in his home city by an orthopedist for "a crooked back." He had back surgery several years ago. He sleeps well but occasionally has a headache upon awakening in the morning. He had a chest radiograph, lab work, and pulmonary function tests (PFTs) at his local hospital, which are shown below. Results of his sleep study are also shown in the following. Review of systems was positive for allergic rhinitis and back discomfort from severe scoliosis. Past medical history was remarkable for spinal fusion surgery. Currently prescribed medications include steroid nasal spray and ibuprofen as needed for pain.

PHYSICAL EXAM

The patient was alert and interactive. Weight was at the 50th percentile, and height was less than the 5th percentile; arm length was at the 50th percentile. He was afebrile. Blood pressure was 118/75, pulse 100 beats/min, respiratory rate 24 breaths/min, and SpO_2 94%. Tonsils were 1+ and the Mallampati was grade II. Examination of the chest revealed scoliosis with decreased breath sounds at the right base but no crackles, rhonchi, or wheezes. Heart sounds were normal with a regular rate and rhythm. The abdomen was soft with no organomegaly. There was no digital clubbing.

LABORATORY AND SLEEP FINDINGS

Pulmonary Function Tests

Forced vital capacity (FVC) 0.54 L (16% predicted); forced expiratory volume in 1 second (FEV_1) 0.49 L (16% predicted); FEV_1/FVC ratio 91, forced expiratory flow between 25% and 75% of vital capacity (FEF_{25-75}) 0.97 L (26% predicted) (Fig. 48-1).

Electrolytes: Na 141, K 4.1, Cl 98, CO_2 40, BUN 6, creatinine 0.45.

Polysomnography results: Sleep efficiency was 80%. The apnea–hypopnea index was 1.3/h. Baseline SpO_2 was 94% during wakefulness and 85% during sleep, with a nadir of 75% during REM sleep. Baseline end-tidal CO_2 was 52 torr during wakefulness and 68 torr during sleep, with a peak of 73 torr during REM sleep.

Capillary blood gas drawn just after awakening: pH 7.23, PCO_2 76, PO_2 47, bicarb 32.

Chest radiograph: Clear lung fields, severe cervicothoracic scoliosis with evidence of repair (Fig. 48-2).

QUESTION

Why is he hypoxemic during sleep? How should his nocturnal hypoxemia be treated?

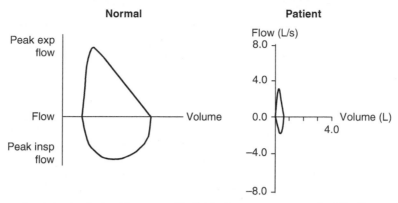

FIGURE 48-1 ■ Flow volume loop of a healthy normal individual person compared with a flow volume loop of our patient. Flow is on the *y*-axis and volume on the *x*-axis. Note the severe decrease in flows and volumes in the patient compared with the healthy subject.

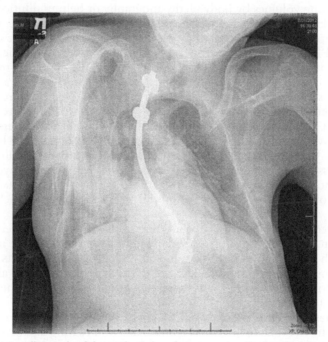

FIGURE 48-2 ■ Chest radiograph of the patient showing severe scoliosis with a surgical rod in place.

ANSWER

The patient has severe restrictive lung disease and hypoventilation because of kyphoscoliosis. One of the causes for hypoxemia is hypoventilation. He should be treated with ventilatory support during sleep.

DISCUSSION

Scoliosis is a common spinal issue in adolescents and children and is characterized by a side-to-side curvature of the spine (Cobb angle) >10 degrees. Adolescent idiopathic scoliosis is more common in girls than in boys, with a prevalence of 0.47% to 5.2%.[1] Adolescent idiopathic scoliosis accounts for 90% of the cases of idiopathic scoliosis in children and usually presents in the 11- to 18-year-old age group.[1] Thoracic curves are the most common.[1] Curves >10% are seen in 2% to 3% of the school population.[2] Upon exam, this young man has severe scoliosis and restrictive lung disease because of his chest wall deformity. His lung function tests show severe decreases in his FEV_1 and FVC, with a normal (relatively high) FEV_1/FVC ratio, which is consistent with a pattern of restrictive ventilatory dysfunction. The FVC is most sensitive to alterations in thoracic cage size and mobility.[2] The total lung capacity (TLC) is reduced in restrictive lung disease; however, the measurement of TLC requires equipment to measure lung volumes by body plethysmography or helium dilution, which may not be available in all settings. However, FVC reductions are proportional to a decrease in TLC if the patient has no obstructive component, and forced vital capacity can be obtained with spirometry, which is more readily available. PFT and overnight oximetry should be considered in patients with moderate to severe scoliosis and before consideration of surgery.[2,3] However, the approach to treatment for most patients is based on the clinical examination, individual patient characteristics, and the measurement of the Cobb angle.[4] This patient's physical examination suggests that extrinsic restrictive dysfunction is present because of the chest wall disorder (kyphoscoliosis). The patient has severe sleep-related hypoventilation. A chest radiograph demonstrated clear lung fields with a 72-degree curvature (Cobb angle). Once patients have a Cobb angle >60 degrees, restrictive lung disease can be detected on PFTs, and nocturnal hypoventilation may be present.[2] Hypoventilation is more likely in those with an upper thoracic curve and/or associated respiratory muscle weakness.[2] The nocturnal hypoxemia is related to hypoventilation, as demonstrated by the elevated CO_2 noted during the sleep study, and confirmed by the capillary blood gas obtained first thing in the morning. His morning headaches are likely related to CO_2 retention.

Most patients with scoliosis have a gradual worsening of the curvature of their back and a gradual decline in lung function. Early in the course of the disease, patients may have normal gas exchange during wakefulness with deterioration of these values during sleep. Sleep results in changes in respiratory mechanics and muscle control, with a decrease in the tone of the upper airway and chest wall muscles. The lung functional residual capacity is decreased in the supine position because of pressure on the diaphragm from the contents of the abdomen.

In patients with moderate to severe scoliosis with a concern for hypoventilation, monitoring should include polysomnography to evaluate nocturnal gas exchange.[5] Treating a patient with long-standing hypercarbia with supplemental oxygen alone is potentially dangerous and should be approached cautiously because such patients may have a blunted response to hypercarbia, and their respiratory drive may be linked to hypoxemia.[6] Consideration should be given to noninvasive nocturnal ventilation to improve oxygenation and normalize levels of CO_2. Approaches can include bi-level noninvasive ventilation, which allows delivery of a minimum expiratory pressure (EPAP) to maintain airway patency and inspiratory pressure (IPAP) adjustment to provide pressure support equal to the difference between the IPAP and EPAP.[7] Additional features include modes (e.g., spontaneous-timed or pressure control) to assure a respiratory rate consistent with adequate ventilation. Another approach is the use of a volume-assured pressure support device, which automatically adjusts the pressure support to deliver a target alveolar ventilation.[7] In patients with chest wall disorders, a high level of pressure support is often needed to deliver an acceptable tidal volume. One may need to use a lower tidal volume and higher respiratory rate to deliver adequate ventilation. This patient was started on nocturnal positive pressure with a volume-assured pressure support device to deliver a specific tidal volume by a nasal mask. On this therapy, his quality of sleep improved, his headaches resolved, and he noted increased energy during the day.

CLINICAL PEARLS

1. Chest wall deformities such as scoliosis or kyphoscoliosis can result in extrinsic restrictive ventilatory dysfunction.
2. Significant restrictive lung disease can result in respiratory insufficiency, which is often worse during sleep, resulting in hypoventilation with hypoxemia and hypercarbia.
3. Measurement of CO_2 is essential for the evaluation of hypoventilation. An elevated CO_2 on routine serum electrolytes (mainly bicarbonate) should raise the suspicion that hypoventilation may be present.
4. Nocturnal hypoventilation should be treated with some form of ventilation because oxygen alone can decrease respiratory drive and worsen hypercarbia.
5. Morning headaches that improve soon upon awakening should raise the suspicion of severe nocturnal hypoxemia or hypercarbia.

REFERENCES

1. Konieczny MR, Senyurt H, Krauspe R. Epidemiology of adolescent idiopathic scoliosis. *J Child Orthop*. 2013 Feb;7(1):3–9.
2. Praud JP, Redding GJ, Farmer M. Chest wall and respiratory muscle disorders. In: Wilmott RW, Boat TF, Bush A, Chernick V, Deterding RR, Ratjen F, eds. *Disorders of the Respiratory Tract in Children*. 8th ed. Philadelphia, PA: Elsevier Saunders; 2012:631–646.
3. Tsiligiannis T, Grivas T. Pulmonary function in children with idiopathic scoliosis. *Scoliosis*. 2012;7(1):7. doi: 1186/1748-7161-7-7.
4. Negrini S, Aulisa AG, Aulisa L, et al. 2011 SOSORT guidelines: orthopaedic and rehabilitation treatment of idiopathic scoliosis during growth. *Scoliosis*. 2012;7(3):1–35. http://dx.doi.org/10.1186/1748-7161-7-3.
5. Aurora RN, Zak RS, Karippot A, et al. Practice parameters for the respiratory indications for polysomnography in children. *Sleep*. Mar 1 2011;34(3):379–388.
6. West JB. Respiratory failure. In: West JB, ed. *Pulmonary Pathophysiology: The Essentials*. 7th ed. Baltimore, MD: Lippincott Williams and Wilkins; 2008:141.
7. Berry RB, Wagner MH. Fundamentals 30. In: Berry RB, Wagner MH, eds. *Sleep Medicine Pearls*. 3rd ed. Philadelphia, PA: Elsevier Saunders; 2014:399–404.

A 6-month-old with chronic lung disease of infancy, intermittent snoring, and failure to thrive

Suzanne E. Beck

CASE PRESENTATION

A 6-month-old ex-preterm infant was evaluated because of intermittent snoring and poor weight gain following a recent respiratory viral illness. One month earlier, he was hospitalized for respiratory syncytial virus bronchiolitis with wheezing. During that admission, he was noted to have intermittent snoring and hypoxemia during sleep that required supplemental oxygen, all of which resolved before discharge. He was sleeping for 10 hours at night, with two 2-hour naps per day. He had a good appetite and was bottle-fed 24 calorie/ounce formula, receiving 140 calories/kg/day without difficulty, but had been gaining weight slowly. Past medical history revealed that he was born after a 26-week gestation, weighing 850 g. He received surfactant at birth and briefly required mechanical ventilation for respiratory distress syndrome, followed by nasal continuous positive airway pressure and subsequently supplemental oxygen via nasal cannula. He was weaned off supplemental oxygen, diuretics, and methylxanthines by age 37 weeks. He had retinopathy of prematurity that resolved, a patent ductus arteriosus that closed with indomethacin treatment, and a normal head ultrasound. Review of systems was negative for coughing, choking and/or congestion with feeds, vomiting, and observed apnea. His only medications were albuterol, fluticasone, and vitamins.

PHYSICAL EXAM

Vital signs: respiratory rate 36 breaths/min; pulse 132 beats/min; blood pressure 86/62 mm Hg; SpO_2 95% at room air; and weight 5.2 kg and length 56.3 cm (both less than 5th percentile corrected for prematurity). The infant was thin and in no apparent distress. His head was mildly dolichocephalic; nares were patent; the palate was mildly high arched; and tonsils were 1+. The chest wall was symmetrical with mild intercostal retractions. Breath sounds were clear with no wheezes or crackles. Heart exam was normal. The abdomen was soft with no visceromegaly. There was no cyanosis, clubbing, or edema. Muscle tone was normal and movements were symmetric.

LABORATORY AND SLEEP FINDINGS

Chest radiograph showed mild parenchymal interstitial changes, with no acute changes compared with previous radiographs. The trachea appeared normal.

Polysomnography (PSG) revealed a total sleep time (TST) of 462 minutes, with sleep efficiency of 87% and 129 min (28% TST) of REM; arousal index 15.2/h; obstructive apnea–hypopnea index (AHI) 1.3/h; central apnea index 4.6/h with a maximum length of central apnea of 10 seconds; periodic breathing 1% TST; SpO_2 <90% for 2% TST and <92% for 30% TST, with a nadir of 81%; peak end-tidal CO_2 39 mm Hg.

QUESTION

What are the next steps in treating this child?

ANSWER

Administer supplemental oxygen during sleep.

DISCUSSION

Our patient has bronchopulmonary dysplasia (BPD) or chronic lung disease of infancy, with hypoxemia during sleep. Chronic lung disease of infancy is a heterogeneous group of respiratory diseases that develop from BPD or any other disorder that produces acute lung injury and/or requires treatment with positive pressure ventilation or high concentrations of oxygen in the newborn period.[1] BPD typically occurs in infants born prematurely and weighing less than 1000 to 1500 g. Its incidence is inversely proportional to birth weight and gestational age. BPD was first described in 1967 by Northway as severe chronic lung disease in preterm infants with severe respiratory distress syndrome who received treatment with 100% O_2 and high inspiratory ventilator pressures.[2] With advances in treatment, such as the use of antenatal steroids, surfactant, and improved ventilatory strategies, the spectrum of BPD has shifted such that it has almost disappeared in larger preterm infants and now typically affects only very-low-birth-weight preterm infants.[2] However, because of improved survival of very-low-birth-weight infants, the incidence of BPD has increased over the years.[3] A new definition of BPD was defined by a National Institutes of Health consensus panel as supplemental oxygen requirement at age 36 weeks or at discharge (whichever came first) in infants born <32 weeks' gestation or oxygen requirement at age >28 days of life or at discharge in infants born ≥32 weeks' gestation.[4]

Infants with chronic lung disease have more difficulty maintaining rate of growth and weight gain compared with healthy infants of the same age. The etiology is multifactorial, including decreased intake as a consequence of swallowing dysfunction, therapeutic fluid restriction, and fatigue; hypoxemia; and/or increased energy requirements because of increased work of breathing or increased metabolic demands.[1]

An important and often under-recognized cause of poor growth in infants with chronic lung disease that may present to the sleep physician is sleep-related hypoxemia. It has been shown that near-term infants with chronic lung disease experience episodes of hypoxemia with sleep despite acceptable awake oxyhemoglobin saturation.[5] Desaturation occurs most often during REM sleep, and time spent with SpO_2 <90% correlates with increased airway resistance.[5] Others have noted that hypoxemic episodes may worsen airway obstruction or alter lung mechanics[6] and lead to impairment of cardiac function.[7] Prolonged episodes of hypoxemia during sleep can also occur in older infants with chronic lung disease despite normal awake oxyhemoglobin saturation.

Supplemental oxygen can be beneficial in children with chronic lung disease. It has been shown that infants with chronic lung disease whose baseline saturation during sleep was >92% showed better growth velocity than did those with prolonged mild hypoxemia (SpO_2 88% to 91%) during sleep despite normal oxyhemoglobin saturations while awake.[8] In infants with chronic lung disease and marginal sleep-related hypoxemia, the addition of supplemental oxygen resulted in improvement in sleep fragmentation and increased REM sleep.[9] Finally, it has been widely cited that infants with chronic lung disease have a higher incidence of sudden infant death syndrome, and infants who die suddenly may have unrecognized periods of hypoxemia or abnormal ventilatory and arousal responses during sleep; therefore, infants with chronic lung disease should be carefully assessed for sleep-related hypoxemia, as well as for safe sleeping environment and position.[1]

Our patient had mild chronic lung disease of infancy because of BPD, with sleep-related hypoxemia accounting for his poor weight gain. PSG revealed that the obstructive AHI was normal; however, the infant spent significant time with oxyhemoglobin saturation <92%, as shown in Figure 49-1. The central apnea index was also elevated because of frequent short central apneas followed by brief desaturation; however, none were pathologically long in duration as shown in Figure 49-2. The pattern of low baseline oxyhemoglobin saturation in the absence of respiratory events, or brief mild-to-moderate desaturations from baseline following short central apneas, is seen in infants and children with underlying lung disease and is an indicator of decreased pulmonary reserve. Although our patient's nutritional status and respiratory medications had been optimized, he had slower than expected weight gain and failure to thrive. Exacerbations of his underlying chronic lung disease, increased metabolic demand related to prematurity, increased work of breathing related to airway inflammation, a compliant chest wall, and decreased pulmonary functional residual capacity led to our patient's sleep-related hypoxemia.

He was treated with 1/8 L/min supplemental oxygen via nasal cannula while asleep, resulting in oxyhemoglobin saturation >95%. The patient demonstrated improved growth and development over the next several months and was successfully weaned from supplemental oxygen by 12 months of age.

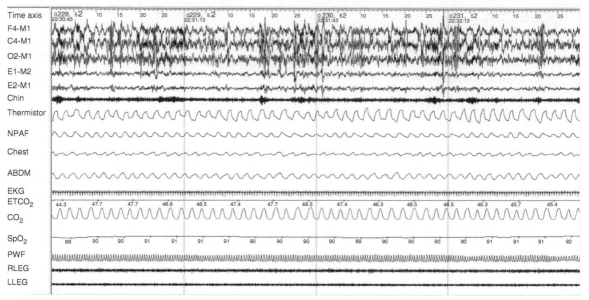

FIGURE 49-1 ■ **Representative 120-second epoch showing mild baseline hypoxemia.** In this sample, the SpO_2 range was 89% to 91% with no respiratory events.

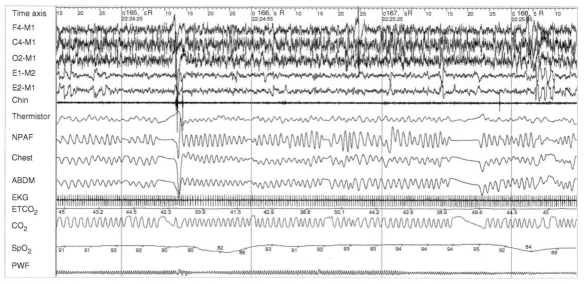

FIGURE 49-2 ■ Representative 120-second epoch demonstrating brief but significant desaturations from baseline following short, physiologic central apneas in REM sleep.

CLINICAL PEARLS

1. An important cause of poor growth in infants with chronic lung disease is sleep-related hypoxemia.
2. In infants with chronic lung disease, oxyhemoglobin saturation during sleep may be low for prolonged periods of time despite normal awake saturation.
3. Eliminating sleep-related hypoxemia in infants with chronic lung disease improves growth and sleep duration and may decrease the risk of sudden infant death.

REFERENCES

1. Allen J, Zwerdling R, Ehrenkranz R, et al. Statement on the care of the child with chronic lung disease of infancy and childhood. *Am J Respir Crit Care Med*. Aug 1 2003;168(3):356–396.
2. Northway Jr WH, Rosan RC, Porter DY. Pulmonary disease following respirator therapy of hyaline-membrane disease. Bronchopulmonary dysplasia. *N Engl J Med*. Feb 16 1967;276(7):357–368.
3. Manktelow BN, Draper ES, Annamalai S, Field D. Factors affecting the incidence of chronic lung disease of prematurity in 1987, 1992, and 1997. *Arch Dis Child Fetal Neonatal Ed*. Jul 2001;85(1):F33–F35.
4. Jobe AH, Bancalari E. Bronchopulmonary dysplasia. *Am J Respir Crit Care Med*. Jun 2001;163(7):1723–1729.
5. Garg M, Kurzner SI, Bautista DB, Keens TG. Clinically unsuspected hypoxia during sleep and feeding in infants with bronchopulmonary dysplasia. *Pediatrics*. May 1988;81(5):635–642.
6. Teague WG, Pian MS, Heldt GP, Tooley WH. An acute reduction in the fraction of inspired oxygen increases airway constriction in infants with chronic lung disease. *Am Rev Respir Dis*. Apr 1988;137(4):861–865.
7. Praud JP, Cavailloles F, Boulhadour K, DeRecondo M, Guilleminault C, Gaultier C. Radionuclide evaluation of cardiac function during sleep in children with bronchopulmonary dysplasia. *Chest*. Sep 1991;100(3):721–725.
8. Moyer-Mileur LJ, Nielson DW, Pfeffer KD, Witte MK, Chapman DL. Eliminating sleep-associated hypoxemia improves growth in infants with bronchopulmonary dysplasia. *Pediatrics*. Oct 1996;98(4 Pt 1):779–783.
9. Harris MA, Sullivan CE. Sleep pattern and supplementary oxygen requirements in infants with chronic neonatal lung disease. *Lancet*. Apr 1 1995;345(8953):831–832.

CASE 50

A 5-year-old boy with obstructive sleep apnea not tolerating continuous positive airway pressure

Lourdes M. DelRosso

CASE PRESENTATION

A 5-year-old boy presented for follow-up of obstructive sleep apnea syndrome (OSAS). A polysomnogram (PSG) (following tonsillectomy and adenoidectomy) had revealed an apnea–hypopnea index (AHI) of 15/h, arousal index of 12/h, and mild desaturation (SpO$_2$ nadir of 87% and 0.1% of total sleep time with SpO$_2$ <90%) without hypoventilation. The patient was placed on continuous positive airway pressure but did not tolerate it despite behavioral psychology support, and the parents wished to discuss other treatment options. The family denied daytime sleepiness or behavioral problems. The patient snored loudly and had labored breathing during sleep. He did not have any other sleep-related concerns or medical problems. His past surgical history was significant for tonsillectomy and adenoidectomy for recurrent tonsillitis at age 4. A PSG was not performed before tonsillectomy. The review of systems was negative for gastroesophageal reflux or allergic rhinitis.

PHYSICAL EXAM

Physical exam revealed an alert and cooperative boy. His vital signs were within the normal range. His height and weight were at the 40th percentile. He had a slightly adenoid facies. He did not have enlarged turbinates. He had a high-arched palate and a cross bite (lateral misalignment of the dental arches). The oropharynx was Mallampati grade III. Tonsils were surgically absent. He did not have micrognathia or retrognathia. The remainder of the exam was normal.

LABORATORY AND SLEEP FINDINGS

Soft tissue lateral neck x-ray did not show adenoid regrowth.

QUESTION

What options would you offer this family?

ANSWER

The options to address this child's OSAS were discussed with the parents and included watchful waiting and rapid maxillary expansion. Other potential options for management of persistent OSAS following adenotonsillectomy include weight loss (this child was not obese), nasal steroids (allergic rhinitis and adenoidal regrowth were not present), mandibular distraction (the patient did not have micrognathia or retrognathia), and management of comorbidities (gastroesophageal reflux or other comorbidities were not present).

DISCUSSION

The Childhood Adenotonsillectomy Trial (CHAT) has provided new evidence about watchful waiting in children aged 5 to 9 years with adenotonsillar hypertrophy and OSAS without prolonged desaturation.[1] For details on the CHAT study, see Case 42: A 7-year old boy with snoring, restless sleep and obstructive sleep apnea Although our patient had a prior tonsillectomy and adenoidectomy, watchful waiting with follow-up PSG is still an option. The patient had symptoms of loud snoring and labored breathing during sleep, and the parents wished to consider other treatment options. The patient had a high-arched palate and irregular dentition on physical exam. A high-arched palate and maxillary constriction can result in nasal obstruction because of elevation of the nasal floor, which in turn can lead to increased nasal resistance, mouth breathing, and a lowered position of the tongue. Treatment of OSAS with rapid maxillary expansion was initiated.

Rapid maxillary expansion is an orthodontic procedure that involves the placement of an expandable device anchored on selected teeth on the upper jaw (Fig. 50-1). The device has a central screw that exerts pressure on the mid-palatal suture, with the goal of opening the suture to increase the transverse diameter of the hard palate. The anchored teeth are commonly the premolars and first molars. Deciduous molars can also be used as long as they are stable. The procedure consists of two phases: a rapid expansion phase, usually lasting up to 20 days, during which the parents turn a key in the device daily (expansion goal of 1 mm a day), and a retention phase, where the device stays in place for approximately 6 months.[2]

Studies have shown an increase in nasal width and a decrease in airway resistance after rapid maxillary expansion in some but not all patients. Computed tomography studies have also shown significant increase in nasopharyngeal volume after completion of the expansion.[3] Rapid maxillary expansion has also improved nocturnal and diurnal symptoms, nasal breathing, and AHI in treated children.[4] The clinical and PSG improvement have been shown to persist over time, as demonstrated by a long-term study (up to 24 months).[5] The American Academy of Sleep Medicine practice parameters for the respiratory indications for PSG in children recommend a repeat PSG after treatment of OSAS with rapid maxillary expansion to assess if additional management for residual OSAS is needed.[6]

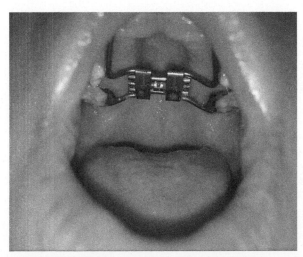

FIGURE 50-1 ■ **Patient with high-arched palate and rapid maxillary expander in place.**

Our patient was successfully treated with rapid maxillary expansion. Nocturnal symptoms improved. A PSG performed after treatment revealed an AHI of 2/h and a SpO$_2$ nadir of 94%.

CLINICAL PEARLS

1. A high-arched palate and maxillary constriction with a cross bite can result in nasal obstruction and mouth breathing.
2. Rapid maxillary expansion may improve OSAS symptoms in patients with these orthodontic abnormalities.
3. A follow-up PSG after treatment with rapid maxillary expansion is recommended to evaluate for residual OSAS.

REFERENCES

1. Marcus CL, Moore RH, Rosen CL, et al. A randomized trial of adenotonsillectomy for childhood sleep apnea. *N Engl J Med*. Jun 20 2013;368(25):2366–2376.
2. Pirelli P, Saponara M, Guilleminault C. Rapid maxillary expansion in children with obstructive sleep apnea syndrome. *Sleep*. Jun 15 2004;27(4):761–766.
3. Ngiam J, Cistulli PA. Dental treatment for paediatric obstructive sleep apnea. *Paediatr Respir Rev*. Jun 2015;16(3):174–181.
4. Villa MP, Malagola C, Pagani J, et al. Rapid maxillary expansion in children with obstructive sleep apnea syndrome: 12-month follow-up. *Sleep Med*. Mar 2007;8(2):128–134.
5. Villa MP, Rizzoli A, Miano S, Malagola C. Efficacy of rapid maxillary expansion in children with obstructive sleep apnea syndrome: 36 months of follow-up. *Sleep Breath*. May 2011;15(2):179–184.
6. Aurora RN, Zak RS, Karippot A, et al. Practice parameters for the respiratory indications for polysomnography in children. *Sleep*. Mar 2011;34(3):379–388.

A child referred for positive airway pressure initiation and titration

Suzanne E. Beck

CASE PRESENTATION

An 8-year-old boy with Trisomy 21 was referred to the sleep center for positive airway pressure (PAP) initiation. He had persistent snoring at night and behavioral problems in school that improved but did not resolve after adenotonsillectomy for severe obstructive sleep apnea syndrome (OSAS). Polysomnography (PSG) 2 months following adenotonsillectomy demonstrated residual severe OSAS with hypoxemia and hypoventilation. Otolaryngologic evaluation revealed glossoptosis and pharyngeal hypotonia. He was evaluated by an interdisciplinary pediatric sleep team, which recommended treatment with continuous positive airway pressure (CPAP).

Past medical history: Well-controlled asthma and allergic rhinitis, chronic otitis media controlled after bilateral myringotomy tubes, hypothyroidism controlled on medication, and a small ventricular septal defect that had closed. He had moderate developmental delay and was receiving speech and occupational therapy in a mainstream school. His medications included cetirizine, salmeterol-fluticasone, and levothyroxine.

PHYSICAL EXAM

Vital signs: respiratory rate 18 breaths/min; heart rate 85 beats/min; blood pressure normal for age; and SpO_2 97% during wakefulness. Weight was at the 30th percentile, height less than 5th percentile (as plotted on the usual growth charts rather than the Down syndrome growth charts), body mass index 90th percentile for age. The child was alert and cooperative and had typical features of Down syndrome. Nasal mucosa was mildly edematous with unobstructed passages. His oropharynx was Mallampati grade IV, with glossoptosis and absent tonsillar tissue. His palate and dentition were normal. Lungs were clear to auscultation. Heart sounds were normal. There was mild generalized hypotonia.

LABORATORY AND SLEEP FINDINGS

PSG after adenotonsillectomy: obstructive apnea–hypopnea index 66.7/h; SpO_2 nadir 77%; peak end-tidal CO_2 58 mm Hg; and end-tidal CO_2 >50 mm Hg for 30% total sleep time.

QUESTIONS

1. Is CPAP indicated in this patient?
2. Describe an approach to initiating CPAP in pediatric patients with developmental delays.

ANSWERS

1. Yes.
2. The multidisciplinary sleep team recommended desensitization to a nasal mask and CPAP pressure before titration. This was accomplished with a step-by-step behavioral approach where the patient wore his nasal interface for short periods during the day and as part of his bedtime routine while awake, incorporating positive reinforcement. Once he tolerated the mask and headgear, pressure was added. A PSG titration study was performed once he was able to fall asleep with the mask and pressure on.

DISCUSSION

CPAP treatment for OSAS is often prescribed for children, including children with Down syndrome, as a second-line treatment for obstructive sleep apnea syndrome (OSAS),[1] although adherence is a concern.[2,3] Significant improvement in neurobehavioral function has been shown in children after 3 months of treatment with CPAP, including children with developmental delays.[4] Therefore, CPAP is recommended in this patient population to maximize the child's potential.[4]

CPAP adherence in children and adolescents is related primarily to family and demographic factors, such as maternal education and family social support, rather than severity of apnea or measures of psychosocial functioning.[5] CPAP adherence can also be influenced by the support provided to the family early in the course of CPAP initiation. For example, incorporating education by a trained respiratory therapist in the use of CPAP in children and behavioral support by an experienced behavioral therapist at the time of the visit significantly improved adherence to CPAP in pediatric patients with OSAS and poor baseline adherence.[6] In adolescents, several factors are associated with increased use of CPAP adherence: (1) stable family structure and routine (e.g., consistent bedtime routine); (2) an authoritative rather than authoritarian parenting style (i.e., gentle reminders were more effective than punishment and threats); (3) desire to please and self-respect; and (4) perceived benefit from use of CPAP (e.g., those with improved daytime sleepiness and less enuresis on CPAP had increased adherence effects).[7]

A family-centered approach in a multidisciplinary setting is recommended to optimize initial and ongoing use of CPAP in the pediatric population. As part of the initial and maintenance visits, the benefits, use, and side effects of CPAP should be discussed. Patient and family psychosocial stressors should be identified and addressed. These issues can be universal (e.g., cleaning and maintenance of equipment or desensitizing to an interface) or individual (e.g., helping with communication style, sleep hygiene, or bedtime routine), and approaches should be tailored to the age and developmental level of the child. Potential side effects of CPAP should be addressed such as dry eyes, nasal congestion, and skin irritation from mask or headgear. It is important to provide ongoing education to the patient and family about CPAP benefits and equipment maintenance and fit, as well as developmentally appropriate behavioral support to optimize the use of CPAP.

In the sleep laboratory, a child may have a more successful titration study if he or she is used to the mask and pressure before the study and may have a better experience in the sleep laboratory if there is a child-friendly approach.[8] Because children may not tolerate introduction of a CPAP mask for the first time in the middle of the night, and because OSAS tends to worsen through the night in children,[9] starting CPAP midway through the night may not be tolerated or allow enough time for adequate titration. Split-night studies may be appropriate in adolescents or children who have used CPAP in the past but, because of the aforementioned factors, are not ideal in young children. In general, CPAP in children may be titrated according to the recommendations of the Positive Airway Pressure Titration Task Force of the American Academy of Sleep Medicine.[10] However, higher CPAP pressures than those recommended by the Task Force may be indicated to relieve obstructive apnea in some children to avoid tracheostomy; the guidelines being based on expert opinion rather than evidence.[11] Other conditions during titration that the technologist should be aware of in infants and small children are that children may not be able to trigger bi-level PAP (BPAP), may need a faster rise time and a shorter inspiratory time (because of a faster respiratory rate), are prone to central apnea on CPAP (see Clinical Pearls in Case 52: An adolescent referred for bi-level positive airway pressure titration awakens with leg cramps), and may also be at risk for hypoventilation.

Our patient was seen in the sleep center before PSG titration where the indications, benefits, and risks of CPAP were discussed. A treatment plan was agreed upon and expectations were set. As part of

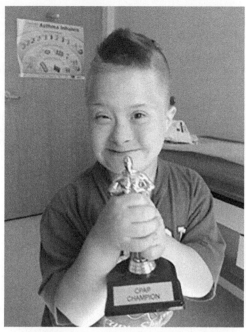

FIGURE 51-1 ■ **Child with a CPAP trophy.**

a multidisciplinary evaluation, a respiratory therapist fit the child for a mask and demonstrated equipment use. A behavioral therapist developed a plan to desensitize the child to the nasal interface and machine pressure by adjusting his bedtime routine and developing a step-wise behavioral modification plan with close monitoring before the titration study.[12] The behavior modification plan included having the child wear the mask alone while watching his favorite video during the daytime, with increasing use of the mask and then the CPAP machine. The family used a sticker chart and small prizes to encourage him at each step. The child had a successful titration PSG and was seen in follow-up to monitor adherence and clinical response to CPAP. He was adherent to CPAP, and positive reinforcement was given in the form of a trophy (obtained cheaply over the Internet) when his adherence goal was reached (Fig. 51-1). His daytime behavior has improved.

CLINICAL PEARLS

1. CPAP treatment for OSAS is often prescribed for children as a second-line treatment for OSAS.
2. CPAP is effective at improving neurodevelopmental performance in children, including atypically developing children, and should be considered in children with residual OSAS to maximize their potential.
3. A family-centered approach in a multidisciplinary setting is recommended to optimize initial and ongoing use of CPAP in the pediatric population.
4. Titration PSG studies should be performed in a child-friendly lab, keeping in mind that children may be at risk for hypoventilation or central apnea.

REFERENCES

1. Marcus CL, Brooks LJ, Draper KA, et al. Diagnosis and management of childhood obstructive sleep apnea syndrome. *Pediatrics*. 2012;130(3):576–584.
2. Marcus CL, Beck SE, Traylor J, et al. Randomized, double-blind clinical trial of two different modes of positive airway pressure therapy on adherence and efficacy in children. *J Clin Sleep Med*. 2012;8(1):37–42.
3. Marcus CL, Rosen G, Ward SL, et al. Adherence to and effectiveness of positive airway pressure therapy in children with obstructive sleep apnea. *Pediatrics*. 2006;117(3):e442–e451.
4. Marcus CL, Radcliffe J, Konstantinopoulou S, et al. Effects of positive airway pressure therapy on neurobehavioral outcomes in children with obstructive sleep apnea. *Am J Respir Crit Care Med*. 2012;185(9):998–1003.
5. DiFeo N, Meltzer LJ, Beck SE, et al. Predictors of positive airway pressure therapy adherence in children: a prospective study. *J Clin Sleep Med*. 2012;8(3):279–286.

6. Jambhekar SK, Com G, Tang X, et al. Role of a respiratory therapist in improving adherence to positive airway pressure treatment in a pediatric sleep apnea clinic. *Respir Care*. 2013;58(12):2038–2044.
7. Prashad PS, Marcus CL, Maggs J, et al. Investigating reasons for CPAP adherence in adolescents: a qualitative approach. *J Clin Sleep Med*. 2013;9(12):1303–1313.
8. Beck SE, Marcus CL. Pediatric polysomnography. *Sleep Med Clin*. 2009;4(3):393–406.
9. Goh DY, Galster P, Marcus CL. Sleep architecture and respiratory disturbances in children with obstructive sleep apnea. *Am J Respir Crit Care Med*. 2000;162(2 Pt 1):682–686.
10. Kushida CA, Chediak A, Berry RB, et al. Clinical guidelines for the manual titration of positive airway pressure in patients with obstructive sleep apnea. *J Clin Sleep Med*. 2008;4(2):157–171.
11. Marcus CL. Concerns regarding the pediatric component of the AASM clinical guidelines for the manual titration of positive airway pressure in patients with obstructive sleep apnea. *J Clin Sleep Med*. 2008;4(6):607. author reply 608–609.
12. King MS, Xanthopoulos MS, Marcus CL. Improving positive airway pressure adherence in children. *Sleep Med Clin*. 2014;9(2):219–234.

An adolescent referred for bi-level positive airway pressure titration awakens with leg cramps

Suzanne E. Beck

CASE PRESENTATION

A 17-year-old girl with spinal muscular atrophy type II was referred to the sleep laboratory for titration of bi-level positive airway pressure (BPAP) before her moving away for college. She had severe scoliosis and respiratory insufficiency and had been on nighttime BPAP for the past 6 years. She used BPAP 20/8 cm H_2O in the spontaneous timed (ST) mode with a backup rate of 20 breaths/min and an inspiratory time of 1 second via nasal interface. She tolerated it well and used it every night. Her last adherence download showed that she was using BPAP every night for an average of 9.5 hours per night. She had recently begun waking early because of cramps and tingling in her legs and sometimes found it difficult to return to sleep in the early morning. She did not endorse leg paresthesia in the evening or difficulty falling asleep at her usual bedtime. A recent cardiology evaluation was normal. She was on no medications. She had lab tests drawn and a polysomnography (PSG) titration study ordered. The technician called from the sleep lab with questions and further instructions regarding the events in Figure 52-1.

PHYSICAL EXAM

Vital signs: respiratory rate was 18 breaths/min; heart rate 90 beats/min; and blood pressure 110/68 mm Hg, SpO_2 96% in room air. Weight was 27 kg (less than 5th percentile). Exam revealed an alert young woman who sat upright in her wheelchair. She had a normal oropharynx with scant tonsillar tissue. Her head and neck were normal. She had marked kyphoscoliosis. Breath sounds were diminished at the bases. Heart sounds were normal. She had atrophy of her limbs and contractures of the lower extremities without edema or digital clubbing.

LABORATORY AND SLEEP FINDINGS

A metabolic panel was normal including calcium 9.8 mg/mL (normal 8.4 to 10.2 mg/L) and serum bicarbonate 20 mmol/L (normal 22 to 30 mmol/L).

PSG: Respiratory data while awake showed a respiratory rate of 18 breaths/min, SpO_2 nadir 95%, and peak end-tidal CO_2 40 mm Hg.

Total recording time 352 minutes; total sleep time (TST) 130 minutes; sleep efficiency 37%; sleep latency 220 minutes; N1 9% of TST; N2 34%; N3 26%; REM 31%; arousal index 21/h; obstructive apnea–hypopnea index (AHI) 0/h; central AHI 2.9/h; longest central apnea 30 seconds (see Fig. 52-1); and SpO_2 nadir 69%; periodic limb movement index 2.1/h. Sleep efficiency was diminished because of a long sleep latency and a long awakening associated with leg cramps.

QUESTIONS

1. What are the respiratory events occurring in Figure 52-1?
2. What is the likely cause of the muscle spasm and the event in Figure 52-1?
3. What should the technician in the sleep lab do next?

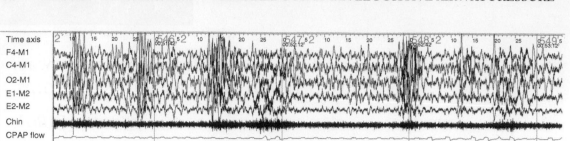

FIGURE 52-1 ■ A 120-second epoch of sleep with the patient on BPAP 20/8 cm H_2O in the ST mode with a rate of 20 breaths/min and inspiratory time of 1 second.

ANSWERS

1. Prolonged central apneas associated with desaturation and arousals.
2. Hyperventilation induced by overtitration.
3. The technician should lower the BPAP rate to restore eucapnia.

DISCUSSION

Noninvasive ventilation with bi-level positive pressure support is commonly used in children and adolescents with respiratory insufficiency and hypoventilation due to neuromuscular weakness and improves quality of sleep and daytime symptoms.[1] The most effective ventilatory strategy uses expiratory pressure (EPAP) to maintain upper airway patency, along with an inspiratory pressure (IPAP) above EPAP, or pressure support, to augment tidal volume. A backup rate in the ST or pressure control (PC) mode is often employed because children and adolescents with neuromuscular disease are typically too weak to trigger the machine or maintain inspiratory time.

Treatment-emergent central apnea is the term used to describe a form of sleep-disordered breathing in which repeated central apneas (>5/h) persist or emerge during the administration of continuous positive airway pressure (CPAP) once obstructive events are extinguished and for which there is not a clear cause for the central apneas, such as central sleep apnea (CSA) caused by a medication or central sleep apnea with Cheyne-Stokes breathing.[2] The proposed mechanism is believed to be instability of sleep maintenance or ventilatory control because of associated oscillations in PCO_2, CPAP-related increased CO_2 elimination, and activation of airway and pulmonary stretch receptors triggering these central apneas, but it is not fully understood.[2] Children may experience transient, self-limited central apneas during CPAP titration, but it is not common to meet the above-mentioned diagnostic criteria in neurologically intact children. When central apneas are long (exceeding 20 to 25 seconds duration), frequent, or associated with hypoxemia or hypoventilation, the use of a backup rate or a switch to PC or timed mode should be considered (for a discussion of different BPAP modes, see the Clinical Pearls section in Case 53: A 3-year-old girl with irregular breathing on bi-level positive airway pressure). Newer modes of noninvasive ventilation are also available for more complex apneas, such as adaptive servo ventilation or volume-assured pressure support.

Our patient did not meet criteria for treatment-emergent central apnea because she had only a few isolated central apneas and did not have obstructive sleep apnea syndrome. In addition, she was on a backup rate. The cause of the central apnea in our patient was overtitration of BPAP. This drove our patient's PCO_2 below her apneic threshold during sleep, eliminating her drive to breathe and resulting in prolonged central apneas (see Fig. 52-1). Theoretically, the backup rate in the ST mode should overcome the central apneas, but in our experience, the ST mode is ineffective at treating prolonged central apnea in children. Hyperventilation and resultant hypocapnia likely caused a respiratory alkalosis (as supported by the low serum bicarbonate). Additionally, note that the transcutaneous PCO_2 values were quite reduced, supporting the concept of excessive ventilation. In normal individuals one would expect values in the low 40s (slightly higher than during wake) but certainly not in the 30 to 35 mmHg range. During alkalosis, hypocalcemia develops because of ion shifts in the blood, and it may cause muscle spasms and leg cramps.

In our patient, decreasing the rate to 16 breaths/min (closer to her awake respiratory rate) restored eucapnia. The IPAP and EPAP pressures remained the same. A high-pressure support was needed to maintain minute ventilation, given our patient's neuromuscular weakness and scoliosis. The mode was switched to PC to ensure that all breaths (patient and device triggered) were device cycled (to ensure an adequate inspiratory time). In the ST mode, only device-triggered breaths have a set inspiratory time. In patients with a stiff chest wall, spontaneously triggered breaths may fail to deliver an adequate tidal volume because BPAP devices may prematurely cycle from IPAP to EPAP. In the current patient, a reduction in backup rate to slightly below the spontaneous rate resulted in a respiratory rate in the 16 to 18 breaths/min range, and the PCO_2 gradually normalized during the rest of the study. Central apnea, arousals, and leg cramps resolved.

CLINICAL PEARLS

1. Treatment-emergent central apnea is often transient and self-limited, and it may not require a backup rate unless it is associated with prolonged central apnea or significant desaturation.
2. Overtitration of CPAP/BiPAP can cause central apnea in children. In these cases, the treatment is to reduce the pressure or rate to maintain eucapnia.
3. It is important to reassess CPAP/BiPAP needs in children because their needs may change as they grow and develop.

REFERENCES

1. Mellies U, Ragette R, Dohna Schwake C, Boehm H, Voit T, Teschler H. Long-term noninvasive ventilation in children and adolescents with neuromuscular disorders. *Eur Respir J*. 2003;22(4):631–636.
2. American Academy of Sleep Medicine; *International Classification of Sleep Disorders*. 3rd ed. Darien, IL: 2014.

A 3-year-old girl with irregular breathing on bilevel positive airway pressure

Carole L. Marcus

CASE PRESENTATION

A 3-year-old girl with cerebral palsy, seizures, developmental delay, general hypotonia, and obstructive sleep apnea syndrome (OSAS) underwent polysomnography (PSG) for routine re-evaluation of her bilevel positive airway pressure (BPAP) requirements (Fig. 53-1). She had been born full-term but was noted to be hypotonic and had seizures while in the neonatal intensive care unit. She was diagnosed with severe OSAS at 2 years of age, with only partial improvement following adenotonsillectomy. She was placed on BPAP (pressure control [PC] mode, inspiratory positive airway pressure [IPAP] of 20 cm H_2O and expiratory positive airway pressure [EPAP] of 10 cm H_2O, rate 16 breaths/min, inspiratory time 0.8 seconds) because of baseline hypercapnia and the need for high pressures to overcome the OSAS. Her last PSG was a year ago. Since then, she has had a hospitalization for aspiration pneumonia and was noted to have intermittent desaturations on her home oximeter. The patient was fed via gastrostomy. Medications included two anticonvulsants, ranitidine, and albuterol.

PHYSICAL EXAM

Physical exam revealed a severely developmentally delayed child in a wheelchair who was in no distress. Pulse was 90 beats/min, and respiratory rate was 16 breaths/min. Height was at the 5th percentile, and weight was at the 3rd percentile. Her facies was not dysmorphic. The oropharynx was Mallampati grade IV, with absent tonsillar tissue. Examination of the thorax revealed mild scoliosis. Lungs were clear to auscultation with normal air exchange. Heart sounds were normal. The abdomen was soft, and a gastrostomy tube was in place. There was hypotonia of the extremities, but no clubbing (Fig. 53-1).

QUESTIONS

1. What is the cause of the unusual pattern on the nasal pressure channel (large arrows)?
2. What adjustments can be made to the BPAP settings to correct this?

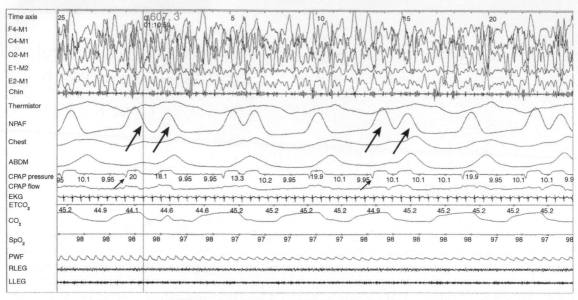

FIGURE 53-1 ■ A 30-second PSG epoch is shown.

ANSWERS

1. The downward deflection on the continuous positive airway pressure (CPAP) pressure channel (thin arrows) indicates a machine-initiated breath. The patient has frequent machine-initiated breaths that often do not result in full chest wall movements and are therefore followed rapidly by spontaneous breaths, leading to the "double hump" appearance on the nasal pressure channel (large arrows). A subtle "double hump" appearance can also be seen on the chest and abdominal effort leads and on one CO_2 waveform. This breathing pattern is occurring because the set inspiratory time is too short for the patient and does not allow for a full inspiration. The child has a respiratory rate of 14 breaths/min so that the duration of each respiratory cycle is 4.3 seconds. A normal inspiratory:expiratory ratio is 1:2, so an inspiratory time of 1.4 seconds would be appropriate in her case. However, the BPAP inspiratory time setting is only 0.8 seconds, resulting in an inspiratory:expiratory ratio close to 1:4.
2. Increase the inspiratory time, for example, to 1.4 seconds.

DISCUSSION

BPAP triggering and cycling problems are frequently encountered when managing pediatric patients requiring ventilatory support because the device algorithms in most machines are designed for adults. To date, standard BPAP machines are not approved by the Food and Drug Administration (FDA) for use in children under 7 years of age or weighing <40 lb (18.2 kg). However, they are frequently used off-label in children to avoid a tracheostomy for invasive mechanical ventilation.

Modern noninvasive ventilators now offer multiple modes for ventilating patients with complex disorders. Our patient had OSAS, as well as baseline hypercapnia, which were most likely because of both upper airway and ventilatory muscle hypotonia. Such patients may benefit from advanced modes of ventilation. The PC mode is both device- and patient-triggered (Table 53-1). It delivers breaths at a set pressure and rate with a fixed inspiratory time; both patient- and device-initiated breaths receive pressure support. In the PC mode, the ventilator cycles to expiration once the pressure has been delivered for a set inspiratory time. The inspiratory:expiratory ratio is typically set at 1:2, unless the patient has severe obstructive disease (in which case a longer expiratory phase may be needed) or difficulty with oxygenation (in which case, a longer inspiratory phase may be needed). Only select home devices have the PC mode available.

The initial approach to treating patients with neuromuscular weakness and sleep disordered breathing, whether because of central apnea, obstructive apnea, or gas exchange abnormalities caused by hypoventilation, is usually to apply noninvasive ventilation during sleep, titrated to optimal settings.[1] Ventilation modalities include BPAP in the spontaneous (S) mode (breaths initiated by the patient only, with no backup rate), spontaneous-timed (ST) mode (a backup rate is available to deliver pressure if the patient does not initiate a breath within a set time window), timed mode (inspiratory time and respiratory rate are fixed, but the patient does not receive pressure support for spontaneously initiated breaths), and PC mode (see Table 53-1).[2] Additional modes, such as adaptive servoventilation for patients with both obstructive and central apneas, and Average Volume Assured Pressure Support (AVAPS) for patients with respiratory insufficiency who would benefit from ventilation with a set tidal volume, are available for patients with more complex ventilatory needs. In our experience, patients

TABLE 53-1. Positive airway pressure modes

Mode	EPAP	IPAP	Rate	Patient-Triggered	Device-Triggered	Patient Cycled	Device Cycled
CPAP	X	—	—	NA	NA	NA	NA
Spontaneous (S)	X	X	—	X		X	
Spontaneous-timed (ST)	X	X	X	X	X (if not initiated by patient within a set time)	X	X (for device-triggered breaths)
Timed (T)	X	X	X	—	X	—	X
Pressure control (PC)	X	X	X	X	X	—	X

with respiratory insufficiency often ventilate better in the PC than the ST mode because the PC mode allows breaths to be triggered by either the patient or the device (thereby improving patient comfort) but ensures that each breath is machine-cycled, thereby allowing for better ventilation. However, when using more advanced modes of ventilation, it is important to ensure that all settings are adjusted appropriately for the patient. Although our patient tolerated the BPAP well, with no sleep disruption and adequate gas exchange, other patients with too-short inspiratory times may have discomfort from ventilator-patient asynchrony or may have inadequate ventilation.

Another problem that may arise in children is inappropriate setting of the rise time, available with certain brands of BPAP equipment. The rise time is the amount of time it takes for the device to reach the prescribed IPAP, and was introduced into BPAP devices primarily as a comfort measure to enable a slower and more physiologic increase in IPAP to full pressure, as compared with an artificial, mechanical "square wave" rise. However, BPAP devices are made for adults, who have a slower respiratory rate than children. Thus, if the rise time is too long, the child may cycle off inspiration before the prescribed IPAP is attained. In younger children who have a rapid respiratory rate, it is therefore advisable to set a short rise time.

CLINICAL PEARLS

1. It is important to set appropriate inspiratory and rise times when using advanced BPAP modes.
2. Most BPAP machines were designed for adult patients who have a slower respiratory rate and different respiratory timing compared with children; thus, triggering and cycling issues may occur in children.
3. Although CPAP and BPAP devices are not approved by the FDA for use in young children, they are often used off-label because of lack of clinical alternatives.

REFERENCES

1. Arens R, Muzumdar H. Sleep, sleep disordered breathing, and nocturnal hypoventilation in children with neuromuscular diseases. *Paediatr Respir Rev*. 2010;11:24–30.
2. Berry RB, Chediak A, Brown LK, et al. Best clinical practices for the sleep center adjustment of noninvasive positive pressure ventilation (NPPV) in stable chronic alveolar hypoventilation syndromes. *J Clin Sleep Med*. 2010;6:491–509.

Why is the continuous positive airway pressure no longer working?

Mary H. Wagner

CASE PRESENTATION

The parent of a 10-year-old followed in the sleep clinic contacts your office because the child is having trouble in school. He has been on continuous positive airway pressure (CPAP) of 7 cm, using a nasal mask for residual obstructive sleep apnea syndrome (OSAS) after adenotonsillectomy for the past year. His apnea–hypopnea index (AHI) after adenotonsillectomy was 8.9 events/h and increased in REM to 19 events/h. On a CPAP titration, his OSAS was well controlled on the 7 cm H_2O. On his initial return visit after starting CPAP, he was doing well and had excellent adherence, with a download of the CPAP machine showing 9 hours of use nightly. His mother is concerned because his school performance has declined over the past couple of months despite his using CPAP every night. He is unable to remember his spelling words, which is a drastic change for him. His teacher has also reported more issues with inattention and aggressive behavior. Mom also reports that the child left his usual mask at his grandmother's house after a visit in the summer, and he is using an old mask that used to belong to his father. He has grown recently, with a weight gain of 4 kg since his CPAP titration. His only medication is a steroid nasal spray, used daily for nasal congestion.

PHYSICAL EXAM

Vital signs: blood pressure 100/60; pulse 72 beats/min; afebrile, respiratory rate 12 breaths/min; SpO_2 98%; weight 90th percentile; height 70th percentile; body mass index 95th percentile. Head, eyes, ears, nose, and throat exam: small mid face; normal jaw; Mallampati grade IV; tonsils surgically absent. The remainder of the exam was normal.

QUESTION

What may be going on with this patient, and what is the best way to figure it out?

ANSWER

Issues to explain ineffective CPAP can include suboptimal CPAP adherence, increased mask leak, CPAP device malfunction, or an increased CPAP pressure requirement. In this situation, a download should be obtained from the CPAP machine to examine CPAP usage, including days of use, duration of use on each day, CPAP leak, and residual AHI. During the clinic visit, the interface fit, mask leak, condition of the mask and device, and any barriers to CPAP use should be assessed. The patient may require a repeat sleep study to re-evaluate pressure requirements because of changes in growth and possibly obesity since his previous sleep study.

Our patient's CPAP device was downloaded (Fig. 54-1). The download showed adequate hours of CPAP usage but with extended periods of leak. This is likely contributing to suboptimal sleep and poorer daytime performance.

DISCUSSION

Children with untreated OSAS may manifest daytime symptoms including overt daytime sleepiness, as well as symptoms involving mood, behavior, and school performance.[1-4] OSAS in children has been linked to many behaviors and symptoms, including aggressiveness, impulsivity, hyperactivity, inattention, poor academic performance, and decreased executive functioning.[1-5] Although studies support the association of these dysfunctional behaviors with OSAS, causality is difficult to prove. However, studies do support improvement in academic performance, attention, and mental processing with treatment of OSAS by adenotonsillectomy.[5-9] In addition, in a group of children using CPAP for OSAS, Marcus et al.[10] demonstrated decreased daytime sleepiness, as measured by a modified Epworth Sleepiness Scale; improved attention-deficit hyperactivity disorder symptoms, as measured by the Conner scale and attention problems subscale of the Child Behavior Checklist; and improved quality of life, rated by both children using CPAP and their caregivers. Only the sleepiness improvement was shown to significantly correlate with duration of CPAP use.[10]

The adherence benchmark established for adequate CPAP adherence in adults is use of the machine for 4 hours per night for at least 70% of nights.[11] Such a benchmark has not been established for children, who sleep for longer periods than adults. In the Marcus study, improvements in daytime sleepiness correlated with increased CPAP use, suggesting that the longer the device was worn, the fewer the symptoms.[10] In addition, it has been shown that parents' recollection of duration of use overestimates objective measures of use by a mean of 2.8 hours per night, demonstrating the need for evaluating objective device downloads.[12]

It is important to evaluate adherence and how individual patients improve on therapy. This can provide a baseline for future comparison, as demonstrated in the patient discussed. Evaluation of leak and residual AHI can also be obtained from machine downloads and can give additional information about machine effectiveness. If the leak is large, the patient's interface should be evaluated for fit, and it is helpful to have the patient demonstrate how he or she puts on his or her mask to troubleshoot over- or undertightening. As children are growing, mask fit will change over time, and fit must be frequently reassessed. Pattern of leak may suggest that the patient is pulling off the mask at a particular time of the night, which can be amenable to intervention. A high residual AHI may give an indication

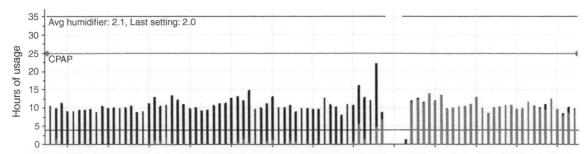

FIGURE 54-1 ■ This graph shows the number of hours of CPAP use per night. It demonstrates that on most nights the patient is having extended hours of leak (black bars; left side of panel). After the mask was replaced, the leak resolved (right side of panel; green bars).

that the machine pressure needs to be adjusted or a repeat polysomnography should be obtained to investigate further residual events. However, it should be noted that the accuracy of the software in detecting AHI in children has not been well studied.[13]

Review of the download in this patient demonstrated good CPAP adherence, with the device being turned on every night (left side of panel of Fig. 54-1; black columns). However, there was a large leak present every night. The patient was able to demonstrate good technique in mask placement during his clinic visit, but the mask was noted to be large for his face, and a large leak was present when the patient was placed on his usual home pressure. His mask was replaced with elimination of the leak (right side of panel; green columns). His mother called 3 weeks after the mask replacement to report that his behavior had improved to his usual good baseline and that his memory for spelling words had also returned to normal.

CLINICAL PEARLS

1. Patients using CPAP should have their machines downloaded to monitor adherence. Evaluations of adherence should include pattern and duration of use.
2. Adequate hours of CPAP use should be judged based on age-related sleep requirements.
3. Leak should be evaluated on the download, including duration and pattern, to help the patient maximize benefit from CPAP use.
4. Children on CPAP should have their pressure requirements re-evaluated, typically on an annual basis, because of ongoing growth and other changes in condition such as weight gain.

REFERENCES

1. Chervin RD, Archibold KH. Hyperactivity and polysomnographic findings in children evaluated for sleep-disordered breathing. *Sleep*. 2001;24:313–320.
2. Chervin RD, Dillon JE, Bassetti C, Ganoczy DA, Pituch KJ. Symptoms of sleep disorders, inattention, and hyperactivity in children. *Sleep*. 1997;20:1185–1192.
3. Gozal D, Pope Jr DW. Snoring during early childhood and academic performance at ages thirteen to fourteen years. *Pediatrics*. 2001;107(6):1394–1399.
4. O'Brien LM, Mervis CB, Holbrook CR, et al. Neurobehavioral implications of habitual snoring in children. *Pediatrics*. 2004;114:44–49.
5. Marcus CL, Moore RH, Rosen CL, et al. A randomized trial of adenotonsillectomy for childhood sleep apnea. *N Engl J Med*. 2013;368:2366–2376.
6. Chervin RD, Ruzicka DL, Giordani BJ, et al. Sleep-disordered breathing, behavior, and cognition in children before and after adenotonsillectomy. *Pediatrics*. 2006;117(4):e769–e778.
7. Gozal D. Sleep-disordered breathing and school performance in children. *Pediatrics*. 1998;102:616–620.
8. Hogan AM, Hill CM, Harrison D, et al. Cerebral blood flow velocity and cognition in children before and after adenotonsillectomy. *Pediatrics*. 2008;122(1):75–82.
9. Landau YE, Bar-Yishay O, Greenberg-Dotan S, et al. Impaired behavior and neurocognitive function in preschool children with obstructive sleep apnea. *Pediatr Pulmonol*. 2012;47(2):180–188.
10. Marcus CL, Radcliffe J, Konstantinopoulou S, et al. Effects of positive airway pressure therapy on neurobehavioral outcomes in children with obstructive sleep apnea. *Am J Respir Crit Care Med*. 2012;185(9):998–1003.
11. Sawyer AM, Gooneratne N, Marcus CL, Ofer D, Richards KC, Weaver TE. A systematic review of CPAP adherence across age groups: clinical and empiric insights for developing CPAP adherence interventions. *Sleep Med Rev*. 2011;15(6):343–356.
12. Marcus CL, Rosen G, Ward SL, et al. Adherence to and effectiveness of positive airway pressure therapy in children with obstructive sleep apnea. *Pediatrics*. 2006;117:e442–e451.
13. Schwab RJ, Badr SM, Epstein LJ, et al. An official American Thoracic Society statement: continuous positive airway pressure adherence tracking systems. The optimal monitoring strategies and outcome measures in adults. *Am J Respir Crit Care Med*. 2013;188(5):613–620.

CASE 55

A 3-year-old girl with Down syndrome, chronic otitis media, and snoring

Suzanne E. Beck

CASE PRESENTATION

A 3-year-old girl with Down syndrome and chronic otitis media was evaluated for snoring. She was referred by an anesthesiologist who noted her history of snoring during a preoperative evaluation for myringotomy tubes planned by her local otolaryngologist. Her parents endorsed snoring, mouth breathing, and restless sleep during colds. Parents reported that her preferred sleeping position was on her side, propped up on three pillows, with her neck hyperextended. There was no gasping, cyanosis, or witnessed apnea, so her parents were not concerned. She had no recent changes in her behavior. She had frequent nasal congestion and chronic otitis media with effusion. The remainder of her history was noncontributory.

PHYSICAL EXAM

Vital signs: pulse 96 beats/min; blood pressure 89/45 mm Hg; respiratory rate 22 breaths/min; SpO_2: 97%; weight 13.2 kg (25th percentile Centers for Disease Control and Prevention [CDC] growth curve and 50th percentile Down syndrome growth curve); height 86.9 cm (less than 5th percentile CDC growth curve and 50th percentile Down syndrome growth curve); body mass index 17.5 kg/(m^2) (90th percentile).

Physical exam revealed an obese girl in no distress. She had dysmorphic features including brachycephaly, down-slanting palpebral fissures, low-set ears with narrow external canals, flattened nasal bridge, and midface hypoplasia. Her oropharynx was narrow, with glossoptosis, dental crowding, and 3+ tonsils. Her lungs were clear to auscultation. Heart sounds were normal. Her fifth finger was curved in. Her muscle tone was slightly decreased.

LABORATORY AND SLEEP FINDINGS

Polysomnography (PSG) revealed a total sleep time (TST) of 510 minutes; SE 93%; REM 122 minutes (26.6%); arousal index 20.7/h; obstructive apnea–hypopnea index (AHI) 26.9/h; central apnea index 0.5/h; SpO_2 nadir 53%; SpO_2 <90% for 12.5% of TST; peak end-tidal CO_2 71 mm Hg; time with end-tidal CO_2 >50 mm Hg 75 % of TST.

QUESTIONS

1. What features of Down syndrome predispose our patient to obstructive sleep apnea syndrome (OSAS)?
2. What is the treatment for OSAS in children with Down syndrome?

ANSWERS

1. Several clinical features of Down syndrome place a child at risk for OSAS, including midface hypoplasia, maxillary hypoplasia, and crowding of the oropharynx because of glossoptosis (posterior displacement of the tongue), lymphoid hyperplasia, adiposity, and hypotonia.
2. The initial treatment of OSAS in the vast majority of children with Down syndrome is adenotonsillectomy, which results in a wider oropharynx. However, because of the above-mentioned anatomic and neuromuscular abnormalities, further treatment (e.g., continuous positive airway pressure (CPAP)) may be needed if the OSAS persists after surgery.

DISCUSSION

Down syndrome, first described in 1866 by John Langdon Down,[1] is the most common genetic cause of intellectual disability. Down syndrome affects individuals of all socioeconomic and racial groups and has a worldwide incidence of 1/600-1000.[2] Down syndrome is due to triplication of chromosome 21 (Trisomy 21) or, rarely, because of an unbalanced translocation or mosaicism. Down syndrome is characterized by multiple comorbidities, including intellectual impairment; characteristic facial features; high rates of cancer; congenital cardiac, gastrointestinal (GI), respiratory, oropharyngeal, orthopedic, and neurologic defects; and early-onset dementia.

Children with Down syndrome are at increased risk of OSAS because of certain features that predispose them to airway obstruction, including a small upper airway and cranium with mid-face and mandibular hypoplasia; crowding of the airway with relative macroglossia or glossoptosis, adiposity, adenotonsillar hyperplasia, and generalized lymphoid hyperplasia; pharyngeal hypotonia; and other skeletal anomalies, including an increased incidence of choanal atresia.[3,4] Hypothyroidism may also contribute. Depending on the age of the population studied and PSG cut-off values used to define OSAS, the estimated prevalence of OSAS in children with Down syndrome varies between 30% and 75%, much greater than the estimated OSAS prevalence of 4% in the general pediatric population (reviewed in detail by Churchill).[5] OSAS is also very common in adults with Down syndrome.[6] Children with Down syndrome also have a high prevalence of other sleep abnormalities, such as insomnia, increased sleep fragmentation and parasomnias, regardless of the presence of OSAS. In addition to being more common, OSAS can be more severe in children with Down syndrome. In a referred population of children with Down syndrome and OSAS matched with typically developing children with a similar AHI, the children with Down syndrome had more severe desaturation and hypercapnia.[7]

Obstructive sleep apnea is also common in very young infants with Down syndrome and may be severe. A retrospective study of infants <6 months of age referred to a Down syndrome clinic obtained PSGs in all infants who were symptomatic. Of those undergoing PSG, 95% had OSAS (31% of the total infants), and 71% were severe.[8] OSAS was more common and more severe in the infants with a history of prematurity, congenital heart disease, dysphagia, gastroesophageal reflux, and other GI and pulmonary disorders.[8] Therefore, it is important to keep in mind these underlying comorbidities when identifying infants at risk for OSAS.

The usual first-line treatment for OSAS in children with Down syndrome is adenotonsillectomy. Further, 10% to 30% of children with Down syndrome have atlantoaxial instability because of laxity between the cervical vertebrae,[9] and therefore caution is required during surgery. Most pediatric patients with Down syndrome show improvement after adenotonsillectomy; however, only about one third will have a normal postoperative sleep study.[10] OSAS may also recur[11] because of recurrence of lymphoid hyperplasia, including development of lingual tonsils or increasing obesity. In these patients, treatment with CPAP with behavioral support can be successful.[12] Treatment of underlying comorbidities such as rhinitis, asthma, and gastroesophageal reflux is important, as is vigilant follow-up. In some patients, tongue-reduction surgery has been performed.

Despite the recognition in pediatrics that infants and children with Down syndrome are at greater risk for development of OSAS, sleep-disordered breathing is often under-recognized by parents as well as clinicians. Parents of children with Down syndrome may consider the child's breathing or sleep patterns as normal or as an acceptable part of their child's syndrome. For example, results of a survey from a Down syndrome center revealed that over 70% of parents of children with Down syndrome reported problems with initiating or maintaining sleep, 125 reported witnessed apnea, and over half reported excessive daytime sleepiness, but only half of the parents were concerned or discussed the issue with a physician.[13] Further, pulmonary, cardiovascular, skeletal, neurologic, and behavioral comorbidities in Down syndrome can overlap with the symptoms or influence the severity of OSAS; therefore, these conditions should be recognized and treated. The American Academy of Pediatrics, guidelines for health supervision of children with Down syndrome recommend that pediatricians review symptoms of OSAS with parents of these children within the first 6 months of life.[14] Anticipatory guidance related to the modifiable risk factors for OSAS should be discussed at subsequent visits, including sleeping position, car-seat position, and risk of cervical spine injury related to atlantoaxial instability and obesity. Referral to a physician with expertise in pediatric sleep disorders is recommended for examination and further evaluation of a possible sleep disorder if any of the above-mentioned symptoms occur. In addition, the American Academy of Pediatrics recommends that all children with Down syndrome undergo PSG by age 4 years.[14]

Our patient had severe OSAS, as evidenced by the PSG findings of an obstructive AHI of 26.9/h, with repeated, severe, primarily REM-related oxyhemoglobin desaturations to a nadir of 53% (Fig. 55-1). The obstructive events were prolonged, with profound hypoxemia and hypoventilation (Fig. 55-2). Our patient was admitted to the intensive care unit and underwent cardiac and pulmonary evaluation before adenotonsillectomy. After surgery, there was resolution of desaturation, but low-grade snoring persisted. Follow-up PSG 8 weeks after surgery revealed intermittent snoring with an obstructive AHI of 2.4/h and minimal desaturation to a nadir of 92%. The child follows closely in the sleep center for recurrence of symptoms.

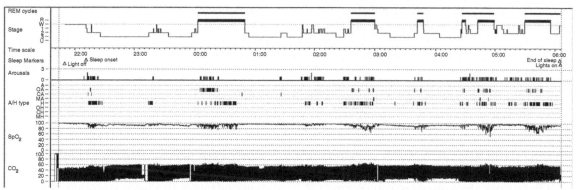

FIGURE 55-1 ■ Hypnogram showing frequent obstructive apneas and obstructive hypopneas with desaturation and hypoventilation, primarily during REM sleep.

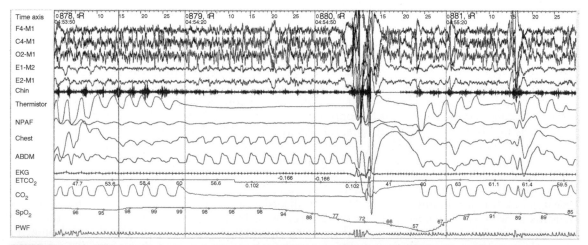

FIGURE 55-2 ■ Hundred and twenty–second epoch showing a 40-second obstructive apnea with profound desaturation and hypercapnia.

CLINICAL PEARLS

1. Infants and children with Down syndrome have a high prevalence of OSAS, primarily because of a small, crowded upper airway, lymphoid hyperplasia, and pharyngeal hypotonia.
2. Adenotonsillectomy is usually beneficial in children, but there is a high risk of recurrence or residual OSAS, and, therefore, follow-up is indicated. Recognition and treatment of other comorbidities, such as rhinitis, asthma, dysphagia, and gastroesophageal reflux in infants, or obesity or hypothyroidism in older children, should be considered. CPAP is often indicated and can be successful with behavioral support.
3. Pulmonary, cardiovascular, skeletal, neurologic, and behavioral comorbidities can overlap with the symptoms of, or influence the severity of, OSAS and should be considered when evaluating and treating a patient with Down syndrome.
4. All caregivers of children with Down syndrome should have a high index of suspicion for OSAS.

REFERENCES

1. Down JL. Observations on an ethnic classification of idiots. 1866. *Ment Retard.* Feb 1995;33(1):54–56.
2. Parker SE, Mai CT, Canfield MA, et al. Updated National Birth Prevalence estimates for selected birth defects in the United States, 2004-2006. *Birth Defects Res A Clin Mol Teratol.* Dec 2010;88(12):1008–1016.
3. de Miguel-Diez J, Alvarez-Sala JL, Villa-Asensi JR. Magnetic resonance imaging of the upper airway in children with Down syndrome. *Am J Respir Crit Care Med.* Apr 15 2002;165(8):1187. author reply 1187.
4. de Miguel-Diez J, Villa-Asensi JR, Alvarez-Sala JL. Prevalence of sleep-disordered breathing in children with Down syndrome: polygraphic findings in 108 children. *Sleep.* Dec 15 2003;26(8):1006–1009.
5. Churchill SS, Kieckhefer GM, Landis CA, Ward TM. Sleep measurement and monitoring in children with Down syndrome: a review of the literature, 1960-2010. *Sleep Med Rev.* Oct 2012;16(5):477–488.
6. Trois MS, Capone GT, Lutz JA, et al. Obstructive sleep apnea in adults with Down syndrome. *J Clin Sleep Med.* Aug 15 2009;5(4):317–323.
7. Lin SC, Davey MJ, Horne RS, Nixon GM. Screening for obstructive sleep apnea in children with Down syndrome. *J Pediatr.* Jul 2014;165(1):117–122.
8. Goffinski A, Stanley MA, Shepherd N, et al. Obstructive sleep apnea in young infants with Down syndrome evaluated in a Down syndrome specialty clinic. *Am J Med Genet A.* Feb 2015;167A(2):324–330.
9. Winell J, Burke SW. Sports participation of children with Down syndrome. *Orthop Clin North Am.* Jul 2003;34(3):439–443.
10. Shete MM, Stocks RM, Sebelik ME, Schoumacher RA. Effects of adeno-tonsillectomy on polysomnography patterns in Down syndrome children with obstructive sleep apnea: a comparative study with children without Down syndrome. *Int J Pediatr Otorhinolaryngol.* Mar 2010;74(3):241–244.
11. Merrell JA, Shott SR. OSAS in Down syndrome: T&A versus T&A plus lateral pharyngoplasty. *Int J Pediatr Otorhinolaryngol.* Aug 2007;71(8):1197–1203.
12. Marcus CL, Beck SE, Traylor J, et al. Randomized, double-blind clinical trial of two different modes of positive airway pressure therapy on adherence and efficacy in children. *J Clin Sleep Med.* Feb 15 2012;8(1):37–42.
13. Rosen D, Lombardo A, Skotko B, Davidson EJ. Parental perceptions of sleep disturbances and sleep-disordered breathing in children with Down syndrome. *Clin Pediatr (Phila).* Feb 2011;50(2):121–125.
14. Bull MJ. Health supervision for children with Down syndrome. *Pediatrics.* Aug 2011;128(2):393–406.

An 18-month-old with snoring and achondroplasia

Lourdes M. DelRosso

CASE PRESENTATION

An 18-month-old male with achondroplasia presented for evaluation of snoring. The parents had noticed loud snoring, gasping, breathing pauses, mouth breathing, and neck hyperextension for the last 2 months. The family denied symptoms of parasomnias. He was born full term via cesarean section without complications from a 29-year-old G3P1 mother. He did not have any other medical problems and did not take any medications.

PHYSICAL EXAM

Physical exam revealed vital signs within normal limits. His weight was 9.505 kg (9th percentile on the Centers for Disease Control and Prevention growth chart), height 68.8 cm (31st percentile on achondroplasia growth chart), and head circumference 51 cm (15th percentile based on achondroplasia growth chart). The patient appeared comfortable and in no distress. Facial features demonstrated frontal bossing and macrocephaly. The oropharynx was Mallampati score IV, and the tonsil size was 3+. Cardiopulmonary exam was normal. Musculoskeletal exam revealed rhizomelia. There was no evidence of kyphosis or lordosis. Neurologic exam revealed normal patellar reflexes with no evidence of clonus and no hypotonia (Fig. 56-1).

LABORATORY AND SLEEP FINDINGS

Polysomnography (PSG) revealed a total sleep time (TST) of 343 minutes; total recording time of 406 minutes; sleep efficiency of 84%; and arousal index of 37/h. The obstructive apnea–hypopnea index was 41.6/h. The central apnea index was 8.4/h. SpO_2 nadir was 71%. The time with end-tidal CO_2 above 50 torr was 68% of TST.

QUESTION

What is the next step in the management of this patient's severe obstructive sleep apnea syndrome (OSAS)?

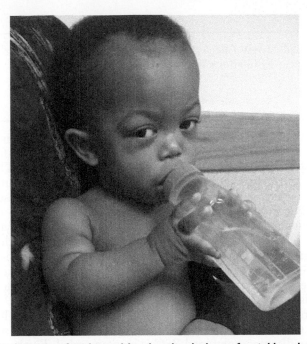

FIGURE 56-1 ■ Characteristic features of patient with achondroplasia are frontal bossing, midface hypoplasia, and rhizomelia.

ANSWER

Tonsillectomy and adenoidectomy (T&A), magnetic resonance imaging for evaluation of foramen magnum stenosis, and repeat PSG after surgery.

DISCUSSION

Achondroplasia is an autosomal dominant condition caused by a mutation in the fibroblast growth factor receptor 3; however, 80% of cases are sporadic. The prevalence is 1:30,000 live births. There is underdevelopment of the long bones formed by endochondral ossification. The main manifestations are short stature, short limbs (rhizomelia), hypotonia, midface hypoplasia, and frontal bossing. The diagnosis is made based on clinical findings, radiologic findings, or genetic testing.[1]

Patients with achondroplasia are at higher risk of OSAS (prevalence up to 32%). Contributing factors include midface hypoplasia with a narrowed nasopharyngeal space, hypotonia, and brainstem compression. Symptoms of sleep-disordered breathing and physical exam of the oropharynx correlate poorly with polysomnographic findings.[2,3] Nocturnal hypoxemia with or without hypoventilation has been reported in up to 44% of affected children. The mechanism may be due to a small thorax with mild restrictive lung disease, thoracolumbar kyphosis (reported in up to 90% of infants with achondroplasia), and hypotonia.[4,5]

Patients with achondroplasia are at risk of craniocervical stenosis, and 35% have been found to have cervicomedullary compression. This can result in central apnea. Evaluation with imaging (magnetic resonance or computerized tomography) and PSG is recommended. Further, 60% of children with achondroplasia have been found to have central apnea on PSG. Note that long central apneas may be a manifestation of brainstem compression, whereas short central apneas with desaturation are probably a manifestation of decreased pulmonary reserve. Imaging of the cervical region may show decreased transverse and sagittal dimensions of the foramen magnum, with or without spinal cord compression. Indications for foramen magnum decompression surgery include signs of upper neuron involvement (clonus and hyperreflexia), central sleep apnea on PSG, or evidence of spinal cord compression on imaging studies. Surgical intervention is controversial in cases of asymptomatic children with a small foramen magnum.[6]

Management of patients with achondroplasia should include a multidisciplinary team with input from pediatrics, sleep medicine, neurology, orthopedics, neurosurgery, and genetics, as appropriate. OSAS may not resolve with T&A, and noninvasive positive pressure ventilation may be needed.[3]

CLINICAL PEARLS

1. Patients with achondroplasia are at higher risk of OSAS.
2. Patients with achondroplasia are at higher risk of central apnea because of cervicomedullary compression.
3. Patients with achondroplasia are at higher risk of nocturnal hypoxemia, with or without hypoventilation, because of thoracolumbar kyphosis, a small thorax, and hypotonia.

REFERENCES

1. Pauli RM. Achondroplasia. In: Pagon RA, Adam MP, Ardinger HH, et al., eds. *GeneReviews(R)*. Seattle, WA: University of Washington; 1993.
2. Afsharpaiman S, Sillence DO, Sheikhvatan M, Ault JE, Waters K. Respiratory events and obstructive sleep apnea in children with achondroplasia: investigation and treatment outcomes. *Sleep Breath*. Dec 2011;15(4):755–761.
3. Julliand S, Boule M, Baujat G, et al. Lung function, diagnosis, and treatment of sleep-disordered breathing in children with achondroplasia. *Am J Med Genet A*. Aug 2012;158A(8):1987–1993.
4. Mogayzel Jr PJ, Carroll JL, Loughlin GM, Hurko O, Francomano CA, Marcus CL. Sleep-disordered breathing in children with achondroplasia. *J Pediatr*. Apr 1998;132(4):667–671.
5. DelRosso LM, Gonzalez-Toledo E, Hoque R. A three-month-old achondroplastic baby with both obstructive apneas and central apneas. *J Clin Sleep Med*. Mar 15 2013;9(3):287–289.
6. King JA, Vachhrajani S, Drake JM, Rutka JT. Neurosurgical implications of achondroplasia. *J Neurosurg Pediatr*. Oct 2009;4(4):297–306.

A 9-month-old girl with Pfeiffer syndrome and snoring

Lourdes M. DelRosso

CASE PRESENTATION

A 9-month-old female was referred for evaluation of snoring. The parent reported that the child had been snoring for 2 months. The patient was born full term, via normal spontaneous vaginal delivery without perinatal complications. The patient was diagnosed with Pfeiffer syndrome and hydrocephalus and was hospitalized for observation. During the admission, there was no evidence of snoring, apnea, bradycardia, or oxyhemoglobin desaturation.

Her surgical history included sagittal sinusectomy at 2 months of age and posterior vault distraction at 7 months of age. Medications included acetazolamide and eye lubricant drops. Review of systems was negative for dysphagia and positive for eye dryness, snoring, and global developmental delay.

PHYSICAL EXAM

The patient is shown in Figures 57-1 and 57-2. Her vital signs were normal, her weight was at the 12th percentile, and her length was at the 47th percentile. The physical exam revealed macrocephaly and proptosis. The auditory canals were small and narrow with tympanic membranes not visible. She had a high-arched palate, and there was no visible tonsil tissue. The remainder of the exam was normal.

LABORATORY AND SLEEP FINDINGS

Polysomnography revealed a sleep efficiency of 97%. The arousal index was 16.4/h. The obstructive apnea–hypopnea index (AHI) was 20/h. The central AHI was 0.1/h. The SpO_2 nadir was 79%, and the end-tidal CO_2 was >50 torr for 8% of total sleep time.

QUESTIONS

What features in Pfeiffer syndrome increase the risk of obstructive sleep apnea syndrome (OSAS)?

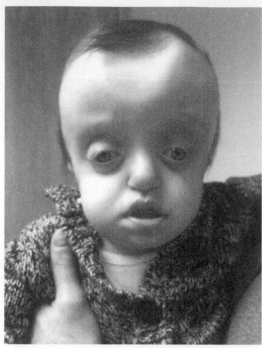

FIGURE 57-1 ■ **Frontal view.** Note macrocephaly and the typical features of Pfeiffer syndrome (proptosis and hypertelorism).

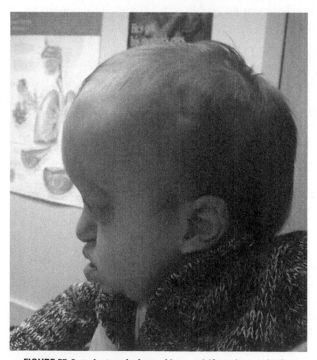

FIGURE 57-2 ■ **Lateral view.** Note midface hypoplasia.

ANSWERS

Midface hypoplasia is the main feature in Pfeiffer syndrome that predisposes patients to OSAS. Other features present in our patient include high-arched palate and increased intracranial pressure.

DISCUSSION

Craniosynostosis syndromes such as Pfeiffer syndrome are characterized by premature fusion of the cranial sutures restricting the normal growth of the skull and facial bones. Pfeiffer syndrome is an autosomal dominant craniosynostosis syndrome caused by several mutations in the fibroblast growth factor receptors 1 and 2 (FGFR1 and FGFR2). A mutation in FGFR2 has also been identified in other craniosynostosis syndromes (Apert and Crouzon). Pfeiffer syndrome has an incidence of 1/100,000 live births. The clinical presentation is variable, but the most common features are broad high forehead, midface hypoplasia, hypertelorism with proptosis, flat nose, and high-arched palate. Limb abnormalities include radially deviated broad toes and partial syndactyly of hands and feet. Increased intracranial pressure, Chiari malformation, and hydrocephalus have been reported. Annual fundoscopic exam for evaluation of papilledema is recommended, and if present, computed tomography or magnetic resonance imaging is recommended.[1,2]

OSAS has been reported in 40% to 85% of children with craniosynostosis syndromes.[3] The cause of OSAS in these children is multifactorial, but the main contributors are midface hypoplasia and central nervous system abnormalities (increased intracranial pressure). Children may develop OSAS at a later age (often during the preschool years) because of growth of adenotonsillar tissue within the constricted skeletal space. The natural course of OSAS in these patients is unknown. In a longitudinal study of 97 children with various craniosynostosis syndromes, children with Apert, Crouzon, and Pfeiffer syndromes had the highest AHI and were least likely to improve over time without intervention.[4] Children with Pfeiffer syndrome have been shown to have more severe OSAS than patients with Crouzon and Apert syndrome do. One study has shown that OSAS may not improve after tonsillectomy and adenoidectomy (T&A) in these patients, likely because of the multiple levels of obstruction and central nervous system involvement.[3]

Early intervention (within the first year of life) with vault expansion may prevent brain damage. This surgery does not affect the fronto-orbital area. Midface advancement (monobloc or Le Font III with distraction) is recommended at an older age (>4 years old) or earlier if severe OSAS or exophthalmos is present. Midface advancement does not always improve the sleep-disordered breathing. Other options for treatment include continuous positive airway pressure and maxillary and mandibular advancements.[5]

CLINICAL PEARLS
1. Patients with craniosynostosis syndromes (Pfeiffer, Crouzon, and Apert) are at high risk of OSAS.
2. The main clinical contributors to OSAS are midface hypoplasia and increased intracranial pressure.
3. Surgical procedures (T&A and distraction) improve OSAS but are not always curative. Close monitoring is recommended.

REFERENCES

1. Junior HM, de Aquino SN, Machado RA, Leao LL, Coletta RD, Burle-Aguiar MJ. Pfeiffer syndrome: clinical and genetic findings in five Brazilian families. *Med Oral Patol Oral Cir Bucal*. 2015;20(1):e52–e58.
2. Kalathia MB, Parikh YN, Dhami MD, Hapani PT. Pfeiffer syndrome. *J Pediatr Neurosci*. Jan 2014;9(1):85–86.
3. Zandieh SO, Padwa BL, Katz ES. Adenotonsillectomy for obstructive sleep apnea in children with syndromic craniosynostosis. *Plast Reconstr Surg*. Apr 2013;131(4):847–852.
4. Driessen C, Joosten KF, Bannink N, et al. How does obstructive sleep apnoea evolve in syndromic craniosynostosis? A prospective cohort study. *Arch Dis Child*. Jul 2013;98(7):538–543.
5. de Jong T, Bannink N, Bredero-Boelhouwer HH, et al. Long-term functional outcome in 167 patients with syndromic craniosynostosis; defining a syndrome-specific risk profile. *J Plast Reconstr Aesthet Surg*. Oct 2010;63(10):1635–1641.

A 3-year-old girl with Prader-Willi syndrome and obesity

Lourdes M. DelRosso

CASE PRESENTATION

A 3-year-old female with Prader-Willi syndrome (PWS) presented for growth hormone supplementation after tonsillectomy and adenoidectomy (T&A) for severe obstructive sleep apnea (OSA). Initial polysomnography (PSG) revealed severe obstructive sleep apnea syndrome (OSAS). She underwent T&A. The parents reported that she used to snore very loudly, but the snoring had resolved after T&A. The parents did not express concern with the patient's sleep patterns. The patient went to bed at 9 PM, slept through the night, and woke up spontaneously at 8 AM. During the day, she did not take naps and did not have symptoms of daytime sleepiness.

There was no other pertinent medical history or surgical history. She did not take any medications. Review of systems was positive for global hypotonia and inability to walk and negative for cough, shortness of breath, swallowing difficulties, and gastroesophageal reflux.

PHYSICAL EXAM

The child is shown in Figure 58-1. Physical exam revealed an obese girl, sleeping comfortably without snoring or increased work of breathing. Her vital signs were within normal range. Her weight was 31 kg (100th percentile), and her height was 97.2 cm (65th percentile). She did not have a high-arched palate, oropharyngeal Mallampati grade was IV, and tonsil size was 0. Her lungs were clear to auscultation. Neurologic exam revealed global hypotonia.

LABORATORY AND SLEEP FINDINGS

Thyroid-stimulating hormone, blood count, electrolytes, and morning cortisol levels were within the normal range.

Preoperative PSG: total sleep time (TST) 406 minutes; obstructive apnea–hypopnea index (AHI) 133/h; central AHI 0.1/h; SpO_2 nadir 68%; and $ETCO_2$ >50 torr for 49% of TST.

QUESTIONS

What is the next step in the evaluation and management of this patient?

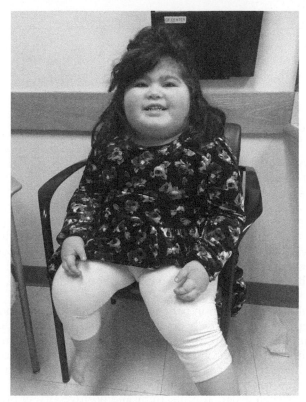

FIGURE 58-1 ■ Patient with Prader-Willi syndrome and obesity.

ANSWERS

The patient is at high risk for residual OSAS because of PWS, obesity, and severe OSA before T&A. Growth hormone is contraindicated in the presence of severe OSA. Post T&A PSG is indicated in this case, before beginning growth hormone therapy.

DISCUSSION

PWS is a genetic disorder that affects approximately 1 in 10,000 to 20,000 children. Of PWS occurrences, 75% are caused by a deletion of the paternal proximal long arm of chromosome 15 (15q11-13), and 25% are caused by maternal disomy, where both chromosomes 15 are derived from the mother. PWS affects boys and girls equally. Newborns and infants with PWS typically present with hypogonadism, severe hypotonia, weak cry, and feeding difficulties. Common subtle facial characteristics include almond-shaped eyes, strabismus, and narrow skull diameter (see Fig. 58-1). Young children (1 to 5 years old) typically present with hyperphagia and rapid weight gain. Older children and adolescents present with delayed puberty, sleep disorders, and complications of obesity (diabetes and hypertension). Adults with PWS present with multiple comorbidities, including hypothyroidism, osteoporosis, pulmonary hypertension, seizure disorder, scoliosis, skin lesions, and mild-to-moderate intellectual disability.[1-4]

Sleep-disordered breathing is common in patients with PWS with or without obesity and can be manifested as central sleep apnea, OSA, or hypoventilation. The mechanism is likely multifactorial, but hypotonia, hypothalamic dysfunction, brainstem immaturity, and abnormal chemosensitivity to CO_2 and O_2 are the main contributors. Infants usually present with both central and obstructive apnea, whereas older children present predominantly with OSA. The central apneas are usually short but associated with desaturation because of decreased pulmonary reserve and have been successfully treated with supplemental oxygen. Adenotonsillectomy and positive airway pressure ventilation continue to be the main treatment options for OSA and hypoventilation.[5,6]

Excessive daytime sleepiness independent of obesity and sleep-disordered breathing has been reported in patients with PWS. Sleep-onset REM periods and cataplexy have also been reported.[7,8] The presence of a sleep latency of <8 minutes and 2 or more sleep-onset REM findings in a Multiple Sleep Latency Test fit *International Classification of Sleep Disorders*, third edition (ICSD-3) diagnostic criteria for narcolepsy. The excessive daytime sleepiness is likely due to hypothalamic dysfunction. A few studies have found decreased levels of hypocretin in the cerebrospinal fluid of patients with PWS, and excessive sleepiness,[9] although a postmortem study in seven patients with PWS did not find a decreased number of hypocretin-producing neurons in the hypothalamus.[10] Modafinil has been reported to improve sleepiness.[11]

Further, 40% to 100% patients with PWS have growth hormone deficiency. Growth hormone supplementation has been shown to improve linear growth, muscle mass, strength, bone density, lipid profile, and cognitive function. However, there has been a temporal association between growth hormone and sudden death during sleep in a few cases. Contraindications to growth hormone supplementation include severe untreated OSAS and severe obesity. PSG should be obtained in all patients before growth hormone initiation. T&A should be pursued if OSA is present as growth hormone supplementation can further stimulate tonsillar and adenoid hypertrophy. PSG should be repeated at 6 weeks, 3 months, and 6 months after growth hormone initiation. Growth hormone should be discontinued if apnea or upper airway obstruction develops after initiation of treatment.[1,12]

CLINICAL PEARLS

1. Patients with PWS are at high risk of sleep-disordered breathing: central sleep apnea, OSA, and central hypoventilation.
2. Patients with PWS are at high risk of excessive sleepiness and narcolepsy.
3. A sleep study must be done before growth hormone treatment and at 6 weeks, 3 months, and 6 months after initiation of growth hormone.

REFERENCES

1. Aycan Z, Bas VN. Prader-Willi syndrome and growth hormone deficiency. *J Clin Res Pediatr Endocrinol*. 2014;6(2):62–67.
2. Emerick JE, Vogt KS. Endocrine manifestations and management of Prader-Willi syndrome. *Int J Pediatr Endocrinol*. 2013;2013(1):14.
3. Laurier V, Lapeyrade A, Copet P, et al. Medical, psychological and social features in a large cohort of adults with Prader-Willi syndrome: experience from a dedicated centre in France. *J Intellect Disabil Res*. May 2015;59(5):411–421.
4. Urquhart DS, Gulliver T, Williams G, Harris MA, Nyunt O, Suresh S. Central sleep-disordered breathing and the effects of oxygen therapy in infants with Prader-Willi syndrome. *Arch Dis Child*. Aug 2013;98(8):592–595.
5. Cohen M, Hamilton J, Narang I. Clinically important age-related differences in sleep related disordered breathing in infants and children with Prader-Willi syndrome. *PLoS One*. 2014;9(6):e101012.
6. Sedky K, Bennett DS, Pumariega A. Prader Willi syndrome and obstructive sleep apnea: co-occurrence in the pediatric population. *J Clin Sleep Med*. Apr 15 2014;10(4):403–409.
7. Weselake SV, Foulds JL, Couch R, Witmans MB, Rubin D, Haqq AM. Prader-Willi syndrome, excessive daytime sleepiness, and narcoleptic symptoms: a case report. *J Med Case Rep*. 2014;8:127.
8. Manni R, Politini L, Nobili L, et al. Hypersomnia in the Prader Willi syndrome: clinical-electrophysiological features and underlying factors. *Clin Neurophysiol*. May 2001;112(5):800–805.
9. Nevsimalova S, Vankova J, Stepanova I, Seemanova E, Mignot E, Nishino S. Hypocretin deficiency in Prader-Willi syndrome. *Eur J Neurol*. Jan 2005;12(1):70–72.
10. Fronczek R, Lammers GJ, Balesar R, Unmehopa UA, Swaab DF. The number of hypothalamic hypocretin (orexin) neurons is not affected in Prader-Willi syndrome. *J Clin Endocrinol Metab*. Sep 2005;90(9):5466–5470.
11. De Cock VC, Dicne G, Molinas C, et al. Efficacy of modafinil on excessive daytime sleepiness in Prader-Willi syndrome. *Am J Med Genet A*. Jul 2011;155A(7):1552–1557.
12. Berini J, Spica Russotto V, Castelnuovo P, et al. Growth hormone therapy and respiratory disorders: long-term follow-up in PWS children. *J Clin Endocrinol Metab*. Sep 2013;98(9):E1516–E1523.

A 12-day-old infant with Pierre Robin sequence and difficulty breathing

Lourdes M. DelRosso

CASE PRESENTATION

A 12-day-old infant was referred for inpatient polysomnography (PSG) during her neonatal intensive care unit admission for evaluation of labored breathing. The infant was born via normal spontaneous vaginal delivery at 40-weeks gestational age. Soon after birth, the infant was found to have cleft palate, micrognathia, and glossoptosis. She was diagnosed with Pierre Robin sequence (PRS).

PHYSICAL EXAM

Physical exam revealed an infant with micrognathia (Fig. 59-1). Her vital signs were normal. Her weight was 3.175 kg (45th percentile), length was 48 cm (10th percentile), and head circumference was 35 cm (60th percentile). Her eyes, ears, and nose were normal. Oral exam revealed a U-shaped cleft palate. Her lungs were clear to auscultation bilaterally, with normal work of breathing while awake and no wheezes, crackles, or rhonchi. Neurologic exam was normal.

LABORATORY AND SLEEP FINDINGS

PSG revealed a total sleep time of 403 minutes, total recording time of 500 minutes, and sleep efficiency of 80%. The obstructive apnea–hypopnea index (AHI) was 60.1/h; the SpO_2 nadir was 78%; and peak end-tidal CO_2 was 59 torr. There were no central events.

QUESTION

What are the treatment options for this patient?

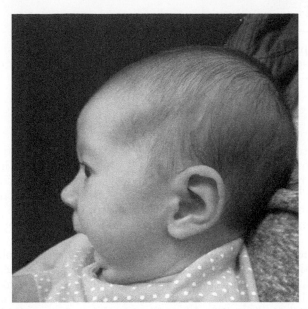

FIGURE 59-1 ■ **Patient with PRS.** Note the micrognathia. (Courtesy of Dr. Christopher Cielo, Pulmonary Medicine, The Children's Hospital of Philadelphia.)

ANSWER

Treatment options for patients with PRS and severe obstructive sleep apnea syndrome (OSAS) include prone positioning, nasopharyngeal airway, tongue-lip adhesion, mandibular distraction osteogenesis, and tracheostomy.

DISCUSSION

PRS has been described as a group of clinical findings that include the triad micrognathia, glossoptosis, and airway obstruction. Cleft palate, often present, is not found in all patients with PRS. The wide variation in reported incidence (1:5000 to 1:80,000) may be secondary to the variability in clinical presentation.[1] Infants with PRS are at increased risk of other anomalies including cardiac, pulmonary, and gastrointestinal abnormalities. Children with PRS who also present with cardiac and pulmonary anomalies have been found to be at increased risk of death compared with children with PRS alone.[2]

Respiratory difficulties can be seen from birth because of oropharyngeal obstruction. The obstruction appears to be multifactorial; however, the main contributor is the posterior displacement of the tongue secondary to micrognathia and retrognathia. The upper airway obstruction may improve from childhood to adulthood as the upper airway grows[3]; however, treatment is needed in the interim to prevent sequelae of OSAS. Feeding difficulties are common in infants with PRS and may persist after correction of the airway obstruction. Gastroesophageal motility disorders and gastroesophageal reflux appear to be contributing factors.[1]

Treatment options are chosen depending on the degree of airway obstruction. Mild obstruction may be relieved with prone positioning or with a nasal or oral airway. Options for management of severe obstruction include nasopharyngeal airway, tongue-lip adhesion, mandibular distraction osteogenesis, and tracheostomy. Tongue-lip adhesion should be reserved for infants with obstruction at the base of the tongue only and is performed less commonly than in the past. Mandibular distraction consists of surgically dividing the mandible and then improving oropharyngeal obstruction by turning screws daily to slowly move sections of the mandible apart and allow bone to fill in the gap (8 to 12 weeks). This procedure has been shown to result in significant improvement in the AHI, gas exchange, and growth, although potential reported side effects may include facial nerve injury, damage to tooth buds, and temporomandibular ankylosis (Fig. 59-2). Tracheostomy is typically reserved for children with life-threatening airway obstruction.

Infants with PRS can benefit from evaluation by a multidisciplinary team that includes plastic surgery, otolaryngology, gastroenterology, speech pathology, genetics, and sleep medicine (Fig. 59-3).

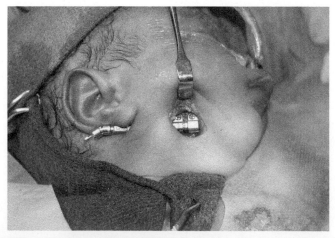

FIGURE 59-2 ■ **Surgical incision reveals mandibular distractor in place.** (Courtesy of Dr. Jesse A. Taylor, Director, Center for Facial Reconstruction, The Children's Hospital of Philadelphia.)

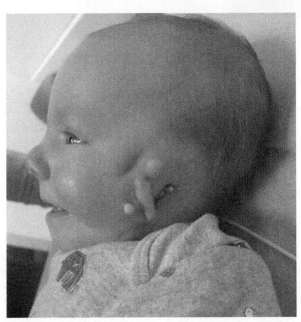

FIGURE 59-3 ■ Six weeks after surgery, the distractor is not visible except for small rods that protrude from behind the mandible, as seen in the picture. (Courtesy of Dr. Jesse A. Taylor, Director, Center for Facial Reconstruction, The Children's Hospital of Philadelphia.)

CLINICAL PEARLS

1. PRS consists of the triad of micrognathia, glossoptosis, and airway obstruction.
2. Infants with PRS are at increased risk of oropharyngeal obstruction and feeding difficulties.
3. There are several surgical procedures available to improve the airway obstruction, including tongue-lip adhesion, mandibular distraction osteogenesis, and tracheostomy.

REFERENCES

1. Cladis F, Kumar A, Grunwaldt L, Otteson T, Ford M, Losee JE. Pierre Robin sequence: a perioperative review. *Anesth Analg.* Aug 2014;119(2):400–412.
2. Costa MA, Tu MM, Murage KP, Tholpady SS, Engle WA, Flores RL. Robin sequence: mortality, causes of death, and clinical outcomes. *Plast Reconstr Surg.* Oct 2014;134(4):738–745.
3. Staudt CB, Gnoinski WM, Peltomaki T. Upper airway changes in Pierre Robin sequence from childhood to adulthood. *Orthod Craniofac Res.* Nov 2013;16(4):202–213.

A 12-year-old girl with Williams syndrome and frequent nocturnal awakenings

Lourdes M. DelRosso

CASE PRESENTATION

A 12-year-old female with Williams syndrome presented for evaluation of snoring and frequent nocturnal awakenings. The parents reported soft snoring without gasping or witnessed apneas. Her bedtime routine started around 8:00 PM and included taking a bath, brushing her teeth, changing into pajamas, and reading. She usually fell asleep within 60 minutes. During the night, she woke up 3 to 4 times but was able to fall asleep independently within 15 to 30 minutes. She usually got up at 7:00 AM. The family noted excessive daytime sleepiness, difficulty concentrating, and irritability. There was no history of cataplexy, hypnagogic hallucinations, or sleep paralysis. The patient denied symptoms of restless legs or parasomnias.

The patient was born full term without complications. Her past medical history included Williams syndrome, mitral valve regurgitation, attention-deficit hyperactivity disorder (ADHD), and scoliosis. Her past surgical history included tonsillectomy and adenoidectomy at age 4. Her medications included amphetamine and dextroamphetamine 10 mg once a day. Review of systems was positive for strabismus and global developmental delay.

PHYSICAL EXAM

Her vital signs were within normal limits, and her height and weight were both at the 9th percentile. The physical exam revealed a cooperative and cheerful girl with distinctive facial features. She had a narrow face, flattened nasal bridge, and strabismus (Fig. 60-1). The oropharynx was Mallampati class II, and tonsils were surgically absent. She had mild scoliosis. The remainder of the cardiovascular and neurologic exam was normal.

LABORATORY AND SLEEP FINDINGS

Polysomnography (PSG) revealed a total recording time of 560 minutes with a total sleep time (TST) of 423 minutes. Sleep efficiency was 76%. Sleep onset latency was 82 minutes. Arousal index was 14/h. The obstructive apnea–hypopnea index (AHI) was 11/h. The central AHI was 1/h. SpO_2 nadir was 88%. The periodic leg movement index was 4/hr. (PLMI) were 4/h. The end-tidal CO_2 was below 50 torr for 100% of TST.

QUESTION

What sleep complaints are common in patients with Williams syndrome?

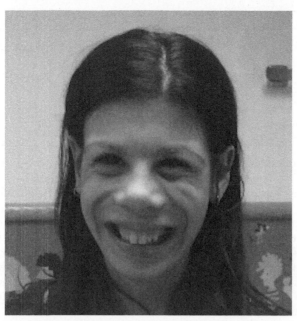

FIGURE 60-1 ■ Typical facial features of a patient with Williams syndrome.

ANSWER

Sleep complaints in children with Williams syndrome include bedtime resistance, shorter night sleep, and sleep anxiety. PSG findings have revealed sleep fragmentation and decreased sleep efficiency. Patients with Williams syndrome are also at increased risk of obstructive sleep apnea syndrome (OSAS).

DISCUSSION

Williams syndrome is a genetic disorder caused by a deletion of approximately 25 genes in the region q11,23 of chromosome 7. The prevalence is estimated to be 1:7500. The majority of cases are sporadic. Physical findings include a distinctive facial appearance commonly called elfin facies (broad forehead, low-set ears, short nose with broad tip, and wide mouth with full lips), small teeth, and strabismus (see Fig. 60-1). Connective tissue abnormalities are common and include cardiovascular complications (supravalvular aortic stenosis and supravalvular pulmonary stenosis), joint hypermobility, soft lax skin, lordosis, scoliosis, and hypotonia. Other complications that may persist through adulthood include hyperacusis, hypercalcemia, hypertension, and gastroesophageal reflux disease. Sudden death has been reported in children with Williams syndrome in association with anesthetic administration. The American Academy of Pediatrics recommends pediatric anesthesia consultation for any child with Williams syndrome referred for surgery.[1]

Children with Williams syndrome usually present with a distinctive cognitive and behavioral profile characterized by visuospatial deficits and relative strength in language development. ADHD is diagnosed in 65% of patients, and mental retardation is diagnosed in about 75% of patients. Although patients with Williams syndrome demonstrate increased sociability and friendliness, they also have increased anxiety and worries.

Sleep complaints are very common in children with Williams syndrome. Parents report bedtime resistance, shorter night sleep, sleep anxiety, and more night waking compared with typically developing children.[2,3] PSG in affected patients has been consistent with increased sleep fragmentation and decreased sleep efficiency. In a study of 35 affected patients, the obstructive AHI was increased as compared with controls. Sleep stage distribution has shown increased slow-wave sleep and decreased REM sleep. The PLMI has not been consistently elevated.[4,5]

A study in 25 children with Williams syndrome found increased bedtime cortisol levels and a decreased rise in melatonin.[6] Therapeutic melatonin supplementation has not been studied in this patient population.

Our patient was initiated on melatonin 3 mg at 8:30 PM. Sleep onset latency improved to 30 minutes. Her obstructive sleep apnea was successfully treated with continuous positive airway pressure.

CLINICAL PEARLS

1. Patients with Williams syndrome can have increased sleep-related anxiety and bedtime resistance.
2. Melatonin may help with delayed sleep onset, but its use has not been studied.
3. Patients with Williams syndrome may be at increased risk of OSAS.
4. The Academy of Pediatrics recommends pediatric anesthesia evaluation for all patients with Williams syndrome undergoing surgery.

REFERENCES

1. Committee on Genetics. American Academy of Pediatrics: health care supervision for children with Williams syndrome. *Pediatrics*. May 2001;107(5):1192–1204.
2. Axelsson EL, Hill CM, Sadeh A, Dimitriou D. Sleep problems and language development in toddlers with Williams syndrome. *Res Dev Disabil*. Nov 2013;34(11):3988–3996.
3. Annaz D, Hill CM, Ashworth A, Holley S, Karmiloff-Smith A. Characterisation of sleep problems in children with Williams syndrome. *Res Dev Disabil*. Jan-Feb 2011;32(1):164–169.
4. Mason TB, Arens R, Sharman J, et al. Sleep in children with Williams syndrome. *Sleep Med*. Oct 2011;12(9):892–897.
5. Gombos F, Bodizs R, Kovacs I. Atypical sleep architecture and altered EEG spectra in Williams syndrome. *J Intellect Disabil Res*. Mar 2011;55(3):255–262.
6. Sniecinska-Cooper AM, Iles RK, Butler SA, Jones H, Bayford R, Dimitriou D. Abnormal secretion of melatonin and cortisol in relation to sleep disturbances in children with Williams syndrome. *Sleep Med*. Jan 2015;16(1):94–100. Epub Sep 19 2014.

A 9-year-old female with Joubert syndrome and breath-holding spells

Lourdes M. DelRosso

CASE PRESENTATION

A 9-year-old female with Joubert syndrome presented with breath-holding spells. Her mother witnessed breath-holding episodes since birth but noted an increased frequency in the last year. The episodes worsened during periods of excitement, with rare reported episodes of lip cyanosis. The mother did not report any problems during sleep; she denied snoring, gasping, witnessed apneas, restless legs, or parasomnias.

The patient was born via normal spontaneous vaginal delivery to a 27-year-old G4P3 mother. She was discharged home on an apnea monitor, which was discontinued at 9 months. The patient's past medical history included Joubert syndrome (common clinical presentation included ataxia, hypotonia, and nystagmus), mental retardation, and global developmental delay. Surgical history was positive for gastrostomy tube placement and eye surgery for ptosis and strabismus. Review of systems was positive for primary enuresis (wears diapers) and ataxia (walks with a walker) and negative for asthma, loss of consciousness, or seizures.

PHYSICAL EXAM

The girl was alert and in no distress. She was nonverbal but followed simple commands. Her respiratory rate ranged from 10 to 28 breaths/min. SpO_2 was 99%. Her weight was at the 33rd percentile, and her height at the 40th percentile. She exhibited horizontal nystagmus bilaterally, more pronounced on lateral gaze. She did not have a high-arched palate; oropharyngeal Mallampati grade was III, and tonsil size was 1+. Her lungs were clear to auscultation. There was global hypotonia. She was able to sit and stand. Gait was ataxic.

LABORATORY AND SLEEP FINDINGS

Brain magnetic resonance imaging (MRI) (Fig. 61-1).

Polysomnography (PSG) showed periods of tachypnea followed by central apnea, while awake and during sleep (Fig. 61-2). The sleep efficiency was 64% (normal is >85%). The central apnea index was 24/h. The obstructive apnea index was 1.7/h. SpO_2 nadir was 82%.

QUESTION

How would you treat this child's breathing pattern during sleep?

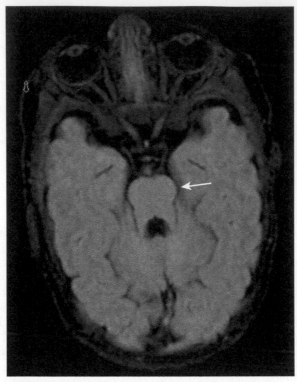

FIGURE 61-1 ■ Axial MRI of the brain reveals "molar tooth" anomaly (*arrow*).

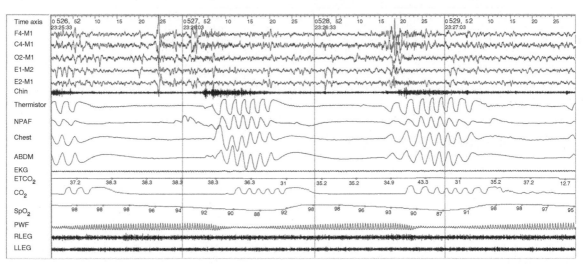

FIGURE 61-2 ■ PSG fragment: a 120-second epoch during N2 showing periodic breathing associated with desaturation.

ANSWER

Assisted noninvasive ventilation with either bilevel positive airway pressure (BPAP) or adaptive servo ventilation (ASV).

DISCUSSION

Joubert syndrome is a rare, heterogeneous, autosomal-recessive disorder with an estimated incidence of 1:80,000 live births. The main abnormalities are agenesis of the cerebellar vermis and failure of decussation in the superior cerebellar peduncles and pyramidal tracts. The clinical presentation includes ataxia, hypotonia, nystagmus, and mental retardation. The mutation affects at least 10 different genes, including NPHP1, AHI1, and CEP290. Some of the affected genes code for a protein of primary cilia in the retina, renal tubules, and neural cell migration. Patients with retinal dysplasia usually have renal disease and have a worse prognosis, and, therefore, ocular screening is recommended in all children with Joubert syndrome. Other features of the syndrome include polydactyly, thyroid dysfunction, and congenital hepatic fibrosis. On MRI of the brain, the diagnostic "molar tooth sign" is created by a thickened superior cerebellar peduncle, widened interpeduncular fossa, and enlarged fourth ventricle (see Fig. 61-1).[1,2]

A typical respiratory pattern of tachypnea followed by central apnea has been seen in up to 71% of patients with Joubert syndrome and is thought to be secondary to involvement of the respiratory centers in the brainstem. Tachypnea of up to 230 breaths/min has been reported. Subsequent central apnea has been seen during both sleep and wakefulness. Periodic breathing and obstructive sleep apnea syndrome have been reported; the latter thought to be associated with hypotonia, large tongue, and obesity.[3,4]

Patients with Joubert syndrome need close evaluation of breathing patterns because prolonged apneas can require assisted ventilation. Newborns and infants are particularly at risk of life-threatening apneic events, but breathing abnormalities can persist beyond childhood.[5] Nocturnal PSG is indicated. Treatment of sleep-disordered breathing has not been thoroughly studied, but case reports have used BPAP and ASV with varying degrees of success.[3]

CLINICAL PEARLS

1. Patients with Joubert syndrome may have periodic breathing while awake and asleep.
2. Patients with Joubert syndrome may be at risk for obstructive apnea.
3. Treatment with ASV or BPAP may successfully treat the breathing abnormalities in patients with Joubert syndrome.

REFERENCES

1. Karegowda LH, Shenoy PM, Sripathi S, Varman M. Joubert syndrome. *BMJ Case Rep*. Mar 2014;20:2014.
2. Nag C, Ghosh M, Das K, Ghosh T. Joubert syndrome: the molar tooth sign of the mid-brain. *Ann Med Health Sci Res*. Apr 2013;3(2):291–294.
3. Wolfe L, Lakadamyali H, Mutlu GM. Joubert syndrome associated with severe central sleep apnea. *J Clin Sleep Med*. Aug 15 2010;6(4):384–388.
4. Kamdar BB, Nandkumar P, Krishnan V, Gamaldo CE, Collop NA. Self-reported sleep and breathing disturbances in Joubert syndrome. *Pediatr Neurol*. Dec 2011;45(6):395–399.
5. Romani M, Micalizzi A, Valente EM. Joubert syndrome: congenital cerebellar ataxia with the molar tooth. *Lancet Neurol*. Sep 2013;12(9):894–905.

A 4-year-old female with early morning awakenings

Suzanne E. Beck

CASE PRESENTATION

A 4-year-old girl was referred for evaluation of early morning awakenings and disruptive behaviors. The parents noted that the child was tired in the afternoon and started a bedtime routine at 5 PM. She usually fell asleep in 60 minutes. Once asleep, she had two to three night awakenings, typically lasting 15 to 30 minutes each. She woke up at 4:00 AM spontaneously and did not return to sleep. Upon waking, she yelled and screamed in the doorway of her room until her exhausted parents responded. Her behavior often escalated to include emptying her dresser drawers, throwing clothes around, and taking off her clothes. Later bedtimes did not result in her sleeping later in the morning but rather resulted in worsening behavior patterns. She took one scheduled nap daily from 12:00 PM to 1:00 PM at day care. The parents denied snoring, leg discomfort, or parasomnias. During the day, the child exhibited unusual behaviors such as hugging herself, licking things, and turning pages of books repetitively. She had frequent temper tantrums and occasional self-injurious behavior. These behaviors began as a toddler and escalated over time. Her past medical history included mild persistent asthma, eczema, recurrent sinus infections, bilateral sensorineural hearing loss with cochlear implants, a diagnosis of attention-deficit hyperactivity disorder (ADHD), and global developmental delay. Her past surgical history was positive for adenotonsillectomy at 3 years of age for recurrent tonsillitis. Her family history was unremarkable for sleep disorders or genetic syndromes.

PHYSICAL EXAMINATION

Vital signs were normal. Weight was14.6 kg (10th percentile); height was 98.1 cm (5th percentile); body mass index was 15.2 (50th percentile). She was in no distress and walked around the exam room, busying herself with page flipping and frequent licking of her book. She had dysmorphic features including brachycephaly (an abnormally short, broad head), small nose with a prominent glabella, broad nasal bridge, midface hypoplasia, tented upper lip, and prominent jaw (prognathism). Tonsils were surgically absent. She had mild hypotonia. The remainder of the physical exam was normal.

LABORATORY AND SLEEP FINDINGS

Sleep diaries are shown in Figure 62-1.

QUESTIONS

1. What is the next step in the care of this patient?
2. What is the diagnosis?

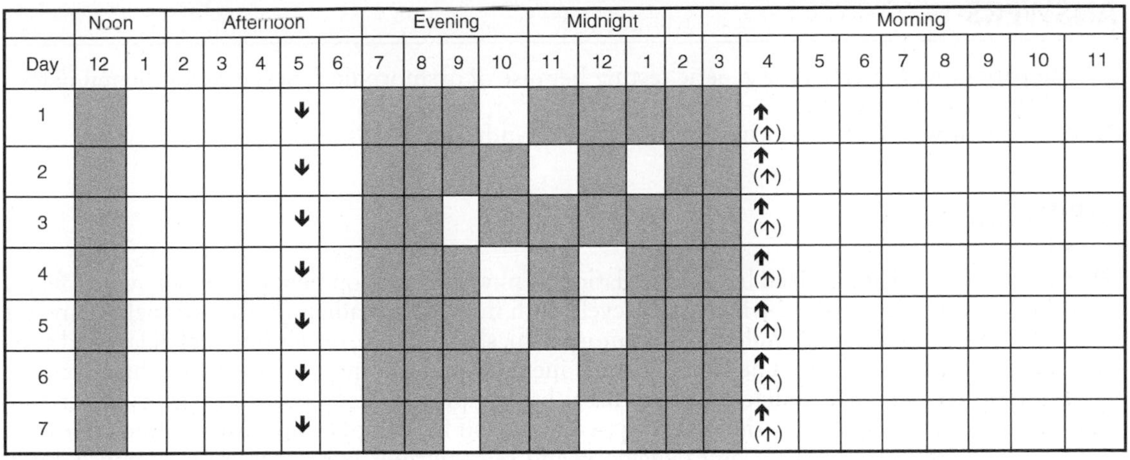

	Noon		Afternoon					Evening				Midnight					Morning						
Day	12	1	2	3	4	5	6	7	8	9	10	11	12	1	2	3	4	5	6	7	8	9	10	11
1						↓											↑ (↑)							
2						↓											↑ (↑)							
3						↓											↑ (↑)							
4						↓											↑ (↑)							
5						↓											↑ (↑)							
6						↓											↑ (↑)							
7						↓											↑ (↑)							

FIGURE 62-1 ■ One-week sleep diary showing a 1-hour nap during the day, long sleep onset latency, night awakenings, and early morning waking for both patient ↑ and family (↑). Sleep is indicated by the gray boxes; onset of bedtime routine by ↓ and waking by ↑.

ANSWERS

1. The patient was referred for genetic testing because of dysmorphic facies, developmental delay, and abnormal behaviors.
2. The patient was diagnosed with Smith-Magenis syndrome (SMS).

DISCUSSION

SMS is a disorder characterized by a constellation of physical, developmental, and behavioral features including disturbance of the 24-hour sleep cycle with inverted circadian rhythm of melatonin secretion. Clinical features include mild facial dysmorphism, short stature, developmental delay, and abnormal, stereotypical behaviors. The facial features include a broad, square-shaped face; brachycephaly; an abnormally broad, flat midface; a broad nasal bridge; prognathism; eyebrows growing across the base of the nose (synophrys); a short, full-tipped nose; and fleshy upper lip with a tented appearance. Temper tantrums, attention-seeking behaviors, and self-injurious behaviors are common. Children with SMS often demonstrate "self-hugging," hand licking, and page-flipping behaviors. SMS is most commonly due to a *de novo* 3.5 Mb interstitial deletion of chromosome 17 band p11.2 and occurs in approximately 1/15,000 to 1/25,000 births.[1]

The severe sleep disturbances and maladaptive daytime behaviors characteristic of SMS have been linked to an abnormal circadian rhythm of melatonin.[2] Children with SMS have an abnormal diurnal melatonin profile, with mean melatonin onset peaking in the morning soon after rising and trough levels occurring at night before bedtime, while both serum cortisol and growth hormone follow a normal circadian secretion pattern.[3] The inverted melatonin secretion that occurs in SMS distinguishes the sleep disturbance in SMS from that seen in other children with developmental disabilities; however, recent case reports in SMS associated with an atypically large deletion and a more normal endogenous melatonin rhythm suggest that the sleep disturbances in SMS may not be solely attributed to abnormal diurnal melatonin.[4]

Considering SMS is a rare syndrome, information regarding pharmacologic interventions in controlled trials is sparse; however, small pilot studies and preliminary case reports show that beta blockers, mood stabilizers, and melatonin[5] may improve both sleep patterns and disruptive behaviors in individuals with SMS. Melatonin has been shown to be effective at improving sleep onset latency in children with an array of neurodevelopmental problems by a mean of 45 minutes in one randomized, double-blind, placebo-controlled trial,[6] and it is used quite commonly in this population.

Other medical problems more frequent in children with SMS include hearing loss, chronic sinusitis and respiratory problems, constipation, feeding difficulties, poor growth, cardiac abnormalities, renal problems, and seizures.[7] Maladaptive behaviors can be extreme and may escalate in adolescence. Nearly all patients with SMS show developmental delay ranging from moderate to borderline functioning, with intelligence quotients in the range of 20 to 78, and many have receptive and expressive language problems.[7] Social skills develop at a higher level than cognitive skills, and many individuals develop communicative personalities with a sense of humor. Most individuals with SMS require some level of supervision throughout their lives.

Many of the features of SMS are subtle in infancy and early childhood and become more apparent in later childhood or adolescence. The behavioral phenotype may mimic ADHD, be attributed to hearing loss or developmental delay, and may be overlooked in young children. Careful evaluation of symptoms along with clues provided by the facial dysmorphisms can lead to the diagnosis, which can be confirmed by genetic testing, and make a significant difference in treatment approach.

In our patient, controlled release melatonin was initiated at 5 PM. A behavioral plan was implemented, which included a "good morning" light on a timer, which was gradually set to 6:30 AM to indicate when it was okay for the child to alert her parents that she was awake, and training the child to occupy herself with quiet activities in her room until the light went on. Repetitive activities such as throwing socks into a basket were recommended. The treatment plan was successful in that the family's sleep was less disrupted and the child had less anxiety during early morning awakenings. The patient played quietly in her room for 2 hours each morning upon awakening, rather than disturbing her parents, and had less night waking (Fig. 62-2); however, she continued to have behavior problems during the day.

	Noon	Afternoon						Evening				Midnight			Morning									
Day	12	1	2	3	4	5	6	7	8	9	10	11	12	1	2	3	4	5	6	7	8	9	10	11
1						*	↓											↑		(↑)				
2						*	↓											↑		(↑)				
3						*	↓											↑		(↑)				
4						*	↓											↑		(↑)				
5						*	↓											↑		(↑)				
6						*	↓											↑		(↑)				
7						*	↓											↑		(↑)				

FIGURE 62-2 ■ One-week sleep diary following administration of melatonin at 5 PM and a "good morning" light set for 6:30 AM. The diary shows a shorter sleep latency, improved night waking, and early morning waking for the patient ↑ but not for family (↑). Sleep is indicated by the gray box, onset of bedtime routine by ↑, and waking by ↑. Melatonin administration is indicated by (*)

CLINICAL PEARLS

1. SMS should be considered in a child with characteristic facial features, developmental delay, and sleep disturbance.
2. The inverted melatonin secretion that occurs in most patients with SMS distinguishes the sleep disturbance in SMS from that seen in other children with developmental disabilities.
3. Children with SMS may benefit from pharmacotherapy including melatonin in addition to behavioral management.

REFERENCES

1. Smith AC, McGavran L, Robinson J, et al. Interstitial deletion of (17)(p11.2p11.2) in nine patients. *Am J Med Genet*. 1986;24(3):393–414.
2. Potocki L, Glaze D, Tan DX, et al. Circadian rhythm abnormalities of melatonin in Smith-Magenis syndrome. *J Med Genet*. Jun 2000;37(6):428–433.
3. Gropman AL, Duncan WC, Smith AC. Neurologic and developmental features of the Smith-Magenis syndrome (del 17p11.2). *Pediatr Neurol*. May 2006;34(5):337–350.
4. Boudreau EA, Johnson KP, Jackman AR, et al. Review of disrupted sleep patterns in Smith-Magenis syndrome and normal melatonin secretion in a patient with an atypical interstitial 17p11.2 deletion. *Am J Med Genet A*. Jul 2009;149A(7):1382–1391.
5. Bruni O, Alonso-Alconada D, Besag F, et al. Current role of melatonin in pediatric neurology: clinical recommendations. *Eur J Paediatr Neurol*. Mar 2015;19(2):122–133.
6. Appleton RE, Jones AP, Gamble C, et al. The use of MElatonin in children with Neurodevelopmental Disorders and impaired Sleep: a randomised, double-blind, placebo-controlled, parallel study (MENDS). *Health Technol Assess*. 2012;16(40):i–239.
7. Smith ACM, Boyd KE, Elsea SH, et al. Smith-Magenis syndrome. In: Pagon RA, Adam MP, Ardinger HH, et al., eds. *GeneReviews [Internet]*. Seattle, WA: University of Washington; 1993.

CASE 63

A 6-year-old girl who goes to school while sleeping

Lourdes M. DelRosso

CLINICAL PRESENTATION

A 6-year-old girl presented for evaluation of sleepwalking. The symptoms started at age 5 and occurred four nights a week, usually within the first hours of sleep. Her mother noticed that the child also talked in her sleep, and some nights she sat on a table during the sleepwalking episodes and behaved as if she were in school. During these episodes, her eyes were open, but she was not aware of her surroundings and she did not have recollection of the events in the morning. She used to have night terrors from 2 to 5 years of age, but these resolved. She snored and was a restless sleeper but denied symptoms of restless leg syndrome. Her bedtime was 8:30 PM. She fell asleep within 5 minutes. Her mother woke her up at 7:30 AM. She did not take naps and did not have daytime sleepiness. Her past medical and surgical history were negative. Her family history was positive for sleepwalking in her mother and paternal aunt. The review of systems was negative for seizure disorder or anxiety.

PHYSICAL EXAM

The child was alert and cooperative. Her vital signs were within normal range. Her weight and height were at the 90th percentile. She did not have an adenoid facies. Oropharyngeal Mallampati grade was IV; tonsil size was 2+; and she did not have a high-arched palate. She did not have micrognathia or retrognathia. The remainder of the physical exam was normal.

LABORATORY AND SLEEP FINDINGS

Polysomnography (PSG) revealed a sleep efficiency of 68%. The obstructive apnea–hypopnea index (AHI) was 1.3/h, central AHI was 0/h, and nadir SpO_2 94%. The periodic leg movement index was were 0.9/h. There was no evidence of hypoventilation. The patient had several spontaneous arousals (Fig. 63-1).

QUESTION

What is the diagnosis in this child?

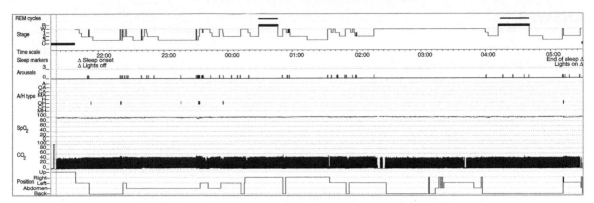

FIGURE 63-1 ■ PSG hypnogram; note several arousals from N3.

ANSWER

The events are characterized by ambulation, talking, and complex behaviors during sleep, occurring a couple of hours after sleep onset. The patient is not aware of her surroundings and has no recollection in the morning. These characteristics are consistent with sleepwalking. The mother's history of sleepwalking further strengthens the diagnosis. A nocturnal PSG was ordered to rule out sleep-disordered breathing in view of the history of snoring and the physical exam findings. The hypnogram seen in Figure 63-1 reveals frequent arousals from N3, which is characteristic of disorders of arousal.

DISCUSSION

Disorders of arousal are NREM parasomnias that occur commonly in childhood and are characterized by sudden partial awakening from NREM sleep (usually N3), nocturnal behaviors, and amnesia after the event. During these episodes, the patient is usually unresponsive to the environment as he or she engages in activities that resemble wakefulness. Disorders of arousal share common pathophysiologic and genetic patterns among each other but differ in their clinical manifestations. There are three common types of disorders of arousal: sleepwalking, night terrors, and confusional arousals. More than one type of disorder of arousal can occur in the same patient.[1] The pathophysiology is the same in all three disorders: failure of the brain to fully awaken after an arousal. Neuroimaging during NREM parasomnias has confirmed activation of motor and cingulate cortices and persistence of delta activity in the frontoparietal cortices, consistent with the presentation of motor behaviors seen during slow-wave sleep.[2]

The *International Classification of Sleep Disorders*, third edition (ICSD-3) criteria for arousal disorders include recurrent episodes of partial awakening from sleep, partial or complete amnesia, absent responsiveness to others, limited or no associated cognition, and that the episodes are not better explained by another sleep disorder, medication use, drug use, psychiatric disorder, or medical disorder. Confusional arousals must also include in the diagnosis confusion during the episode while the patient is in bed. Night terrors are discussed in detail in Clinical Pearls in Case 64: A 3-year-old girl with disruptive nocturnal awakenings. Sleepwalking is associated with complex behaviors and ambulation.

Confusional arousals affect up to 50% of children, mainly toddlers. Sleepwalking usually affects older children (15% of 5 to 12-year-olds).[1] Sleepwalking has a strong familial pattern; one study found that first-degree relatives of sleepwalkers have at least a tenfold increase in risk of sleepwalking.[3] Sleep disruption because of sleep-disordered breathing or periodic limb movements of sleep have been associated with an increased risk of sleepwalking.[4] Other risk factors include sleep deprivation, medications (sedative-hypnotics, antidepressants, some antipsychotics such as olanzapine and quetiapine, lithium, and topiramate), and medical conditions (febrile illnesses, encephalitis, and migraines).[2]

PSG is not routinely indicated in the evaluation of typical, uncomplicated, noninjurious parasomnias but may be considered for forensic evaluation (in the event of personal injury or trauma). PSG is indicated when there is suspicion of other sleep disorders such as obstructive sleep apnea syndrome (OSAS), periodic limb movement disorder (PLMD), or nocturnal epilepsy.[5] Nocturnal frontal lobe epilepsy (NFLE) in particular is difficult to differentiate from NREM parasomnias. NFLE is peculiar in that it occurs exclusively during sleep, presents with complex motor behaviors, can have an autosomal dominant mode of inheritance, and the ictal and interictal electroencephalogram (EEG) is often normal.[6] A video-EEG study on 23 patients with parasomnia and 21 patients with NFLE demonstrated that both events usually started with an arousal from NREM sleep; coherent speech was common in NREM parasomnias and rare in NFLE; and 88% of seizures ended in wakefulness. Features that favored parasomnia over NFLE included failure to fully arouse after the event, physical or verbal interaction, waxing and waning pattern, and prolonged duration (>2 minutes).[7]

Treatment of disorders of arousals is usually not necessary other than securing the environment. Parents should be advised to keep a safe environment, locking doors and windows and placing door alarms. Other recommendations include keeping a consistent bedtime routine, avoidance of sleep deprivation, minimizing the use of medications that can predispose to parasomnia, and management of comorbidities that could predispose to increased arousals such as OSAS, PLMD, gastroesophageal reflux, or eczema. On rare occasions when parasomnias are frequent and result in injuries, clonazepam can be used.[8]

CLINICAL PEARLS

1. The ICSD-3 criteria for disorders of arousal include recurrent episodes of partial awakening from sleep, partial or complete amnesia, absent responsiveness to others, and limited or no associated cognition.
2. Disorders of arousal from NREM sleep include sleepwalking, night terrors, and confusional arousals.
3. When evaluating disorders of arousal, a PSG is not usually necessary but may be indicated in injurious parasomnias or if comorbid sleep disorders or nocturnal seizures are suspected.
4. Pharmacologic treatment is usually not necessary.

REFERENCES

1. Provini F, Tinuper P, Bisulli F, Lugaresi E. Arousal disorders. *Sleep Med*. Dec 2011;12(suppl 2):S22–S26.
2. Howell MJ. Parasomnias: an updated review. *Neurotherapeutics*. Oct 2012;9(4):753–775.
3. Licis AK, Desruisseau DM, Yamada KA, Duntley SP, Gurnett CA. Novel genetic findings in an extended family pedigree with sleepwalking. *Neurology*. Jan 4 2011;76(1):49–52.
4. Cao M, Guilleminault C. Families with sleepwalking. *Sleep Med*. Aug 2010;11(7):726–734.
5. Kushida CA, Littner MR, Morgenthaler T, et al. Practice parameters for the indications for polysomnography and related procedures: an update for 2005. *Sleep*. Apr 2005;28(4):499–521.
6. Bisulli F, Vignatelli L, Provini F, Leta C, Lugaresi E, Tinuper P. Parasomnias and nocturnal frontal lobe epilepsy (NFLE): lights and shadows–controversial points in the differential diagnosis. *Sleep Med*. Dec 2011;12(suppl 2):S27–S32.
7. Derry CP, Harvey AS, Walker MC, Duncan JS, Berkovic SF. NREM arousal parasomnias and their distinction from nocturnal frontal lobe epilepsy: a video EEG analysis. *Sleep*. Dec 2009;32(12):1637–1644.
8. Markov D, Jaffe F, Doghramji K. Update on parasomnias: a review for psychiatric practice. *Psychiatry (Edgmont)*. Jul 2006;3(7):69–76.

A 3-year-old girl with disruptive nocturnal awakenings

Lourdes M. DelRosso

CASE PRESENTATION

A 3-year-old girl was referred for evaluation of disruptive nocturnal awakenings. Her mother reported a bedtime of 10 PM. The child fell asleep within 10 minutes. Every other night she woke up around midnight with a loud scream. During these awakenings, she appeared scared and agitated but did not respond to her mother's attempts to console her. Her mother noticed fast breathing and sweaty palms. The episodes lasted for 10 to 30 minutes, after which the child returned to sleep. She woke up at 7 AM without recollection of the event. The episodes usually occurred once a night. The child napped from 1 PM until 2 PM daily, without awakenings. There was no history of snoring, sleepwalking, or sleep talking. Her mother reported that the child had leg kicking and restless sleep. There was no past medical or surgical history. She did not take any medications. Her review of systems was negative.

PHYSICAL EXAMINATION

The patient was alert and playful. She had normal development. The physical exam was noncontributory.

LABORATORY AND SLEEP FINDINGS

A polysomnogram (PSG) was ordered to evaluate for possible periodic leg movements of sleep contributing to the nocturnal awakenings. The sleep efficiency was 90%. All stages of sleep were represented. One episode of awakening associated with crying and a scared appearance occurred at 11:46 PM (epoch shown in Fig. 64-1). There were no abnormal respiratory events or periodic leg movements.

QUESTION

What is the diagnosis in this patient?

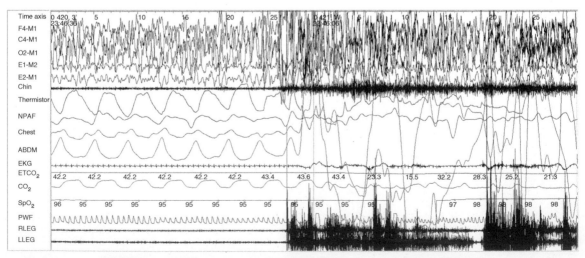

FIGURE 64-1 ■ **Thirty-second epoch representative of nocturnal awakenings.**

ANSWER

Sleep terrors.

DISCUSSION

Sleep terrors are characterized by abrupt awakening, usually with a loud scream and intense fear, accompanied by signs of autonomic activation: diaphoresis, tachycardia, tachypnea, and mydriasis (Boxes 64-1 and 64-2). To fit *International Classification of Sleep Disorders*, third edition (ICSD-3) criteria for sleep terrors, the disorder must also meet the general criteria for a NREM disorder of arousal (see Box 64-1).

Sleep terrors are common in young children, with a prevalence of up to 19% in children aged 4 to 9 years. The prevalence of sleep terrors decreases with age, occurring in 3.8% of children aged 11 and in <1% of adults.[1] Sleep terrors may be precipitated by sleep deprivation, infections, or acute stressful events. Many medications can trigger sleep terrors; the more common ones are antihistamines, stimulants, neuroleptics, and hypnotics.[2] Sleep terrors are usually more prominent during the first hours of sleep and commonly arise from N3, but can also arise from N2 sleep.

The diagnosis of sleep terrors is based on history. Home videos can also assist in the diagnosis. PSG is not indicated in the evaluation of typical noninjurious parasomnia. PSG is indicated in the evaluation or frequent parasomnias when an underlying sleep disorder is suspected (obstructive sleep apnea syndrome or periodic limb movements of sleep). An extended electroencephalogram montage may be used when seizures are suspected in patients with atypical or potentially injurious parasomnias.[3] Sleep

---

BOX 64-1   *INTERNATIONAL CLASSIFICATION OF SLEEP DISORDERS*, THIRD EDITION GENERAL DIAGNOSTIC CRITERIA FOR DISORDERS OF AROUSAL FROM NON-RAPID EYE MOVEMENT SLEEP

General Diagnostic Criteria for Disorders of Arousal

Criteria a-e must be met

a. Recurrent episodes of incomplete awakening from sleep.[1]
b. Inappropriate or absent responsiveness to efforts of others to intervene or redirect the person during the episode.
c. Limited (e.g., a single visual scene) or no associated cognition or dream imagery.
d. Partial or complete amnesia for the episode.
e. The disturbance is not better explained by another sleep disorder, mental disorder, medical condition, medication, or substance use.

Notes

1. The events usually occur during the first third of the major sleep episode.
2. The individual may continue to appear confused and disoriented for several minutes or longer following the episode.

(American Academy of Sleep Medicine. *International Classifications of Sleep Disorders*. 3rd ed. Darien, IL: American Academy of Sleep Medicine; 2014.)

BOX 64-2   *INTERNATIONAL CLASSIFICATION OF SLEEP DISORDERS*-3 DIAGNOSTIC CRITERIA FOR SLEEP TERRORS (ALL MUST BE MET)[5]

Diagnostic Criteria

Criteria a-c must be met

a. The disorder meets general criteria for NREM disorders of arousal.
b. The arousals are characterized by episodes of abrupt terror, typically beginning with an alarming vocalization such as a frightening scream.
c. There is intense fear and signs of autonomic arousal, including mydriasis, tachycardia, tachypnea, and diaphoresis during an episode.

(American Academy of Sleep Medicine. *International Classifications of Sleep Disorders*. 3rd ed. Darien, IL: American Academy of Sleep Medicine; 2014.)

terrors are commonly mistaken with nightmare disorder. Nightmares usually arise from REM sleep and occur during the second half of the night. In contrast to sleep terrors, children with nightmares usually remember the dream content after awakening and respond to parental comfort.[2]

Management of sleep terrors consists of establishing an adequate sleep routine, preventing sleep loss or sleep disruption, avoiding precipitating factors, and resisting trying to awaken and comfort the child, because this interference is likely to prolong the episode.[4] Parents should be reassured that the child does not recall the events, and there do not seem to be any long-term deleterious effects. Sleep terrors are not associated with daytime sleepiness.

Our patient's total sleep time was 10 hours/day. This is below the total amount of sleep recommended for her age (approximately 12 hours a day). The parents were reassured that the events were benign in nature. Behavioral interventions included sleep extension and consistent bedtime routine. These interventions decreased the frequency of sleep terrors to once a week.

CLINICAL PEARLS

1. Sleep terrors are NREM parasomnias that usually arise from N3 sleep.
2. Sleep terrors are benign and resolve spontaneously in the majority of children.
3. Sleep terrors are exacerbated by sleep deprivation, infection, and stress.
4. PSG is not routinely indicated for the evaluation of sleep terrors.
5. Management includes reassurance and avoidance of precipitating factors.

REFERENCES

1. Nguyen BH, Perusse D, Paquet J, et al. Sleep terrors in children: a prospective study of twins. *Pediatrics*. Dec 2008;122(6):e1164–e1167.
2. Mason 2nd TB, Pack AI. Sleep terrors in childhood. *J Pediatr*. Sep 2005;147(3):388–392.
3. Aurora RN, Lamm CI, Zak RS, et al. Practice parameters for the non-respiratory indications for polysomnography and multiple sleep latency testing for children. *Sleep*. Nov 2012;35(11):1467–1473.
4. Provini F, Tinuper P, Bisulli F, Lugaresi E. Arousal disorders. *Sleep Med*. Dec 2011;12(suppl 2):S22–S26.
5. American Academy of Sleep Medicine. *International Classifications of Sleep Disorders*. 3rd ed. Darien, IL: American Academy of Sleep Medicine; 2014.

An 11-year-old boy with obesity and secondary enuresis

Lourdes M. DelRosso

CASE PRESENTATION

An 11-year-old boy presented for evaluation of nocturnal enuresis. After being continent for years, he started wetting the bed during the last 3 months, at least 3 times a week. He did not have daytime incontinence. The patient reported slowly gaining approximately 7 kg in the past 6 months. He snored, but the parents had not noticed gasping or witnessed apnea. The family denied excessive daytime sleepiness, restless legs, or sleepwalking. He did not have any other medical problems and did not take any medications. He lived with both parents and one sibling; He attended sixth grade and was an honor roll student. Review of systems was positive for obesity and negative for polydipsia, polyuria, constipation, seizure disorder, depression, and anxiety.

PHYSICAL EXAM

Physical exam revealed an obese boy. His blood pressure was 138/59; pulse 106; height and weight at the 100th percentile. He had a slight adenoid facies. His nose had mildly enlarged inferior turbinates. He did not have a high-arched palate. His throat was Mallampati grade IV. Tonsil size was 2+. He did not have micrognathia or retrognathia. The remainder of the cardiovascular and neurologic exam was normal.

LABORATORY AND SLEEP FINDINGS

Urinalysis: normal.

Soft-tissue lateral neck x-ray showed significant adenoid hypertrophy (Fig. 65-1).

A nocturnal polysomnogram (PSG) showed severe obstructive sleep apnea (OSA), with an apnea–hypopnea index of 102/h and SpO_2 nadir of 43%.

QUESTIONS

What is the next step in the management of this patient's enuresis?

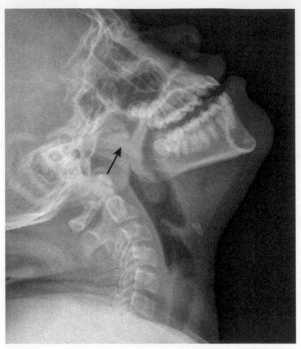

FIGURE 65-1 ■ Obstructive adenoid hypertrophy (*arrow*).

ANSWERS

The patient has severe OSA, obesity, adenoid hypertrophy, and secondary enuresis. The next step is evaluation by an ears, nose, and throat specialist for possible tonsillectomy and adenoidectomy (T&A). Because of OSA severity and the persistence of an underlying risk factor (obesity), a PSG should be repeated 6 to 8 weeks after T&A to evaluate for residual OSA. Weight loss would be beneficial but is difficult to accomplish.

DISCUSSION

Sleep enuresis is a parasomnia defined by the *International Classification of Sleep Disorders*, third edition (ICSD-3)[1] as recurrent and involuntary voiding that occurs during sleep, at least twice a week, for a minimum of 3 months in a child older than 5 years. Sleep enuresis is divided into primary, if the child has never been consistently dry during sleep, or secondary, if the child has been dry during sleep for at least 6 months. Primary and secondary enuresis are two different conditions with different underlying pathophysiology.

Primary sleep enuresis spontaneously decreases with age. It is estimated to be present in 30% of 4-year-olds, 10% of 6-year-olds, 3% of 12-year-olds, and 1% of 15-year-olds.[2] Sleep enuresis is 3 times more common in boys than in girls. Secondary enuresis has been associated with constipation, diabetes, bladder dysfunction, OSA, and, rarely, seizure disorder. The evaluation of sleep enuresis includes a thorough history and physical exam and a urinalysis to rule out infection.[3]

Although not consistently duplicated, some studies have found sleep enuresis to be more common among obese children than among normal weight children. The pathophysiology linking both conditions could be associated with unhealthy diet, hyperglycemia, and psychological distress found in obese children and adolescents. Similarly, several studies have found that children with obstructive sleep apnea syndrome (OSAS) are at increased risk of sleep enuresis. The negative intrathoracic pressure caused by the apneic episodes produces cardiac distention, resulting in release of atrial natriuretic peptide, with subsequent increase in water excretion and inhibition of vasopressin. This, in combination with increased intra-abdominal pressure and frequent arousals, may result in nocturnal enuresis.[4,5] Treatment of the sleep-disordered breathing improves or resolves secondary enuresis in a large number of children with OSAS who undergo T&A.[6,7] Persistence of enuresis after T&A is associated with obesity, severe enuresis before T&A, history of familial enuresis, and arousal difficulties.[8] Children with sleep enuresis have reported other sleep-related problems, in particular bedtime resistance, sleep anxiety, and daytime sleepiness.[2,9]

Treatment of nocturnal enuresis consists of treatment of the underlying precipitating factor, in this case, treatment of OSAS with T&A resolved nocturnal enuresis. When no etiology is found, treatment options include fluid restriction, scheduled night waking, bedwetting alarms, or intranasal desmopressin.

CLINICAL PEARLS

1. Sleep enuresis is considered in a child older than 5 years of age.
2. OSA may be a contributor to sleep enuresis.
3. Management of OSAS can resolve or decrease the frequency of sleep enuresis.

REFERENCES

1. American Academy of Sleep Medicine. *International Classification of Sleep Disorders*. 3rd ed. Darin, IL: American Academy of Sleep Medicine; 2013.
2. Abou-Khadra MK, Amin OR, Ahmed D. Association between sleep and behavioural problems among children with enuresis. *J Paediatr Child Health*. Feb 2013;49(2):E160–E166.
3. Ramakrishnan K. Evaluation and treatment of enuresis. *Am Fam Physician*. Aug 15 2008;78(4):489–496.
4. Weintraub Y, Singer S, Alexander D, et al. Enuresis—an unattended comorbidity of childhood obesity. *Int J Obes (Lond)*. Jan 2013;37(1):75–78.
5. Barone JG, Hanson C, DaJusta DG, Gioia K, England SJ, Schneider D. Nocturnal enuresis and overweight are associated with obstructive sleep apnea. *Pediatrics*. Jul 2009;124(1):e53–e59.
6. Weissbach A, Leiberman A, Tarasiuk A, Goldbart A, Tal A. Adenotonsilectomy improves enuresis in children with obstructive sleep apnea syndrome. *Int J Pediatr Otorhinolaryngol*. Aug 2006;70(8):1351–1356.

7. Basha S, Bialowas C, Ende K, Szeremeta W. Effectiveness of adenotonsillectomy in the resolution of nocturnal enuresis secondary to obstructive sleep apnea. *Laryngoscope*. Jun 2005;115(6):1101–1103.
8. Kovacevic L, Jurewicz M, Dabaja A, et al. Enuretic children with obstructive sleep apnea syndrome: should they see otolaryngology first? *J Pediatr Urol*. Apr 2013;9(2):145–150.
9. Cohen-Zrubavel V, Kushnir B, Kushnir J, Sadeh A. Sleep and sleepiness in children with nocturnal enuresis. *Sleep*. Feb 2011;34(2):191–194.

A 13-year-old boy with Moebius sequence and violent nocturnal behaviors

Lourdes M. DelRosso

CASE PRESENTATION

A 13-year-old male presented for evaluation of nocturnal screaming and violent movements that started about a year ago. The episodes occurred 2 to 3 times a week between 3 and 5 AM. His mother noted that the boy screamed and moved his arms and legs violently for a few minutes but never injured himself. If awoken during the episodes, he remembered having a nightmare. These episodes usually occurred once a night. His bedtime was 9:30 PM on weekdays and 10:30 PM on weekends; he usually fell asleep within 20 minutes. He woke up at 6 AM on weekdays and at 9 AM on weekends. He did not nap during the day and did not have daytime sleepiness. He reported rare episodes of sleep paralysis but denied hypnagogic hallucinations, cataplexy, or symptoms of restless legs. There was no snoring or sleepwalking. He did not drink caffeine. His past medical history was positive for Moebius sequence (absence or hypoplasia of multiple cranial nerves). His past surgical history was negative.

PHYSICAL EXAM

The patient was an alert and cooperative young boy, well nourished, well developed, and in no acute distress. His vital signs were within normal limits. His speech was dysarthric but intelligible. He had decreased right ocular adduction, bilateral ptosis, and was unable to close his eyelids completely. He had a right facial paresis. Tongue, palate, and uvula were midline, although he had tongue atrophy bilaterally. The remainder of the physical exam was normal.

LABORATORY AND SLEEP FINDINGS

Nocturnal polysomnography (PSG) revealed sleep efficiency of 96%. The obstructive apnea–hypopnea index (AHI) was 0.4/h; the central AHI was 0/h; the SpO$_2$ nadir was 94%; and the End-tidal CO$_2$ was below 50 torr for 100% of total sleep time. The leg movements per hour of sleep were 1/h. Video monitoring revealed episodes of repetitive motor behaviors and muscle twitches during REM sleep. A characteristic epoch during REM is seen in Figure 66-1.

QUESTION

What is the diagnosis?

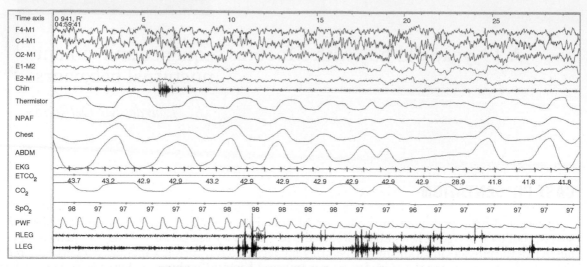

FIGURE 66-1 ■ Thirty-second epoch during REM sleep.

ANSWER

Figure 66-1 reveals an epoch that meets criteria for REM sleep without atonia (see discussion). REM sleep behavior disorder (RBD) was diagnosed in the setting of motor behaviors during REM sleep as seen on video-PSG monitoring, evidence of REM sleep without atonia, and nocturnal vocalization (screaming).

DISCUSSION

The *International Classification of Sleep Disorders*, third edition (ICSD-3) diagnostic criteria for RBD include sleep-related episodes of vocalizations and/or complex motor behaviors, PSG-documented REM sleep without atonia, and documented behaviors during REM sleep or presumed to be during REM sleep by clinical history. The mechanism of RBD is based on loss of the normal muscle atonia seen during REM sleep, manifested on PSG as either tonic or phasic REM sleep without atonia. Chin electromyogram (EMG) with sustained elevation for more than 50% of the epoch qualifies that epoch for tonic REM without atonia. To qualify for phasic REM sleep without atonia, an epoch must be divided into 10 3-second mini epochs. If bursts of transient muscle activity are present on either the chin EMG or the tibialis anterior EMG on more than 50% of the mini epochs, the epoch qualifies for phasic REM sleep without atonia. Time-synchronized video-PSG monitoring is necessary for diagnosis and usually reveals dream enactment or movements.

REM sleep is generated in the brainstem. REM atonia is modulated by neurons in the sublaterodorsal tegmentum nucleus (SLD). These are considered "REM on" cells because they are activated during REM sleep. These cells synthesize glutamate and activate γ-aminobutyric acid (GABA)- and glycine-containing neurons in the gigantocellular reticular nucleus, which inhibit skeletal motor neurons, resulting in muscle atonia. Bilateral lesions in the SLD or disruption in the inhibitory neurotransmitters (GABA and glycine) can produce REM without atonia. Lesions in the brainstem due to tumors, surgery, ischemia, or neurodegenerative conditions can manifest as RBD.[1]

Although seen across all ages and in both sexes, RBD is typically thought to be a disease of older men. More than 80% of adults with RBD eventually develop a synucleinopathy (Parkinson's disease, multiple system atrophy, or dementia with Lewy body). RBD is rarely seen in children. A case series of 13 children diagnosed with RBD found that motor behaviors varied from restless sleep to frank violent movements.[2] Vocalization was common and consisted of yelling rather than the more common talking, crying, or mumbling observed in NREM parasomnias *other than sleep terrors*. In this case series, five of nine patients who had brain magnetic resonance imaging (MRI) were found to have structural lesions that predisposed them to brainstem dysfunction, including central nervous system tumors. One child in this series had Moebius sequence. Case reports have associated RBD in adolescents with *narcolepsy*, juvenile onset Parkinson's disease, and Tourette syndrome.[3]

There are very few reports of treatment options for RBD in children; most used clonazepam or melatonin with various results.[2]

Moebius sequence is a rare condition that affects about 2 to 20 children per one million births. Moebius sequence is characterized by underdevelopment of cranial nerves VI and VII (abducens and facial), but other cranial nerves may be affected, including IX and X, which may result in swallowing dysfunction, vocal cord paralysis, and upper airway obstruction. Moebius sequence may be associated with micrognathia, limb malformations, and hypotonia. The etiology of the sequence is unclear, but one theory is that it is due to brainstem dysfunction secondary to ischemia during the first trimester of pregnancy. Most cases are sporadic, but an autosomal dominant inheritance has been reported.[4]

Our patient had a brain MRI that revealed findings consistent with Moebius sequence (nonvisualization of the cisternal segments of the bilateral cranial nerves VI and VII) with flattening of the dorsal surface of the pons. The family was presented with several options for treatment, but because symptoms were mild, they elected observation without medication.

CLINICAL PEARLS

1. RBD is rarely seen in children.
2. RBD in children has been associated with brainstem lesions including tumors, narcolepsy, juvenile onset Parkinson's disease, and Tourette syndrome.
3. A limited number of reports concerning treatment of RBD in children have been published. Symptoms appear to be modestly responsive to clonazepam and melatonin.

REFERENCES

1. Brooks PL, Peever JH. Identification of the transmitter and receptor mechanisms responsible for REM sleep paralysis. *J Neurosci*. Jul 18 2012;32(29):9785–9795.
2. Lloyd R, Tippmann-Peikert M, Slocumb N, Kotagal S. Characteristics of REM sleep behavior disorder in childhood. *J Clin Sleep Med*. Apr 15 2012;8(2):127–131.
3. Stores G. Rapid eye movement sleep behaviour disorder in children and adolescents. *Dev Med Child Neurol*. Oct 2008;50(10):728–732.
4. Matsui K, Kataoka A, Yamamoto A, et al. Clinical characteristics and outcomes of Mobius syndrome in a children's hospital. *Pediatr Neurol*. Dec 2014;51(6):781–789.

Brain tumor presenting as somnambulism in an adolescent*

*Priya S. Prashad, Carole L. Marcus, Lawrence W. Brown,
Dennis J. Dlugos, Tamara Feygin, Brian N. Harding,
Gregory G. Heuer, and Thornton B. Alexander Mason*

INTRODUCTION

Somnambulism is a common, benign, and self-limited parasomnia of childhood, and onset beyond early childhood is unusual.[1] Affected individuals may also have other symptoms along with a spectrum of arousal parasomnias that include confusional arousals and sleep terrors (*pavor nocturnus*).[1] Because arousal parasomnias normally occur out of stage 3, NREM or slow wave sleep, sleepwalking episodes typically occur in the first third of the major sleep period. Although most children have events unassociated with other sleep disturbances, events can be precipitated by conditions that disrupt this vulnerable sleep state, such as obstructive apnea, periodic limb movements, environmental noise, and so forth.

The differential diagnosis of somnambulism includes REM behavior disorder presenting as sleep terrors and epileptic seizures, particularly those arising from the frontal lobe. Most sleepwalkers usually remain calm and do not have agitated, rhythmic, stereotypical, or repetitive behaviors unlike those with nocturnal seizures. If these features are present, further investigation is warranted including polysomnography (PSG) or electroencephalography (EEG).[1] We describe a teenage boy who presented with new-onset sleepwalking-like behaviors that were found to be complex partial seizures in the presence of a brain tumor.

CASE REPORT

A previously healthy 15-year-old boy presented with nightly episodes of apparent sleepwalking that began abruptly 1 month earlier. The first episode occurred after the patient fell asleep in the living room while watching a movie with his family. He suddenly bolted up from the sofa and ran upstairs; his parents found him confused and agitated when they tried to converse with him. He subsequently had nightly episodes approximately 1.5 hours after falling asleep, between 11:30 PM and 12:30 AM. He would jump out of his bed, run into his parents' bedroom, and stand in front of his parents holding his comforter. His parents noted agitation, prominent sweating, and a distant gaze. He was minimally interactive during episodes and gave monosyllabic answers to his parents' questions. Within a few minutes he would walk slowly to his room and return to sleep. The patient had no immediate or subsequent recall of the episodes.

His parents did not describe any posturing of extremities, head or eye deviation, rhythmic twitching, tongue biting, or enuresis. No symptoms of sleep-disordered breathing or restless legs syndrome were reported. He denied any use of alcohol or illicit drugs or any incidents of trauma or abuse. He attended ninth grade with stable academic and athletic performance. There was no history of parasomnias in any family members. Physical examination showed a well-developed and nondysmorphic boy, and a detailed neurological examination was normal. PSG, including an extended 16-channel EEG, was obtained because of the unusual presentation of these episodes, namely the sudden onset of nightly, sleepwalking-like behaviors in adolescence, with no history of arousal parasomnias in early childhood. Further, there was suspicion of seizures because all spells were brief and stereotypical

*This entire chapter is taken from Prashad PS, Marcus CL, Brown LW, et al. Brain tumor presenting as somnambulism in an adolescent. *Pediatr Neurol*. 2013;49:209-212.

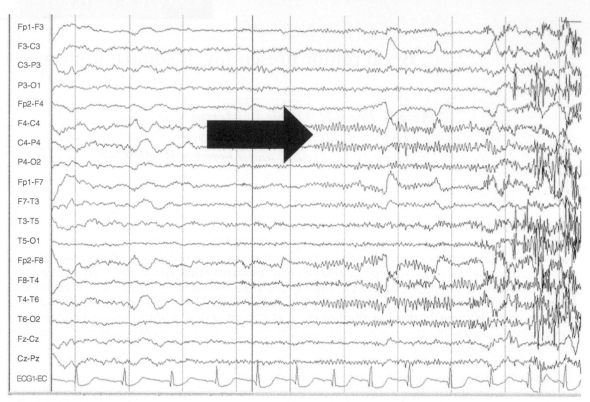

FIGURE 67-1 ■ An episodic nocturnal awakening out of stage 2 NREM sleep, which began with repetitive spikes in the right frontal central temporal regions (*arrow*), maximal at P4-T4 (parietal temporal) before violent agitation obscured the EEG; expanded EEG montage with standard 10 to 20 electrode placement using a 16-channel longitudinal bipolar montage; electrode sites used (Fp1, Fp2, F7, F3, F4, F8, T3, C3, C4, T4, T5, P3, P4, T6, O1, and O2); *F*, Frontal; *Fp*, frontopolar; *C*, central; *O*, occipital; *P*, parietal; *T*, temporal.

(involving either a sudden, dramatic rise from bed with running or agitation or standing next to his bed with a vacant stare).

The PSG was normal from a respiratory standpoint, and no periodic limb movements were recorded. The expanded EEG montage, however, showed occasional right parietal-temporal sharp waves during wakefulness, which activated during NREM sleep. Almost 2 hours after sleep onset, he had an unprovoked arousal from stage 3 NREM sleep.

The initial 20 seconds appeared to be a simple arousal without EEG abnormalities; he suddenly became violently agitated, with initial synchronous spiking in all leads and then mainly in the right hemisphere. A second clinical electrographic seizure occurred in stage 2 NREM sleep (Fig. 67-1) beginning with repetitive spikes in the right frontal central temporal region maximal at EEG channels P4-T4 (parietal-temporal) for 4 seconds before violent agitation again obscured the EEG. At no time did he have focal tonic or clonic activity, bicycling, or pelvic thrusting typical of frontal seizures. The patient was urgently reevaluated in the sleep center and prescribed oxcarbazepine. That night he experienced his first generalized seizure. A few days later, a magnetic resonance imaging (MRI) scan of the brain with contrast revealed a well-circumscribed, lobulated, cortically based mass involving the right parasagittal superior parietal lobe (Fig. 67-2, *A*), with a small focus of ring enhancement along the inferior aspect (see Fig. 67-2, *B*).

He continued on oxcarbazepine therapy, but surgery was delayed for family reasons. During that time he had no further parasomnia-like events, but he did have another tonic-clonic seizure and one episode during basketball practice (described as aimless wandering around the court). In the 6 months following surgery, there were no further paroxysmal events of any kind.

Gross total resection of the lesion was performed. The final pathology report showed a 1- to 1.5 cm dysembryoplastic neuroepithelial tumor (DNET), World Health Organization histologic grade I (see Fig. 67-2, *C*). His treatment plan included continuing pharmacotherapy for at least 1 year, depending on resolution of seizures and EEG abnormalities.

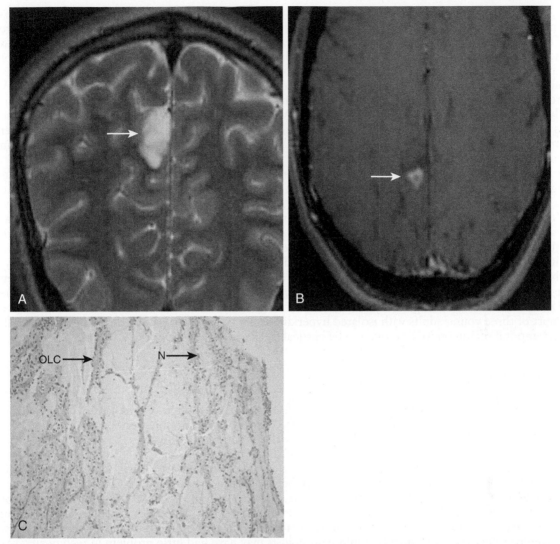

FIGURE 67-2 ■ MRI of DNET. **A,** Coronal T2-weighted MRI shows a well-circumscribed, lobulated mass (*arrow*) in the right parasagittal superior parietal lobe. **B,** Axial T1-weighted postcontrast MRI shows minimal peripheral enhancement of the lesion (*arrow*), which is an unusual feature of this benign tumor. **C,** Stained with hematoxylin and eosin, the photomicrograph shows a mucinous background studded with groups of uniform small cells and oligodendrocyte-like cells (*OLC arrow*), adhering to thin-walled blood vessels, and isolated mature neurons (*N arrow*), which appear to float in the acellular areas, characteristic findings in DNET.

DISCUSSION

DNETs comprise cortical dysplasia and multiple cell lineages of neuronal, astrocytic, and oligodendrocytic components.[2] They are primarily found in children and are associated with complex partial seizures. Seizures typically remit following surgical resection. This boy is unusual because his tumor at presentation was not associated with any symptoms other than sleepwalking-like episodes.

Pediatric brain tumors presenting with seizures as the only clinical sign are rare, and those with exclusively nocturnal seizures mimicking parasomnias are seldom encountered.[3] The differential diagnosis of agitated sleepwalking includes nocturnal frontal epilepsy, which can present as paroxysmal arousals, paroxysmal dystonia, or episodic nocturnal wanderings (ENW). These seizures can defy what defines partial epilepsy: lack of an aura, to and fro movements, rhythmic twitching, focal signs, and a postictal phase. Further, EEGs may not be helpful because interictal discharges are often lacking, and ictal abnormalities are obscured by movement and muscle artifact.

The most common manifestation of the three patterns of nocturnal frontal epilepsy is the paroxysmal arousal from sleep, a brief, recurrent arousal with stereotyped movements and dystonic posture of the limbs. Nocturnal paroxysmal dystonia presents with abrupt arousals accompanied by a complex and bizarre sequence of movements. In ENW, the patient suddenly awakens with abnormal motor features, followed by agitated somnambulism.[4] ENW resembles parasomnias as both involve nocturnal ambulation, altered consciousness during an episode, and retrograde amnesia. However, ENW predominantly occurs in adolescents and young adults, is responsive to antiepileptic drugs, and is usually associated with complex, violent behaviors. Although epileptiform abnormalities may be found on EEG,[5,6] ictal and interictal EEGs are uninformative in many patients.[7,8] Brain tumors can trigger parasomnias or seizures resembling parasomnias. A third possibility is that a seizure could cause an arousal, which in turn triggers a parasomnia.

Among the few reports of ENW in the literature, Huang and Chu[6] described adult-onset sleepwalking and daytime visual hallucinations responsive to carbamazepine in a 25-year-old man. EEG showed an epileptic abnormality in the left temporal lobe on single photon emission computed tomography. Mendez[9] described a 15-year-old boy with apparent night terrors associated with a fourth ventricular brainstem glioma that remitted with clonazepam. Di Gennaro et al.[10] reported a 48-year-old woman with night terrors and neuroradiologic evidence of a right thalamic lesion whose episodes remitted with alprazolam. Duffau et al.[11] described a 38-year-old woman with refractory sleep-related epilepsy whose seizures resolved after surgical resection of a right temporal-insular low-grade glioma. As seen in the case reports, the seizure focus for ENW can originate from other brain regions besides the frontal lobe. Other etiologies beyond tumors can produce the same pattern of seizures; there is a report of three young adults with isolated hyperkinetic paroxysmal arousals associated with lesions in the temporal region on MRI, proven to be cortical dysplasia on resection.[12]

CONCLUSION

Although this boy had some features expected with sleepwalking, there were red flags that should have alerted clinicians, both child neurologists and sleep specialists, to a more serious etiology.[13] These include sudden nightly events, an older patient with no parasomnia history, the exceptionally brief duration (<3 minutes), and stereotyped nature of the episodes. Our patient illustrates the need for vigilance in considering sleep-related epilepsy as a cause for unusual nocturnal behavior. When seizures are suspected, sleep clinicians must remember to include an extended EEG montage for definitive diagnosis. Even if the EEG is unremarkable, consider a brain MRI with contrast to assess for an underlying lesion. As in this patient, further evaluation and management of an associated lesion should involve a multidisciplinary team of sleep medicine, neurology, neurosurgery, neuropathology, and neuro-oncology professionals. Child neurologists may have had little problem in recognizing the possibility of a structural lesion in this boy but should be alert to the various sleep disturbances that can precipitate parasomnias.

REFERENCES

1. Mason TBA, Pack AI. Pediatric parasomnias. *Sleep*. 2007;30:141–151.
2. Daumas-Duport CSB, Chodkiewicz J-P, Laws ER, Vedrenne C. Dysembryoplastic neuroepithelial tumor: a surgically curable tumor of young patients with intractable partial seizures. Report of thirty-nine cases. *Neurosurgery*. 1988;23:545–556.
3. Fattal-Valevski ANN, Kramer U. Seizures as the clinical presenting symptom in children with brain tumors. *J Child Neurol*. 2013;28:292–296.
4. Provini F, Plazzi G, Lugaresi E. From nocturnal paroxysmal dystonia to nocturnal frontal lobe epilepsy. *Clin Neurophysiol*. 2000;111(suppl 2):S2–S8.
5. Pedley TA, Guilleminault C. Episodic nocturnal wanderings responsive to anticonvulsant drug therapy. *Ann Neurol*. 1977;2:30–35.
6. Huang Y-Z, Chu N-S. Episodic nocturnal wandering and complex visual hallucination. A case with long-term follow-up. *Seizure*. 1998;7:67–71.
7. Provini F, Plazzi G, Tinuper P, Vandi S, Lugaresi E, Montagna P. Nocturnal frontal lobe epilepsy: a clinical and polygraphic overview of 100 consecutive cases. *Brain*. 1999;122:1017–1031.
8. Raizen DM, Mason TBA, Pack AI. Genetic basis for sleep regulation and sleep disorders. *Semin Neurol*. 2006;26:467–483.
9. Mendez MF. Pavor nocturnus from a brainstem glioma. *J Neurol. Neurosurg Psychiatry*. 1992;55:860.
10. Di Gennaro G, Autret A, Mascia A, Onorati P, Sebastiano F, Paolo Quarato P. Night terrors associated with thalamic lesion. *Clin Neurophysiol*. 2004;115:2489–2492.
11. Duffau H, Kujas M, Taillandier L. Episodic nocturnal wandering in a patient with epilepsy due to a right temporoinsular low-grade glioma: relief following resection. *J Neurosurg*. 2006;104:436–439.
12. Nobili L, Cossu M, Mai R, et al. Sleep-related hyperkinetic seizures of temporal lobe origin. *Neurology*. 2004;62:482–485.
13. Tinuper P, Bisulli F, Provini F. The parasomnias: mechanisms and treatment. *Epilepsia*. 2012;53:12–19.

A 9-year-old boy with snoring and leg movements

Lourdes M. DelRosso

CASE PRESENTATION

A 9-year-old boy presented for evaluation of snoring without gasping or witnessed apnea. The family denied nocturnal enuresis, morning headaches, or parasomnias. The patient did not report leg discomfort at bedtime. The parents noted kicking in his sleep. His bedtime was 8:30 PM. He fell asleep within 15 minutes. His mother woke him up at 7:00 AM. He did not take naps. He did not have nocturnal awakenings. The parents reported significant daytime sleepiness; a modified Epworth sleepiness score was 13/24. Review of systems was positive for nasal congestion. His past medical history was significant for allergic rhinitis. His medications included mometasone nasal spray.

PHYSICAL EXAM

Physical exam revealed a cooperative boy in no distress. His height was at the 50th percentile, and his weight was at the 40th percentile. He had a slight adenoid facies. His nose had mildly enlarged inferior turbinates. He did not have a high-arched palate. Oropharyngeal Mallampati grade was II, and the tonsil size was 1+. He did not have micrognathia or retrognathia. The remainder of the cardiovascular and musculoskeletal exam was normal.

LABORATORY AND SLEEP FINDINGS

Polysomnography (PSG) revealed a normal sleep latency of 15 minutes. The sleep efficiency was 92%. The arousal index was 12/h. The obstructive apnea–hypopnea index (AHI) was 0.9/h. The central AHI was 0/h. The Periodic Leg Movement index was (PLMI) 11/h (Figs. 68-1 and 68-2).

QUESTION

What is the diagnosis in this patient?

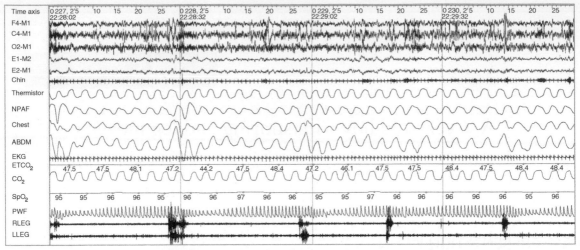

FIGURE 68-1 ■ Two-minute epoch demonstrating PLMS.

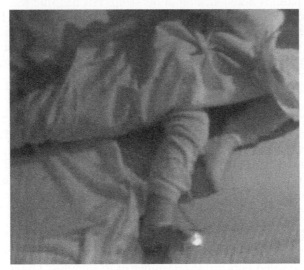

FIGURE 68-2 ■ Leg movement seen demonstrates typical toe extension and ankle flexion. The pulse oximeter sensor is on the toe.

ANSWER

Periodic leg movement disorder (PLMD).

DISCUSSION

Periodic leg movements of sleep (PLMS) are characterized by stereotypic (extension of the toe and flexion of the ankle, knee, and hip) and repetitive movements of the legs during sleep (see Figs. 68-1 and 68-2). PLMS are rare in normal children but are found in up to 80% of those with symptoms of restless leg syndrome (RLS); therefore, when PLMS are seen on PSG, the sleep physician must evaluate for the presence of RLS symptoms.[1] PLMS are also elevated in obstructive sleep apnea syndrome (OSAS), narcolepsy, attention-deficit hyperactivity disorder (ADHD), and Tourette syndrome. Medications found to increase RLS and PLMS include selective serotonin reuptake inhibitors, tricyclic antidepressants, antihistamines, and antipsychotics. The pathophysiology of both RLS and PLMS is related to dopamine dysfunction, which results in increased sympathetic activity. Iron is a cofactor in the rate-limiting step in dopamine synthesis; therefore, iron deficiency indirectly leads to dopamine dysfunction, resulting in RLS and PLMS. Ferritin levels <50 ng/mL are correlated with decreased iron stores.[2]

PLMS are scored according to the following American Academy of Sleep Medicine Scoring Manual 2.1 guidelines:

1. It takes a minimum of four consecutive PLMS to form a series.
   a. A minimum interval of 5 seconds between PLMS
   b. A maximum interval of 90 seconds between PLMS
   c. Must not be within 0.5 second of a respiratory event
   d. Arousal must be within 0.5 second to be considered associated with the movement
2. Each PLM must last at least 0.5 seconds in duration and be no longer than 10 seconds.
3. The onset is defined by an 8 μV increase in electromyogram (EMG) above baseline, and the ending is when the EMG drops to no more than 2 μV for 0.5 seconds.

PLMS can result in sleep fragmentation and can be associated with sleep complaints of insomnia or daytime sleepiness. PLMD in children is diagnosed by *International Classification of Sleep Disorders*, third edition (ICSD-3) criteria: the PLMI is >5/h, symptoms of daytime impairment are present, and medical, neurologic, mental, or sleep disorders are excluded. The daytime impairment symptoms usually include excessive sleepiness, fatigue, and difficulty waking in the morning but can also include poor attention, irritability, aggression, hyperactivity, and impulsivity.[3]

A study of 570 children who underwent PSG evaluation for suspected sleep-disordered breathing, excessive daytime sleepiness, and restless sleep revealed that 10% met criteria for PLMD, and among children with ADHD, the prevalence of PLMD was higher (up to 64%).[4] PSG studies on children with PLMD have shown a high night-to-night variability.[2] Actigraphy results in children overestimate nocturnal movements and, therefore, do not correlate with PLMS.[5] Treatment of PLMD in children includes caffeine avoidance, good sleep hygiene, and iron supplementation. Dopaminergic drugs, benzodiazepines, anticonvulsants, and opioids have been used off-label but have not been studied in children.[6]

Our case demonstrates a 9-year-old child with excessive daytime sleepiness, no symptoms of RLS, and elevated PLMI on PSG. The patient was diagnosed with PLMD. The ferritin level was 13 ng/mL. Iron supplementation was initiated.

CLINICAL PEARLS

1. Of children with RLS, 80% have PLMS.
2. PLMD cannot be diagnosed in the presence of RLS, OSAS, or another sleep or medical disorder.
3. Iron supplementation is the main therapy for PLMD in children who have low ferritin levels.

REFERENCES

1. Becker PM, Novak M. Diagnosis, comorbidities, and management of restless legs syndrome. *Curr Med Res Opin*. Aug 2014;30(8):1441–1460.
2. Durmer JS, Quraishi GH. Restless legs syndrome, periodic leg movements, and periodic limb movement disorder in children. *Pediatr Clin North Am*. Jun 2011;58(3):591–620.
3. Khatwa U, Kothare SV. Restless legs syndrome and periodic limb movements disorder in the pediatric population. *Curr Opin Pulm Med*. Nov 2010;16(6):559–567.
4. Crabtree VM, Ivanenko A, O'Brien LM, Gozal D. Periodic limb movement disorder of sleep in children. *J Sleep Res*. Mar 2003;12(1):73–81.
5. Montgomery-Downs HE, Crabtree VM, Gozal D. Actigraphic recordings in quantification of periodic leg movements during sleep in children. *Sleep Med*. Jul 2005;6(4):325–332.
6. Simakajornboon N. Periodic limb movement disorder in children. *Paediatr Respir Rev*. 2006;7(suppl 1):S55–S57.

A 5-year-old girl with a rush of energy at bedtime

Lourdes M. DelRosso

CASE PRESENTATION

A 5-year-old girl presented for evaluation of difficulty falling asleep. Her symptoms had started, insidiously, 4 months ago, and were getting progressively worse. The patient had a bedtime routine that started at 8:30 PM. After a bedtime story, she got up and walked around her room or started running around. She settled down by 9 PM and fell asleep independently within 20 minutes. She kicked in her sleep. When asked about symptoms of leg discomfort, the patient replied, "I feel like running." The patient did not snore. Her mother denied night terrors, sleepwalking, or nightmares. During the day, the child was very active and "could not sit still for more than 5 minutes." She did not have any significant past medical history. Her past surgical history was significant for typanostomy tube placement at age 3. She did not take any medications. Review of systems was negative for pain. Her mother had restless legs syndrome (RLS) during pregnancy.

PHYSICAL EXAM

The physical exam revealed a cooperative girl in no distress. Her vital signs were within normal range. The neurologic and neuromuscular exam were normal.

LABORATORY AND SLEEP FINDINGS

Polysomnography (PSG) revealed a total recording time of 549 minutes with a total sleep time of 269 minutes. Sleep efficiency was 49%. Sleep onset latency was 62 minutes. The arousal index was 8/h. The obstructive apnea–hypopnea index (AHI) was 0.2/h. The central AHI was 0.3/h. SpO_2 nadir was 96%. The Periodic leg movement index was (PLMI) 11/h.

Ferritin level was 15 ng/mL (normal 10 to 70 ng/mL).

QUESTION

What is the diagnosis in this child?

ANSWER

RLS.

DISCUSSION

RLS is a sleep-related movement disorder that can adversely affect sleep. The prevalence of RLS in children is thought to be about 2%.[1] Children with RLS have a high incidence of comorbidities. Attention-deficit hyperactivity disorder (ADHD), oppositional defiant disorder, anxiety, depression, or parasomnia is found in approximately 20% of children with RLS.[2] Up to 80% of children with RLS have a positive parental history of RLS, and in 16% of affected children, both parents have a positive history of RLS. Studies in adults have reported an association with gene variants BTBD9 (chromosome 6), MEIS1, and MAP2K5/LBXCOR. The presence of heterozygous alleles on BTBD9 doubles the risk of RLS with periodic limb movements during sleep (PLMS), whereas homozygosity quadruples the risk.[3] Iron deficiency has been associated with RLS. Brain magnetic resonance imaging studies in patients with RLS have demonstrated low iron. Iron is a cofactor in dopamine synthesis, and iron deficiency produces an alteration in dopamine, which can manifest as RLS.[4] Positron emission tomography has demonstrated decreased membrane-bound dopamine transporter in the striatum of patients with RLS (Fig. 69-1).[5]

The symptoms of sleep disturbance often precede the diagnosis of RLS, and the final diagnosis is often delayed by many years. In a study of 18 children diagnosed with RLS, the mean age of presentation to a sleep clinic was 10 years; the mean age of diagnosis was 14 years; and the mean age of onset of sleep disturbance was 3 years. The sleep disturbances included sleep onset difficulty, sleep maintenance problems, and restless sleep. All children had gradual progression of symptoms.[6] Typical descriptions of the sensory symptoms of RLS by children were ants or spiders in the legs, funny feelings in the legs, legs with too much energy, or legs that wanted to kick.[7]

The *International Classification of Sleep Disorders*, third edition (ICSD-3) diagnostic criteria for RLS include the urge to move the legs during periods of rest and in the evening. The symptoms are relieved by movement and must produce sleep disturbances or daytime impairment. Approximately 80% of children with RLS will have PLMS on PSG. A periodic limb movement index >5/h in children and >15/h in adults is required to make a diagnosis of the periodic limb movement disorder (PLMD). The diagnosis of PLMD also requires that sleep disturbance or impairment in functioning is present and not better explained by another disorder. A diagnosis of PLMD is not made if a diagnosis of RLS is present. Making a diagnosis of RLS is often difficult in children (they may not be able to verbalize

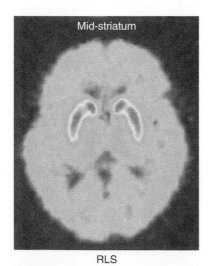
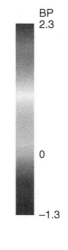
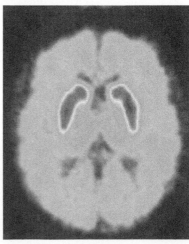

FIGURE 69-1 ■ Examples of DAT binding in the striatum of patients with RLS (*left*) and a control subject (*right*). *BP,* Binding potential; *DAT,* DA transporter; *RLS,* restless legs syndrome. (Reprinted with permission from Earley CJ, Connor J, Garcia-Borreguero D, et al. Altered brain iron homeostasis and dopaminergic function in restless legs syndrome (Willis-Ekbom disease). *Sleep Med.* Nov 2014;15(11):1288-1301.)

symptoms), and some patients are given a diagnosis of PLMD. When they are older, a diagnosis of RLS can be made. Of note, a PLM index of 11/h as noted in the current patient would not be uncommon in an adult (usually asymptomatic) but is distinctly abnormal in children.

The treatment of RLS in children includes iron supplementation if the ferritin level is below 50 ng/mL. Currently, there are no pharmacologic agents approved by the Food and Drug Administration for the treatment of RLS in children; when used, these medications are used off-label.[4] A study of seven children with RLS, PLMS, and ADHD demonstrated improved arousals, symptoms of RLS, PLMS, and subjective and objective symptoms of ADHD with dopaminergic monotherapy.[8] Another study of seven children with ADHD and RLS demonstrated improvement in RLS symptoms, sleep quality, and restorative sleep with the use of levetiracetam.[9] Clonidine and gabapentin have been successfully used in children with RLS who presented with sleep onset disturbances.[2]

Our patient presented with sleep onset disturbance and vague symptoms of RLS. The presence of elevated PLMI on the PSG aided in the diagnosis of RLS. His ferritin level was low, and iron supplementation was implemented with improvement of symptoms 6 weeks later.

CLINICAL PEARLS

1. RLS is present in about 2% of children.
2. Patients with RLS have a high incidence of comorbidities (ADHD, oppositional defiant disorder, anxiety, depression, and parasomnia).
3. A PSG with PLMI >5/h can aid in the diagnosis of RLS in children with nonspecific symptoms (restless sleep or sleep onset or maintenance insomnia).
4. Iron supplementation is the main treatment of RLS in children.

REFERENCES

1. Picchietti D, Allen RP, Walters AS, Davidson JE, Myers A, Ferini-Strambi L. Restless legs syndrome: prevalence and impact in children and adolescents—the Peds REST study. *Pediatrics*. Aug 2007;120(2):253–266.
2. Becker PM, Novak M. Diagnosis, comorbidities, and management of restless legs syndrome. *Curr Med Res Opin*. Aug 2014;30(8):1441–1460.
3. Picchietti MA, Picchietti DL. Advances in pediatric restless legs syndrome: iron, genetics, diagnosis and treatment. *Sleep Med*. Aug 2010;11(7):643–651.
4. Khatwa U, Kothare SV. Restless legs syndrome and periodic limb movements disorder in the pediatric population. *Curr Opin Pulm Med*. Nov 2010;16(6):559–567.
5. Earley CJ, Connor J, Garcia-Borreguero D, et al. Altered brain iron homeostasis and dopaminergic function in restless legs syndrome (Willis-Ekbom disease). *Sleep Med*. Nov 2014;15(11):1288–1301.
6. Picchietti DL, Stevens HE. Early manifestations of restless legs syndrome in childhood and adolescence. *Sleep Med*. Oct 2008;9(7):770–781.
7. de Weerd A, Arico I, Silvestri R. Presenting symptoms in pediatric restless legs syndrome patients. *J Clin Sleep Med*. Oct 15 2013;9(10):1077–1080.
8. Walters AS, Mandelbaum DE, Lewin DS, Kugler S, England SJ, Miller M. Dopaminergic therapy in children with restless legs/periodic limb movements in sleep and ADHD. Dopaminergic Therapy Study Group. *Pediatr Neurol*. Mar 2000;22(3):182–186.
9. Gagliano A, Arico I, Calarese T, et al. Restless leg syndrome in ADHD children: levetiracetam as a reasonable therapeutic option. *Brain Dev*. Jun 2011;33(6):480–486.

A 4-year-old boy with tooth grinding during sleep

Lourdes M. DelRosso

CASE PRESENTATION

A 4-year-old boy presented for evaluation of tooth grinding during sleep. The parents reported tooth grinding every night, several times a night. He slept for 10 hours a night from 9 PM to 7 AM, without nocturnal awakenings. He did not report morning headaches or mandibular pain. The family denied frequent nocturnal awakenings, snoring, leg movements, sleepwalking, and daytime sleepiness. He did not consume caffeine. There was no significant past medical or surgical history. He did not take any medications. The review of systems was negative for anxiety and depression.

PHYSICAL EXAM

The physical exam revealed a cooperative boy in no distress. His weight and height were at the 45th percentile. His vital signs were within normal limits. He did not have an adenoid facies. The oropharynx was Mallampati class I. His tonsils were size 1+. He did not have tooth wear, and dentition appeared normal with no malocclusion. There was no temporomandibular joint tenderness. The remainder of the physical exam was normal.

QUESTIONS

Is polysomnography (PSG) indicated in this patient?

ANSWERS

No, PSG is not indicated in the evaluation of bruxism.

DISCUSSION

Bruxism is commonly seen in children, affecting up to 45% of preschoolers.[1] The etiology is unknown, but contributing factors include genetic predisposition, increased arousability, autonomic sympathetic activation, psychosocial factors (anxiety), drugs, and medications.[2]

The *International Classification of Sleep Disorders*, third edition (ICSD-3) classifies sleep-related bruxism under movement disorders. The diagnostic criteria include reported tooth-grinding sounds during sleep and the presence of clinical signs (either tooth wear, temporal headache, or jaw muscle pain). Our patient did not report any associated symptoms and, therefore, does not meet criteria for diagnosis.

In one study of 120 (8-year-old) children with bruxism reported by parents, compared with 240 age-matched children without reported sleep bruxism, there was a statistically significant difference in reported headaches, mouth breathing, object biting (pencils or pens), nail biting, teeth clenching while awake, and canine wear between both groups, with a higher prevalence of symptoms in the bruxism group.[3]

Evidence of tooth wear on physical exam in the absence of tooth-grinding sounds during sleep should not be assumed to be secondary to bruxism because tooth wear is common in children. Younger children are more susceptible to tooth wear because the primary teeth are not as strong as the permanent teeth are. A 3-year longitudinal study of 572 children demonstrated a 22% prevalence of erosive wear on upper incisors, and 15% prevalence of erosive wear on first lower molars.[4] The etiology was likely multifactorial but included carbonated soft drink intake, gastroesophageal reflux, vomiting, and tooth grinding.[4, 5] However, mouth guards are rarely prescribed by dentists because the primary teeth are not permanent.

PSG is not routinely indicated in the evaluation of sleep bruxism, but it is indicated if there is suspicion of sleep-disordered breathing, periodic leg movements of sleep, or frequent NREM parasomnias.[6] Scoring bruxism is optional. The scoring manual criteria recommend scoring bruxism as either phasic or tonic when the elevation of the chin electromyogram (EMG) is twice the amplitude of the background EMG. Phasic bruxism is depicted in Figure 70-1. Tonic bruxism is scored when the EMG elevation lasts longer than 2 seconds. Recording of audio aids in the scoring of bruxism during PSG, and at least two audible tooth-grinding episodes are required for a diagnosis. A PSG study on children with bruxism demonstrated that 66% of bruxism episodes were associated with arousals.[7] Similarly to bruxism in adults, sleep bruxism in children occurs predominantly in N2 and REM sleep.[7]

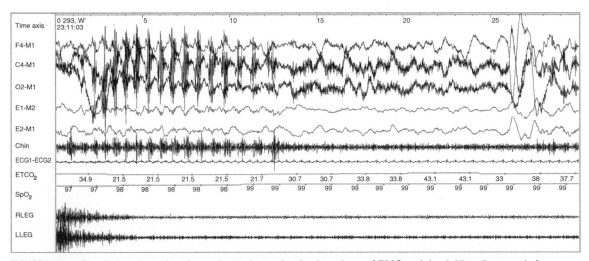

FIGURE 70-1 ■ Phasic bruxism showing at least three phasic elevations of EMG activity 0.25 to 2 seconds in duration.

A longitudinal study on 320 children with bruxism, followed up after 20 years, revealed that 32% had received some kind of orthodontic treatment in childhood. There was no statistically significant difference in bruxism frequency, headaches, or temporomandibular discomfort between the treated group and the nontreated group.[8]

In conclusion, bruxism is commonly seen in children and is associated with increased arousals. Our patient did not require any intervention because symptoms were not present.

CLINICAL PEARLS

1. The diagnosis of sleep-related bruxism requires tooth-grinding sounds and clinical signs (tooth wear, temporal headaches, or jaw muscle pain).
2. PSG is not routinely indicated in the evaluation of sleep bruxism, and scoring of bruxism is optional.
3. Sleep bruxism occurs predominantly in N2 and REM sleep (but it can occur in any sleep stage).
4. Mouth guards are rarely prescribed for children with primary dentition.

REFERENCES

1. Petit D, Touchette E, Tremblay RE, Boivin M, Montplaisir J. Dyssomnias and parasomnias in early childhood. *Pediatrics.* May 2007;119(5):e1016–e1025.
2. Lavigne GJ, Khoury S, Abe S, Yamaguchi T, Raphael K. Bruxism physiology and pathology: an overview for clinicians. *J Oral Rehabil.* Jul 2008;35(7):476–494.
3. Serra-Negra JM, Paiva SM, Auad SM, Ramos-Jorge ML, Pordeus IA. Signs, symptoms, parafunctions and associated factors of parent-reported sleep bruxism in children: a case-control study. *Braz Dent J.* 2012;23(6):746–752.
4. Aidi HE, Bronkhorst EM, Huysmans MC, Truin GJ. Factors associated with the incidence of erosive wear in upper incisors and lower first molars: a multifactorial approach. *J Dent.* Aug 2011;39(8):558–563.
5. Carvalho TS, Lussi A, Jaeggi T, Gambon DL. Erosive tooth wear in children. *Monogr Oral Sci.* 2014;25:262–278.
6. Aurora RN, Lamm CI, Zak RS, et al. Practice parameters for the non-respiratory indications for polysomnography and multiple sleep latency testing for children. *Sleep.* Nov 2012;35(11):1467–1473.
7. Herrera M, Valencia I, Grant M, Metroka D, Chialastri A, Kothare SV. Bruxism in children: effect on sleep architecture and daytime cognitive performance and behavior. *Sleep.* Sep 2006;29(9):1143–1148.
8. Carlsson GE, Egermark I, Magnusson T. Predictors of signs and symptoms of temporomandibular disorders: a 20-year follow-up study from childhood to adulthood. *Acta Odontol Scand.* Jun 2002;60(3):180–185.

A 5-year-old boy with repetitive nocturnal movements

Lourdes M. DelRosso

CASE PRESENTATION

A 5-year-old boy presented for evaluation of abnormal nocturnal movements. The movements started when the child was 2 years old. Usually the episodes occurred at bedtime. The episodes also occurred when the child was asleep; he would suddenly reposition himself, turn on his hands and knees, and move his body back and forth for a few minutes at a time throughout the night. The family had to cushion the bed frame to prevent head injuries. He snored softly, but the parents had not noticed gasping or witnessed apnea. The family did not report excessive daytime sleepiness, restless legs, night terrors, sleep talking, or sleepwalking. He did not have any other medical problems and did not take any medications. Review of systems was negative for headaches, seizure disorder, depression, anxiety, and behavioral problems. He was developmentally appropriate.

PHYSICAL EXAM

Physical exam revealed a cooperative boy in no distress. His vital signs were within normal limits. His weight was 24.6 kg (62nd percentile), and his height was 119 cm (24th percentile). He did not have an adenoid facies or a high-arched palate. His oropharynx was Mallampati grade II. Tonsil size was 1+. He did not have micrognathia or retrognathia. The remainder of the cardiovascular and neurologic exam was normal.

LABORATORY AND SLEEP FINDINGS

Polysomnography (PSG) revealed a sleep efficiency of 90%, with a total sleep time of 508.5 minutes; total recording time 562 minutes; apnea–hypopnea index 0.8/h; and SpO_2 98%. Periodic leg movements index was 1/h. There was no evidence of hypoventilation. During N2, the patient turned on his hands and knees (Fig. 71-1) and moved back and forth repetitively (Figs. 71-2 and 71-3).

QUESTION

What is the diagnosis?

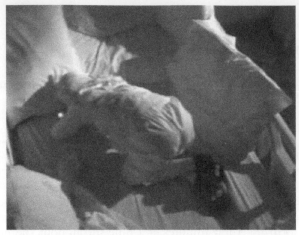

FIGURE 71-1 ■ The patient's position on his hands and knees as he moves repetitively.

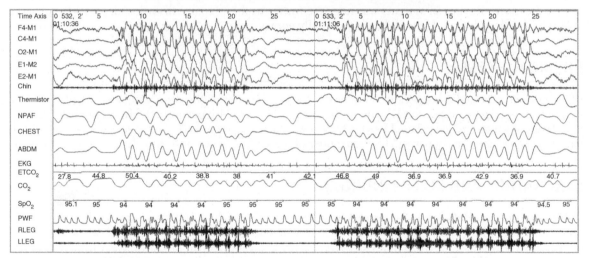

FIGURE 71-2 ■ PSG findings during the repetitive movements, 60-second epoch.

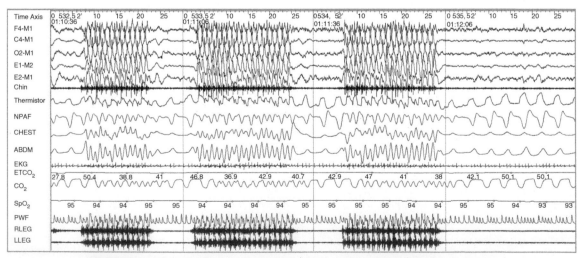

FIGURE 71-3 ■ PSG findings during the repetitive movements, 120-second epoch.

ANSWER

Rhythmic movement disorder (RMD), body-rocking subtype.

DISCUSSION

The *International Classification of Sleep Disorders*, third edition (ICSD-3) describes RMD as repetitive, stereotypic and rhythmic movements that involve large muscle groups and occur during sleep. *To fit criteria, the movements must interfere with sleep, impair daytime alertness, or place the patient at risk of bodily injury.* RMD must not be better explained by seizure disorder or by another movement disorder. RMD can manifest in different subtypes; in body rocking, as seen in our patient, the child usually rocks his body while on his hands and knees. In head banging, the child usually strikes his head against an object. In head rolling, the child moves his head side to side while supine. The PSG characteristics of RMD as described in the scoring manual include a minimum of four repetitive movements with frequencies between 0.5 and 2 Hz, with burst amplitude of at least twice the amplitude of the background electromyogram. The PSG diagnostic criteria include movements seen in time-synchronized video monitoring.

RMD is commonly seen in infants and children and usually remits spontaneously after the fifth year of life, with 5% prevalence in adolescents and adults. The onset is usually during the first year of life, with up to 66% of 9-month-olds exhibiting some rhythmic activity.[1] RMD has been reported in wakefulness and in all stages of sleep, but usually it occurs during early drowsiness and after arousals[2]; episodes thought by parents to be occurring during sleep are usually post arousal. Unlike a seizure disorder, the movement can be stopped upon waking the child.[3] The pathophysiology of RMD has been hypothesized to be secondary to immature motor pathways, vestibular self-stimulation, or disorder of wake-sleep transition. Although often seen in typically developing children, RMD has an increased prevalence in children with autism or developmental delays. RMD has been seen with other sleep disorders such as obstructive sleep apnea syndrome (OSAS). Of interest in adults, when RMD is associated with OSAS, case reports suggest that continuous positive airway pressure (CPAP) can improve RMD.[4-6]

RMD is usually diagnosed by history. Nocturnal PSG is not necessary to diagnose RMD unless a comorbid sleep disorder or seizure disorder is suspected. Management aims at injury prevention. Pharmacological treatment is usually not necessary.

CLINICAL PEARLS

1. RMD is characterized by repetitive, stereotypic, rhythmic movements that occur during wakefulness or sleep.
2. Rhythmic movements are very common in infants and young children but can persist into adulthood. A diagnosis of RMD requires some adverse consequences associated with the movements.
3. In adults, RMD has been seen in association with arousals during OSAS, and two case reports suggest that RMD improves with CPAP treatment.

REFERENCES

1. Gupta R, Goel D, Dhyani M, Mittal M. Head banging persisting during adolescence: a case with polysomnographic findings. *J Neurosci Rural Pract*. Oct 2014;5(4):405–408.
2. Anderson KN, Smith IE, Shneerson JM. Rhythmic movement disorder (head banging) in an adult during rapid eye movement sleep. *Mov Disord*. Jun 2006;21(6):866–867.
3. Walters AS. Clinical identification of the simple sleep-related movement disorders. *Chest*. Apr 2007;131(4):1260–1266.
4. Kohyama J, Matsukura F, Kimura K, Tachibana N. Rhythmic movement disorder: polysomnographic study and summary of reported cases. *Brain Dev*. Jan 2002;24(1):33–38.
5. Chirakalwasan N, Hassan F, Kaplish N, Fetterolf J, Chervin RD. Near resolution of sleep related rhythmic movement disorder after CPAP for OSA. *Sleep Med*. Apr 2009;10(4):497–500.
6. Gharagozlou P, Seyffert M, Santos R, Chokroverty S. Rhythmic movement disorder associated with respiratory arousals and improved by CPAP titration in a patient with restless legs syndrome and sleep apnea. *Sleep Med*. Apr 2009;10(4):501–503.

CASE 72

A patient with sickle cell disease and a low baseline sleeping oxygen saturation*

Mary H. Wagner and Richard B. Berry

An 11-year-old African American male with sickle cell disease (SCD) was referred for evaluation of suspected sleep apnea. Nocturnal symptoms included restlessness, diaphoresis, snoring, kicking, and increased work of breathing. The family reported occasional excessive daytime sleepiness and napping after school. The patient had a history of vaso-occlusive crisis episodes requiring transfusion. Medications at the time of the study included methylphenidate (Metadate), hydroxyurea, penicillin V potassium (Pen VK), and folic acid.

PHYSICAL EXAM

Bilaterally enlarged tonsils.

LABORATORY STUDY

Hematocrit 26%.

SUMMARY OF SLEEP STUDY RESULTS

Apnea–hypopnea index: 14.2 events/h with two obstructive apneas, two central apneas, 87 hypopneas, and a minimum arterial oxygen saturation (SaO_2) of 84%. The 30-second tracing shown in Figure 72-1 was typical for non-rapid eye movement sleep (NREM) (see Fig. 72-1).

QUESTION

What is the explanation for the low SaO_2 during apparently stable breathing?

ANSWER

Low SpO_2 because of an abnormal oxygen hemoglobin dissociation curve.
 The SaO_2 is measured noninvasively using pulse oximetry (SpO_2) to detect arterial oxygen desaturation and hypoxemia. The SaO_2 is usually defined as the amount of oxyhemoglobin (O_2Hb) divided by the sum of the O_2Hb and the deoxygenated or reduced hemoglobin (RHb).

$$SaO_2\% = (O_2Hb) \times 100/(O_2Hb + RHb) \tag{72-1}$$

---

*This entire chapter is taken from Wagner MH, Berry RB. A patient with sickle cell disease and a low baseline sleeping oxygen saturation. *J Clin Sleep Med* 2007;3(3):313-315.

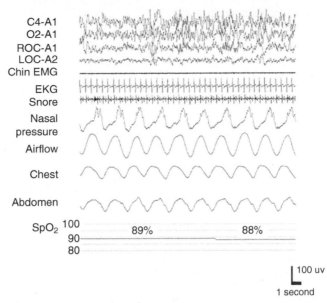

FIGURE 72-1 ■ A 30-second tracing is shown during NREM sleep. The ventilation appears normal, but the pulse oximetry (SpO$_2$) value is reduced. *EKG*, Electrocardiogram; *EMG*, electromyogram; *LOC*, left outer canthus electrooculogram; *ROC*, right outer canthus electrooculogram.

At normal arterial oxygen levels, only a small amount of oxygen is dissolved in the blood, and most of the oxygen-carrying capacity depends on the amount of hemoglobin bound to oxygen.

However, determining the oxygen-carrying capacity of hemoglobin is complicated because both carboxyhemoglobin (COHb) and methemoglobin (metHb) are forms of circulating hemoglobin that do not bind to oxygen. The true fraction of hemoglobin bound to oxygen (FO$_2$Hb) then depends on the fraction (%) of carboxyhemoglobin (FCOHb) and methemoglobin (FMetHb), as well as the fraction of reduced hemoglobin (FRHb).

$$FO_2Hb + FRHb + FCOHb + FMetHb = 100\% \qquad (72\text{-}2)$$

For example, if the FO$_2$Hb = 85%, FCOHb = 8%, and FMetHb = 1%, then the FRHb is 6%. Using these numbers, the SaO$_2$ equals $85 \times 100/(85 + 6)$ or 93%, which is considerably higher than an FO$_2$Hb of 85%. The FO$_2$Hb and the amount of hemoglobin are the main determinants of the oxygen-carrying capacity of the blood. The difference between the SaO$_2$ and the FO$_2$Hb is primarily determined by the amount of COHb and MetHb. The FO$_2$Hb is sometimes called the fractional saturation, and the SaO$_2$, the functional or effective saturation. The four fractions of hemoglobin can be accurately measured by co-oximeters that measure the absorption of four or more wavelengths of electromagnetic radiation by a sample of arterial blood.[1] This is possible because the four forms of hemoglobin differ in their absorption for the different wavelengths of radiation. In contrast, pulse oximetry[1] uses only two wavelengths, 660 nm (red) and 940 nm (infrared), to measure the O$_2$Hb and RHb. The absorption of radiation at 660 nm is much greater with RHb than with O$_2$Hb, whereas O$_2$Hb absorbs more radiation at 940 nm (Fig. 72-2, *A*). Pulse oximetry is based on the empiric observation that the ratio (R) of absorbance at the two wavelengths is related to the oxygen saturation (see Fig. 72-2, *B*). This relationship (calibration curve) is determined experimentally by determining R at varying oxygen saturations. To determine the specific absorbance of arterial blood, the AC (pulse added absorbance) at each wavelength is divided by the DC (background absorbance) to account for the effect of the absorption of the radiation by venous blood and tissue. Carboxyhemoglobin has about the same absorbance at 660 as oxyhemoglobin does and, if present, it increases the measured SpO$_2$ value. In normal individuals, FCOHb is 2% or less but can be 8% or more in cigarette smokers. Patients with SCD often have FCOHb values of 4% or more because of production of carbon dioxide from chronic hemolysis. Based on a canine experiment,[1] it has been estimated that a pulse oximeter sees COHb as 90% O$_2$Hb and 10% RHb. For example, from the values (FO2Hb = 85%, COHb = 4%, MetHb = 0%, and RHb = 11%), one can estimate the SpO$_2$ as 88.6% $(85 + 0.9 \times 4)$. This is essentially the same as the SaO2 computed from Eq. 72-1 for these values. SpO$_2$ measurements in

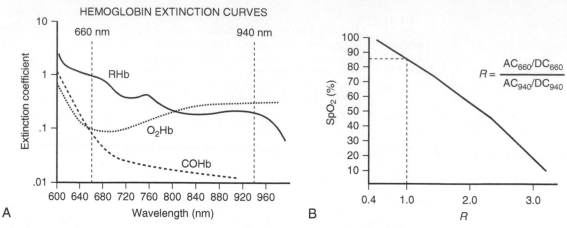

FIGURE 72-2 ■ **A,** Hemoglobin extinction curves for RHb, O_2Hb, and COHb at different wavelengths of light. Note that the *y*-axis is a log scale. **B,** Empirical curve of the ratio of absorption of radiation at wavelengths of 660 and 940 nm. The AC is the pulse added absorption, and DC the steady state or background absorbance. (Adapted from Temper KK, Barker SJ. Pulse oximetry. *Anesthesiology.* 1989;70:98-108).

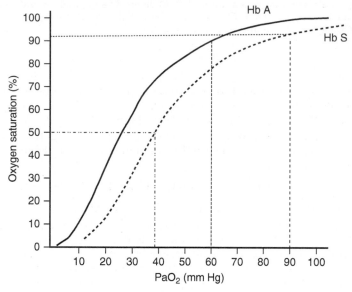

FIGURE 72-3 ■ The oxygen hemoglobin dissociation curve showing the values for hemoglobin (Hb) A (*solid line*) and a patient with Hb S (*dashed line*). For the patient with Hb S, the P50 is 38 mm Hg, and an SaO_2 value of 92% corresponds to a PO_2 of 90 mm Hg.

patients with SCD who have carboxyhemoglobinemia often show fairly good agreement with the SaO_2 but overestimate the FO_2Hb.

Inference about the arterial oxygen pressure (PaO_2) based on the SaO_2 requires knowledge of the factors that can affect the oxyhemoglobin dissociation curve (Fig. 72-3). The oxyhemoglobin dissociation curve is shifted to the right with increases in body temperature, $PaCO_2$, 2-3DPG (a product of glycolysis), or H^+ ion concentration (acidemia). The opposite changes in the factors shift the curve to the left. CO can not only bind a portion of the Hb (preventing oxygen binding) but also shift the oxyhemoglobin dissociation curve of the remaining Hb to the left. Variant hemoglobin can shift the position of the curve to the left or right from that associated with normal hemoglobin (Hb A). In dilute solution, sickle hemoglobin (Hb S) has similar affinity for oxygen as Hb A does. (They differ by only a single peptide.) However, at the higher hemoglobin concentration present in red cells, deoxygenated Hb S forms polymers that have a low affinity for oxygen.[2,3] The net effect is a rightward shift in the oxyhemoglobin dissociation curve for Hb S (see Fig. 72-3). The position of the oxyhemoglobin dissociation curve is often defined by the P50, which is the PO_2 corresponding to a SaO_2 of 50%. For Hb A, the P50 is 26 mm Hg but is 42 to 56 mm Hg in patients with SCD.[3] This means that, for a given SaO_2, the PaO_2 is higher in patients with SCD than would be expected based on the normal oxyhemoglobin dissociation curve. The amount of right shift varies considerably among patients with SCD and can be influenced by transfusion with blood (Hb A).

Given the similar structures of Hb A and Hb S, one might expect similar absorption at the wavelengths of electromagnetic radiation used for oximetry. A number of studies have assessed the ability of pulse oximetry (SpO_2) to estimate the SaO_2 and to detect hypoxemia in patients with SCD. In general, the SpO_2 exceeds the FO_2Hb but is fairly close to the SaO_2. Craft et al.[4] found that the SpO_2 exceeded the FO_2Hb by a mean of approximately 7%. Ortiz et al.[5] studied 22 patients with SCD admitted with a vaso-occlusive episode. The mean SpO_2 exceeded the FO_2Hb (90.4% vs. 87.1%) but approximated the SaO_2 (91.5%). In this study, the COHb was 3.8%, and the P50 was 35 mm Hg. Blaisdell et al.[6] found that 33% of a group of patients with SCD who were predicted to be hypoxemic with SpO_2 measurements less than 93% actually had PaO_2 values >70 mm Hg. Bromberg and Jensen[7] studied nine patients with SCD with SpO_2 values ranging from 75% to 90%, and none had an arterial PO_2 <70 mm Hg. In the current patient, an arterial blood gas was obtained at the end of the study, while the patient was awake and breathing room air. The values were a pH of 7.44, a $PaCO_2$ of 37 mm Hg, a PaO_2 of 90 mm Hg, and a HCO_3 of 25.3 mmol/L. The SpO_2 measurement at same time was 92%. Co-oximetry was not performed on the sample, but prior measurements had shown FCOHb and FMetHb values of 4% and 1%, respectively. Given the high PO_2 corresponding to an SpO_2 of 92%, one can conclude that the low SpO_2 in Figure 72-1 was not due to hypoxemia but rather to the patient's abnormal hemoglobin.

CLINICAL PEARLS

1. The SpO_2 is often greater than the oxygenated fraction of hemoglobin as measured by a co-oximeter in patients with SCD (primarily because of elevated carboxyhemoglobin).
2. The oxyhemoglobin dissociation curve for Hb S is shifted to the right, compared to Hb A. Therefore, a given SaO_2 corresponds to a higher PaO_2 than would be predicted based on Hb A.
3. Lower-than-normal SpO_2 values during sleep in patients with SCD may not represent hypoxemia. If clinically indicated, an arterial blood gas reading can be obtained for precise determination of the arterial PO_2.
4. In patients with significant amounts of carboxyhemoglobinemia, to determine accurately the fraction of hemoglobin that is bound to oxygen, use co-oximetry of a sample of arterial blood rather than pulse oximetry.

REFERENCES

1. Temper KK, Barker SJ. Pulse oximetry. *Anesthesiology*. 1989;70:98–108.
2. Blaisdell Carol J. Sickle cell disease and breathing during sleep. In: Loughlin GM, Carroll JL, Marcus C, eds. *Sleep and Breathing in Children. A Developmental Approach*. New York: Marcel Dekker, Inc; 2000:755–763.
3. Seakins M, Gibbs WN, Milner PF, et al. Erthyrocyte Hb-S concentration—an important factor in low oxygen affinity of blood in sickle cell anemia. *J Clin Invest*. 1973;52:422–432.
4. Craft JA, Alessandrini E, Kenney LB, et al. Comparison of oxygenation measurements in pediatric patients during sickle cell crises. *J Pediatr*. 1994;24:93–95.
5. Ortiz FO, Aldrich TK, Nagel RL, Benjamin LJ. Accuracy of pulse oximetry in sickle disease. *Am J Respir Crit Care Med*. 1999;169:447–451.
6. Blaisdell CJ, Goodman S, Clark K, et al. Pulse oximetry is a poor predictor of hypoxemia in stable children with sickle cell disease. *Arch Pediatr Adolesc Med*. 2000;154:900–903.
7. Bromberg PA, Jensen WN. Arterial oxygen unsaturation in sickle cell disease. *Am Rev Respir Dis*. 1967;96:400–407.

A 5-month-old baby who wakes and spits up through the night

Lourdes M. DelRosso

CASE PRESENTATION

A 5-month-old infant presented for evaluation of frequent nocturnal awakenings. The parents stated that during his first month of life he was fed formula on demand every 3 to 4 hours. During the night, he was fed consistently at approximately 10 PM, 1 AM, and 4 AM. He slept between feedings. By 3 months of age, he was fed at 10 PM and slept through the night until 5 AM. At 4 months of age, he started waking up several times during the night. The parents noticed that he cried, grimaced, and arched his back during these awakenings. They also noticed a couple of episodes of choking at night and a few diurnal and nocturnal episodes of spitting up of formula during feedings. The parents were afraid to introduce new foods because of these episodes. The parents did not notice snoring, apneic episodes, forceful vomiting, or gagging. He had daily bowel movements.

The infant was born full term via normal spontaneous vaginal delivery. He did not have any perinatal complications. His mother, a 27-year-old G1P1 woman, received full prenatal care. His birth weight was 3.5 kg and birth length was 49 cm (50th percentile). He was fed formula exclusively. There was no other significant past medical or surgical history.

PHYSICAL EXAM

Physical exam revealed a well-developed infant with adequate milestones for age. His vital signs were within normal range, and his weight and length were at the 50th percentile. He did not have a high-arched palate. Oropharyngeal exam was normal. His lungs were clear to auscultation. His abdomen was not distended and without organomegaly or masses. The remainder of the exam was normal.

LABORATORY AND SLEEP FINDINGS

Nocturnal polysomnography (PSG) with pH probe monitoring (hypnogram shown in Fig. 73-1) revealed total sleep time 456 minutes, sleep efficiency 80%, arousal index 16/h, periodic leg movement index 2.2/h, and apnea–hypopnea index 0.4/h. The results of the pH probe monitoring during the sleep study are shown in Table 73-1.

QUESTION

What is the diagnosis in this infant?

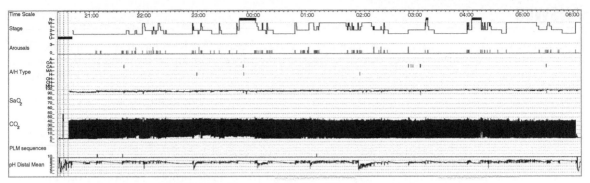

FIGURE 73-1 ■ **Hypnogram with pH probe monitoring.**

TABLE 73-1.	pH was <4 for 0.4% of total recording time; the lowest pH was 3.2							
pH	0-1	1-2	2-3	3-4	4-5	5-6	6-7	7-8	8-9
Min	0	0	0	2	5	16	225	294	14
% total recording time	0.0	0.0	0.0	0.4	0.9	2.8	40.5	52.9	2.5

ANSWER

The infant was diagnosed with gastroesophageal reflux disease (GERD) based on symptoms. The pH monitoring was not diagnostic of acid reflux, and, therefore, acid suppressant medication was not started; non-acid reflux was diagnosed. Thickening the formula with cereal and keeping him upright after feedings improved his symptoms.

DISCUSSION

Gastroesophageal reflux (GER), defined as the passage of gastric contents into the esophagus, is found in over 75% of healthy infants; it constitutes a normal physiologic process resulting from episodic brief relaxations of the lower esophageal sphincter, in contrast to GERD, which is far less common and associated with bothersome symptoms and medical complications.[1]

The mechanism of GER is different during the day versus night. During the day, GER is related to transient lower esophageal sphincter relaxation in combination with postprandial abdominal distention. During the night, gastric acid secretion peaks between 10 PM and 2 AM. With sleep onset, there is decreased peristalsis and swallowing, making sleep periods particularly vulnerable to GER. Because of the frequency of feedings, the refluxate in infants mainly consists of buffered gastric contents. These reflux episodes produce frequent arousals and awakenings as a protective mechanism because swallowing is decreased during sleep.[2] Preterm infants, children with neurologic disorders, and obese children are at higher risk of GERD.

GERD is often diagnosed based on clinical presentation. GERD in infants is most common at 4 months of age, with symptoms including dysphagia, arching of the back during feedings, respiratory symptoms, and failure to thrive. The prevalence of GERD declines in older children, with symptoms including vomiting, heartburn, abdominal pain, anorexia, and respiratory symptoms. If reflux reaches the pharynx, dysphonia, chronic cough, dysphagia, and laryngeal spasm may occur. Arytenoid, postglottic and/or vocal fold edema may be present on laryngoscopy.[3]

The following studies can be used to aid in the diagnosis of GERD: Esophageal pH monitoring calculates reflux index (the percentage of time with esophageal pH <4). It is abnormal when >12% in infants up to 11 months old and >6% in older children and adults.[4] pH monitoring has not been shown to correlate with severity of symptoms in infants, possibly because of the higher prevalence of non-acid reflux as opposed to acid reflux. Multiple intraluminal impedance can measure the volume of reflux, regardless of acid content, and is, therefore, more useful than pH monitoring is in infants. Both tests combined can be useful to determine a temporal relationship with apnea or cough. Upper endoscopy and esophageal biopsy allow for direct visualization and histologic evaluation of the esophageal mucosa. Other tests that can be performed during wakefulness include a barium swallow, which has less sensitivity and specificity but is less invasive and can also evaluate for anatomic abnormalities of the gastrointestinal tract, and nuclear scintiscan.

Although the American Academy of Sleep Medicine does not recommend the routine use of simultaneous pH monitoring during PSG, infants with unexplained nocturnal respiratory events may benefit from pH or impedance monitoring. The limitation of combining pH monitoring with PSG includes underestimation of GER when compared with 24-hour pH monitoring and inability to detect non-acid reflux. Complications of pH probe insertion in infants include apnea and bradycardia.[5]

Management of GERD can be pharmacological and nonpharmacological. In formula-fed infants, a thickened formula is recommended. It is also recommended to keep the infant in an upright position after feeding. In older children, lifestyle modifications include weight loss (in obese patients) and avoidance of caffeine, chocolate, and spicy foods. Pharmacological management includes acid suppressants (antacids, H_2 receptor antagonists, and proton pump inhibitors) and prokinetics (metoclopramide, bethanechol, baclofen, and erythromycin). Surgical options include gastric fundoplication.[1]

CLINICAL PEARLS

1. GER is common in infants.
2. GER in infants mainly consists of non-acid reflux of gastric contents.
3. Frequent nocturnal arousals and awakenings are common in infants with GER.

REFERENCES

1. Lightdale JR, Gremse DA. Gastroesophageal reflux: management guidance for the pediatrician. *Pediatrics*. May 2013;131(5):e1684–e1695.
2. Machado R, Woodley FW, Skaggs B, Di Lorenzo C, Splaingard M, Mousa H. Gastroesophageal reflux causing sleep interruptions in infants. *J Pediatr Gastroenterol Nutr*. Apr 2013;56(4):431–435.
3. Baudoin T, Kosec A, Cor IS, Zaja O. Clinical features and diagnostic reliability in paediatric laryngopharyngeal reflux. *Int J Pediatr Otorhinolaryngol*. Jul 2014;78(7):1101–1106.
4. Vandeplas Y, Rudolph C. Pediatric gastroesophageal reflux clinical practice guidelines: joint recommendation of the North American Society for Pediatric Gastroenterology, Hepatology, and Nutrition (NASPGHAN) and the European Society for Pediatric Gastroenterology, Hepatology and Nutrition (ESPGHAN). and committee members. *J Pediatr Gastroenterol Nutr*. 2009;49(4):498–547.
5. Greenfeld M, Tauman R, Sivan Y. The yield of esophageal pH monitoring during polysomnography in infants with sleep-disordered breathing. *Clin Pediatr (Phila)*. Sep 2004;43(7):653–658.

A 3-year-old boy with trisomy 21 and unchanged apnea–hypopnea index after tonsillectomy and adenoidectomy

Lourdes M. DelRosso

CASE PRESENTATION

A 3-year-old boy with Trisomy 21 underwent tonsillectomy and adenoidectomy (T&A) for obstructive sleep apnea syndrome (OSAS). The repeat polysomnography 8 weeks after T&A showed only a slight improvement (Table 74-1). His mother reported snoring with gasping and breathing pauses. The patient's past medical history included Trisomy 21 and hypothyroidism diagnosed at birth. His past surgical history included repaired atrial septal defect, ventricular septal defect, and patent ductus arteriosus, as well as myringotomy tube placement and T&A. He took levothyroxine 25 µg daily for a couple of years, but his mother discontinued the medication because she thought he did not need it anymore. The review of systems was positive for global developmental delay, nasal congestion, recurrent otitis media, dry skin, and constipation.

PHYSICAL EXAM

The child appeared in no distress. His weight was 14.1 kg (80th percentile, Down syndrome growth chart), and his height was 89 cm (75th percentile, Down syndrome growth chart). The vital signs were within normal limits. He had up-slanting palpebral fissures and a large-appearing tongue. The oropharynx Mallampati grade was IV, and tonsils were surgically absent. The thyroid gland could not be palpated on neck exam. His cardiovascular exam was normal. He had dry skin. There was no edema.

LABORATORY AND SLEEP FINDINGS

Thyriod-stimulating hormone (TSH): 12.6 mIU/L (normal range: 0.5 to 3.8 mIU/L).
Free T4: 0.8 ng/dL (normal range: 1.0 to 2.7 ng/dL).

QUESTION

What would you treat first in this patient, hypothyroidism or OSAS?

TABLE 74-1. **Summary of polysomnography results**

	Total Sleep Time (TST)	Total Recording Time	Sleep Efficiency (%)	Apnea–Hypopnea Index	SpO$_2$ Nadir (%)	ETCO$_2$ >50 torr (%TST)
Pre T&A	432	497	87	13/h	89	2.3
Post T&A	527	572	92	11/h	90	0.3

ANSWER

Both conditions must be treated. Management of OSAS should not be delayed until after normalization of TSH.

DISCUSSION

Up to one third of children with Down syndrome have hypothyroidism. The American Academy of Pediatrics (AAP) recommends testing T4 and TSH levels at birth in children with Down syndrome and retesting TSH at 6 months, 12 months, and annually, thereafter.[1] Laboratory testing is particularly important in this patient population because some of the symptoms of childhood hypothyroidism, such as hypotonia, macroglossia, feeding difficulties, developmental delay, and mental retardation, are difficult to distinguish from the symptoms of Down syndrome, making the clinical diagnosis of hypothyroidism particularly challenging.[2]

Congenital hypothyroidism in the general population is a preventable cause of mental retardation. The AAP recommends checking T4 and TSH levels in all newborns. Infants with low T4 and high TSH should be referred to a pediatric endocrinologist. Symptoms of congenital hypothyroidism include constipation, prolonged jaundice, poor feeding, and decreased activity level. Acquired hypothyroidism can present with delayed growth, constipation, lethargy, and OSAS.

Hypothyroidism can cause or worsen OSAS by several proposed mechanisms: deposition of mucoproteins in the upper airway, neuropathy affecting the pharyngeal muscles, and depression of the respiratory centers; however, the incidence of hypothyroidism in patients with OSAS is not higher than in the general population. Screening for hypothyroidism in patients with OSAS is not routinely recommended. Both OSAS and hypothyroidism share similar symptoms: fatigue, sleepiness, decreased cognitive function, obesity, and depressed mood. Further evaluation should be pursued if either condition is suspected.[3] Treatment of hypothyroidism has not shown to resolve OSAS consistently; therefore, initiation of CPAP should not be delayed until after normalization of TSH. L-thyroxine is the treatment of choice for congenital and acquired hypothyroidism.[4]

CLINICAL PEARLS

1. Up to one third of children with Trisomy 21 have hypothyroidism.
2. The AAP recommends testing T4 and TSH at birth in patients with Trisomy 21, with retesting at 6 months, 12 months, and annually, thereafter.
3. Hypothyroidism can worsen OSAS.
4. Management of OSAS should not be delayed in patients with hypothyroidism.

REFERENCES

1. Bull MJ. Health supervision for children with Down syndrome. *Pediatrics*. Aug 2011;128(2):393–406.
2. Purdy IB, Singh N, Brown WL, Vangala S, Devaskar UP. Revisiting early hypothyroidism screening in infants with Down syndrome. *J Perinatol*. Dec 2014;34(12):936–940.
3. Bahammam SA, Sharif MM, Jammah AA, Bahammam AS. Prevalence of thyroid disease in patients with obstructive sleep apnea. *Respir Med*. Nov 2011;105(11):1755–1760.
4. Rosen D. Severe hypothyroidism presenting as obstructive sleep apnea. *Clin Pediatr (Phila)*. Apr 2010;49(4):381–383.

A 10-year-old with snoring and hypoxemia

Lourdes M. DelRosso

CASE PRESENTATION

A 10-year-old boy presented for evaluation of snoring. The parents stated that he snored softly without gasping or witnessed apneas. The parents denied nocturnal awakenings, enuresis, or parasomnias. During the day, he did not have excessive sleepiness or behavioral problems. His past medical history was significant for hypoplastic left heart syndrome (underdevelopment of the left ventricle). His past surgical history was significant for Fontan procedure with fenestration. His medications included enalapril and aspirin. The review of systems was negative for nasal congestion, shortness of breath, or gastroesophageal reflux.

PHYSICAL EXAM

Physical exam revealed a smiling, happy boy in no acute distress, with a height at the 15th percentile and weight at the 20th percentile. His pulse oximeter reading was 90%; heart rate 108 beats/min; respiratory rate 24 breaths/min; and blood pressure 104/63 mm Hg. There was no cyanosis or clubbing noted. He did not have adenoid facies. The oropharynx was Mallampati grade II. Tonsil size was 1+. Lungs were clear to auscultation. Cardiac exam revealed a normal S1, a single S2, and a 3/6 systolic murmur at the left midsternal border. There was no peripheral edema.

LABORATORY AND SLEEP FINDINGS

An echocardiogram revealed an unobstructed Fontan pathway with a good size fenestration with right-to-left shunting.

Polysomnography revealed a sleep efficiency of 85%, with normal sleep stage distribution. The apnea–hypopnea index was 1/h. The mean SpO_2 during wakefulness was 90%, and, during sleep, it was 87%. The SpO_2 nadir was 85% (Fig. 75-1). There was no evidence of hypoventilation ($ETCO_2$ was <50 torr for the entire study). The periodic leg movements index was 0/h.

QUESTION

What is your next intervention in this patient?

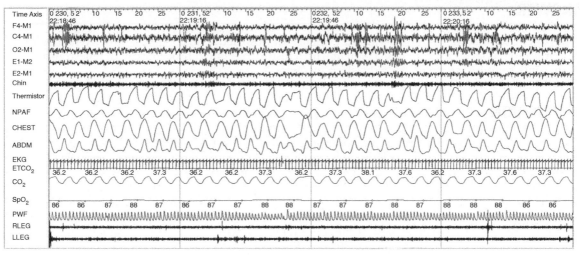

FIGURE 75-1 ■ Two-minute representative epoch during N2 sleep.

ANSWER

The patient has habitual snoring without evidence of obstructive sleep apnea. The oxyhemoglobin saturation was at levels expected for a patient with a history of Fontan procedure with fenestration. No further intervention is needed from the sleep medicine perspective.

DISCUSSION

The Fontan procedure is a surgical intervention that bypasses venous blood from the right atrium to the pulmonary arteries. It is usually indicated in infants with single ventricle or complex congenital heart disease. In the absence of a ventricle, the flow to the pulmonary circulation is passive, and cardiac output is particularly sensitive to changes in intrathoracic pressure and pulmonary vascular resistance. Cardiac output decreases with higher intrathoracic pressure.[1] Patients with marginal ventricular function may benefit from fenestration, which creates a right-to-left shunt through the atrial baffle to improve cardiac output. A drawback of the fenestrated Fontan is that it leaves the patient with systemic oxyhemoglobin saturations in the 80% to 90% range.[2, 3] Lower saturation is compensated by erythropoiesis, resulting in higher than normal hematocrit levels (at least 45%); in fact, the lower the saturation, the higher the hematocrit level required to maintain adequate oxygenation. Supplemental oxygen may not be very effective in raising a low saturation because of the presence of a shunt.[4]

Obstructive sleep apnea syndrome (OSAS) in patients with fenestrated Fontan further contributes to hypoxemia, leading to pulmonary vasoconstriction and increased pulmonary vascular resistance, both of which can decrease cardiac output and contribute to hemodynamic instability. The use of continuous positive airway pressure can also compromise cardiac output by increasing intrathoracic pressure. In a case series of four adults with OSAS and Fontan procedures for complex congenital heart disease, cardiac catheterization was performed while the patients were on continuous positive airway pressure (CPAP) to evaluate the safest CPAP pressure to treat OSAS. Hemodynamic values were recorded at each CPAP pressure. The CPAP threshold was defined as the pressure at which the pulmonary capillary wedge pressure and mixed venous oxygenation remained stable. Using this technique, safe CPAP pressures were determined for three of the patients, and the fourth was managed with subtherapeutic CPAP plus supplemental oxygen. Similar studies have not been performed in children.[5] If significant OSAS is present, options for treatment other than CPAP should be considered. These include tonsillectomy and adenoidectomy, oral appliances, maxillary expansion, mandibular distraction, and tracheostomy.

Our patient was clinically stable with SpO_2 at 90% during wakefulness. SpO_2 was expected to decrease to the mid-80s% during sleep, exercise, and infections. No further intervention was needed.

CLINICAL PEARLS

1. Cardiac patients who have undergone the Fontan procedure with fenestration have low SpO_2, while awake and asleep.
2. CPAP can decrease cardiac output by increasing intrathoracic pressure, and thus, must be considered with caution in cardiac patients with Fontan procedure.
3. Other options for management of significant OSAS in patients who have undergone Fontan procedure with fenestration should be considered before CPAP. These include tonsillectomy and adenoidectomy, oral appliances, maxillary expansion, mandibular distraction, and tracheostomy.

REFERENCES

1. Al-Eyadhy A. Mechanical ventilation strategy following Glenn and Fontan surgeries: on going challenge!. *J Saudi Heart Assoc*. Jul 2009;21(3):153–157.
2. Goff DA, Blume ED, Gauvreau K, Mayer JE, Lock JE, Jenkins KJ. Clinical outcome of fenestrated Fontan patients after closure: the first 10 years. *Circulation*. Oct 24 2000;102(17):2094–2099.
3. Thompson LD, Petrossian E, McElhinney DB, et al. Is it necessary to routinely fenestrate an extracardiac fontan? *J Am Coll Cardiol*. Aug 1999;34(2):539–544.
4. McRae ME. Long-term issues after the Fontan procedure. *AACN Adv Crit Care*. Jul-Sep 2013;24(3):264–282. quiz 283–264.
5. Watson NF, Bushnell T, Jones TK, Stout K. A novel method for the evaluation and treatment of obstructive sleep apnea in four adults with complex congenital heart disease and Fontan repairs. *Sleep Breath*. Nov 2009;13(4):421–424.

A 13-year-old girl with multiple nocturnal awakenings

Lourdes M. DelRosso

CASE PRESENTATION

A 13-year-girl presented for evaluation of difficulty with sleep onset and multiple nocturnal awakenings. Her mother reported that the child had never been a good sleeper. Usually she went to bed at 9 PM but could not fall asleep for up to 2 hours. The patient reported that during this time, she tossed and turned and did not feel comfortable. She did not identify symptoms of restless legs. Once asleep, she woke up several times during the night but was able to fall back to sleep within minutes. In the morning, she woke up with an alarm at 7 AM to go to school. She dozed off during classes. The family denied snoring, cataplexy, sleep paralysis, hypnagogic hallucinations, sleep walking, or dream enactment. She did not take naps during the day. Her modified Epworth sleepiness scale was 15/24. Her past medical history was significant for eczema. Her medications included fexofenadine, montelukast, and vitamin D.

PHYSICAL EXAM

Physical exam revealed a cooperative girl in no distress. Her vital signs were within normal limits. Her skin was dry and scaly, with some darkened and scarred areas over her arms and neck. The remainder of the physical exam was normal.

LABORATORY AND SLEEP FINDINGS

Polysomnography revealed a sleep latency of 104 minutes. Sleep efficiency was 51% (normal >85%). REM sleep was not achieved. The arousal index was 18.2/h (normal is <15/h). The obstructive apnea–hypopnea index (AHI) was 0.3/h, and the central AHI was 0/h. The periodic leg movements index was 3/h. The hypnogram is shown in Figure 76-1. An epoch representative of her arousals is shown in Figure 76-2.

QUESTION

What is the cause of this child's nocturnal disruption and daytime sleepiness?

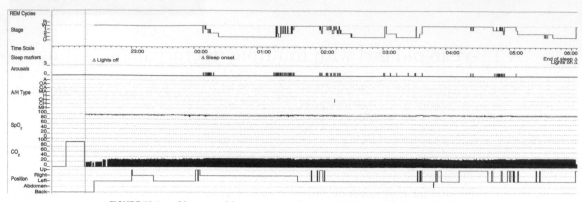

FIGURE 76-1 ■ Nocturnal hypnogram demonstrates multiple awakenings.

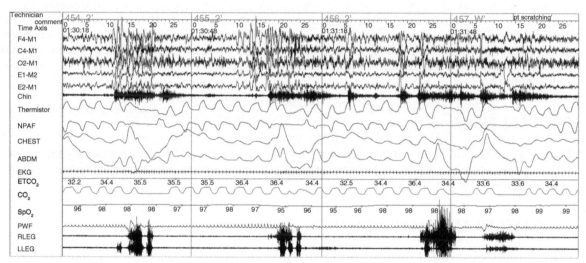

FIGURE 76-2 ■ Two-minute epoch representative of the patient's arousals and awakenings.

ANSWER

The hypnogram in Figure 76-1 demonstrates a long sleep latency and multiple nocturnal awakenings. Figure 76-2 shows the patient's typical arousals. On the right upper corner, the technician comments read "patient scratching." Video monitoring confirmed that most awakenings were associated with scratching. The cause of this child's sleep disruption was eczema. The cause of the daytime sleepiness was sleep disruption and insufficient sleep secondary to eczema.

DISCUSSION

Eczema is a chronic inflammatory skin disease that affects 13% of children, and it is commonly associated with other comorbidities including asthma, allergic rhinitis, and food allergy. Eczema can affect the quality of life of the child and the family, and it is associated with increased healthcare use, recurrent infections, and sleep impairment.[1] Studies have demonstrated that up to 60% of children with eczema experience disturbed sleep. This percentage increases to up to 83% during times of eczema exacerbation.[2] A study of 77 children with eczema, aged 6 to 16 years, revealed that younger age and lower socioeconomic status were associated with increased sleep disturbances because of eczema. As compared with healthy controls, children with eczema were found to have more difficulty settling at night and maintaining sleep, while during the day, they exhibited excessive daytime sleepiness and higher attention-deficit hyperactivity and oppositional defiant scores.[3]

The mechanism of the sleep disturbance in eczema is thought to be secondary to itching. Vasodilation occurs secondary to neuropeptide release, producing erythema and increases in skin temperature leading to itching. Scratching causes skin damage with further increase in itch, leading to the itch-scratch cycles seen in patients with eczema.[2]

Actigraphy in patients with eczema has shown mixed results; the majority demonstrated difficulty recognizing itch-related movements from non–itch-related movements.[4, 5] Polysomnographic studies in children with eczema have shown that patients with eczema have at least 4 times more disturbed sleep than controls do. Video monitoring revealed significantly decreased sleep efficiency, likely because of itching. Scratching was seen in all stages of sleep, with predominance during N1.[2] Treatment of eczema has been associated with sleep improvement in some studies.[6]

Our patient was referred to dermatology for optimization of the eczema treatment. Topical triamcinolone was applied at bedtime with improvement in sleep latency and daytime symptoms.

CLINICAL PEARLS

1. Children with eczema should be evaluated clinically for sleep disruption.
2. Children with eczema often have prolonged sleep latency and decreased sleep efficiency.
3. Treatment of eczema may improve sleep disruption.

REFERENCES

1. Cipriani F, Dondi A, Ricci G. Recent advances in epidemiology and prevention of atopic eczema. *Pediatr Allergy Immunol.* Nov 2014;25(7):630–638.
2. Camfferman D, Kennedy JD, Gold M, Martin AJ, Lushington K. Eczema and sleep and its relationship to daytime functioning in children. *Sleep Med Rev.* Dec 2010;14(6):359–369.
3. Camfferman D, Kennedy JD, Gold M, Martin AJ, Winwood P, Lushington K. Eczema, sleep, and behavior in children. *J Clin Sleep Med.* Dec 15 2010;6(6):581 588.
4. Wootton CI, Koller K, Lawton S, O'Leary C, Thomas KS. Are accelerometers a useful tool for measuring disease activity in children with eczema? Validity, responsiveness to change, and acceptability of use in a clinical trial setting. *Br J Dermatol.* Nov 2012;167(5):1131–1137.
5. Murray CS, Rees JL. Are subjective accounts of itch to be relied on? The lack of relation between visual analogue itch scores and actigraphic measures of scratch. *Acta Derm Venereol.* Jan 2011;91(1):18–23.
6. Bieber T, Vick K, Folster-Holst R, et al. Efficacy and safety of methylprednisolone aceponate ointment 0.1% compared to tacrolimus 0.03% in children and adolescents with an acute flare of severe atopic dermatitis. *Allergy.* Feb 2007;62(2):184–189.

A 5-year-old with nocturnal cough and daytime fatigue

Suzanne E. Beck

CASE PRESENTATION

A 5-year-old boy was evaluated because of fatigue and coughing during sleep. The parents were concerned that their son had dark circles under his eyes, was more fatigued compared with his peers, and was tired after school. He did not nap or fall asleep in school. He had occasional snoring, with no witnessed apnea, diaphoresis, or restless sleep. He reported coughing several times per night but did not get out of bed. The parents reported hearing him cough about 2 to 3 times per week in the early morning hours. He fell asleep independently by 9 PM and arose to an alarm clock at 7:30 AM. Past medical history revealed he was born full term, had respiratory syncytial virus bronchiolitis and eczema as an infant, and mild intermittent asthma with no hospitalizations or emergency room visits. He used an albuterol metered-dose inhaler with a holding chamber as needed for symptoms with colds or exercise, usually about twice a month. Review of systems revealed seasonal rhinitis treated with an oral antihistamine as needed. There was no wheezing, shortness of breath, recent or recurrent infections, sinusitis, or gastroesophageal reflux. The child was typically developing, growing well, and his school grades were average. There was no family history of sleep apnea or asthma, but the father had seasonal allergies.

PHYSICAL EXAM

Physical exam revealed a healthy prepubertal boy with normal vital signs. Respiratory rate was 18 breaths/min; SpO_2 was 98%. Growth parameters were at the 50th percentiles for weight and height. Physical exam was normal, and lungs were clear to auscultation with good air-exchange bilaterally.

LABORATORY AND SLEEP FINDINGS

Pulmonary function tests were normal: forced vital capacity (FVC) was 1.77 L (118% predicted); forced expiratory volume in 1 second (FEV_1) was 1.42 L (107% predicted); FEV_1/FVC was 80%; forced expiratory flow$_{25-75}$ was 1.23 L/sec (91% predicted); and the shape of the inspiratory and expiratory flow volume curves were normal (Fig. 77-1).

Polysomnography (PSG) revealed a total sleep time (TST) of 512 minutes. Sleep efficiency was 82%. Sleep stage distribution was normal. The arousal index was 22.4/h; obstructive apnea–hypopnea index 0.2/h; SpO_2 nadir 94%; and $ETCO_2$ was >50 torr for 15% of TST. The periodic movement index per hour of sleep was 2.5/h.

QUESTION

What can you do to improve the daytime fatigue in this child?

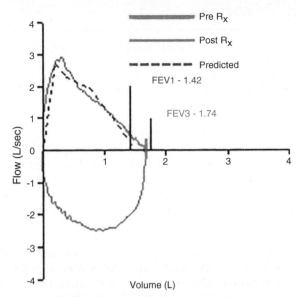

FIGURE 77-1 ■ Normal flow-volume curve.

ANSWER

Improve control of nocturnal asthma. Nocturnal cough is common in children with asthma, but it can also be associated with other conditions such as chronic rhinosinusitis, gastroesophageal disease, or other infections. Bronchial narrowing is increased during the night in patients with asthma as an amplification of the normal circadian response.

DISCUSSION

Children with asthma are at increased risk of daytime sleepiness.[1] Nocturnal cough is a common symptom of asthma and can be associated with poor sleep and daytime sleepiness, even during periods of relative stability.[2] In a population-based sample of children, nocturnal cough was twice as common in children with current asthma (39%) compared with asymptomatic children (19%).[3] In a large study of school-aged children, those with asthma (defined as wheezing in the preceding 12 months) were more likely to have decreased quality of sleep (associated with chronic cough, snoring, rhinitis, and eczema) and daytime sleepiness (associated with chronic cough or rhinitis) compared with non-wheezy controls.[4] In a study of over 1000 children with mild-moderate asthma, nocturnal awakenings occurred in one third of the children during a period of stability, and nocturnal cough was an indicator of more severe asthma and atopy.[5] Also noteworthy, nocturnal dry cough (apart from a cough associated with an infection or a cold) in toddlers without a history of wheezing was an independent risk factor for development of asthma at age 8 years.[6] Because asthma affects over 8% of children,[7] and nocturnal coughing may be the only indicator of asthma, as well as a marker of asthma severity, the presence of nocturnal cough is an important and treatable determinant of sleep quality, and it can be ascertained from a sleep history.

Airway obstruction, inflammation, and bronchial hyper-responsiveness are the three main features of asthma, and all are under a circadian influence, with airway caliber reaching a nadir at 4 AM.[8] In patients with asthma, the fall in lung function during the night reflects an amplification of the normal circadian rhythm in airway caliber because of airway hyper-reactivity and airway inflammation.[9] Thus, lung function has a circadian-based nadir in the early morning, and patients with nocturnal asthma experience a greater than normal diurnal decrease in airway function, independent of sleep. Classic studies have shown that cough during sleep is preceded by arousal,[10] which may be another mechanism of sleep disruption.

Our patient had adequate hours of sleep for his age and did not have evidence of obstructive sleep apnea on PSG but was experiencing disrupted sleep because of nocturnal cough (Fig. 77-2), which was captured during PSG (Fig. 77-3) and confirmed the suspicion of poorly controlled asthma. His clinical picture was that of mild persistent asthma despite normal spirometry (see Fig. 77-1) and lack of perceived daytime symptoms. He was treated with low-dose inhaled corticosteroids to manage mild persistent asthma[11] and an oral antihistamine to manage his rhinitis. His disrupted sleep and daytime fatigue improved.

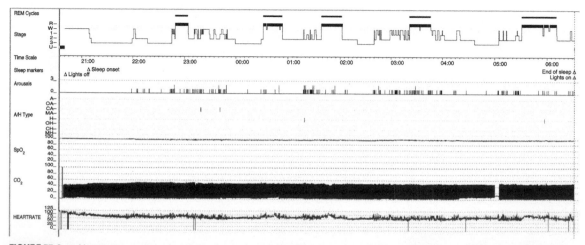

FIGURE 77-2 ■ Hypnogram showing frequent arousals and awakenings. Technician notes indicated awakenings correlated with brief coughing episodes.

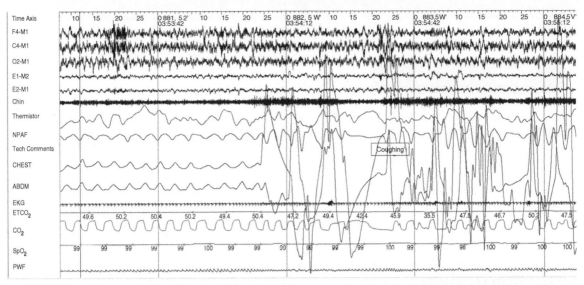

FIGURE 77-3 ■ **Representative 120-second epoch showing an awakening from N2 associated with coughing.**

CLINICAL PEARLS

1. A thorough sleep and medical history can help elucidate whether insufficient sleep versus disrupted sleep is a cause of daytime sleepiness and point toward a specific treatment.
2. Nocturnal cough is an important cause of disrupted sleep and daytime sleepiness in children.
3. Underlying asthma, manifested primarily as nocturnal coughing, is common in children.

REFERENCES

1. Calhoun SL, Vgontzas AN, Fernandez-Mendoza J, et al. Prevalence and risk factors of excessive daytime sleepiness in a community sample of young children: the role of obesity, asthma, anxiety/depression, and sleep. *Sleep.* Apr 2011;34(4):503–507.
2. Horner CC, Mauger D, Strunk RC, et al. Most nocturnal asthma symptoms occur outside of exacerbations and associate with morbidity. *J Allergy Clin Immunol.* Nov 2011;128(5):977–982. e971-e972.
3. Brooke AM, Lambert PC, Burton PR, Clarke C, Luyt DK, Simpson H. Night cough in a population-based sample of children: characteristics, relation to symptoms and associations with measures of asthma severity. *Eur Respir J.* Jan 1996;9(1):65–71.
4. Desager KN, Nelen V, Weyler JJ, De Backer WA. Sleep disturbance and daytime symptoms in wheezing school-aged children. *J Sleep Res.* Mar 2005;14(1):77–82.
5. Strunk RC, Sternberg AL, Bacharier LB, Szefler SJ. Nocturnal awakening caused by asthma in children with mild-to-moderate asthma in the childhood asthma management program. *J Allergy Clin Immunol.* Sep 2002;110(3):395–403.
6. Boudewijn IM, Savenije OE, Koppelman GH, et al. Nocturnal dry cough in the first 7 years of life is associated with asthma at school age. *Pediatr Pulmonol.* Sep 2015;50(9):848–855. Epub 2014 Aug 26.
7. Center for Disease Control and Prevention. *CDC Data Statistics and Surveillence.* http://www.cdc.gov/asthma/asthmadata.htm; 2015 Accessed 20.04.15.
8. Syabbalo N. Chronobiology and chronopathophysiology of nocturnal asthma. *Int J Clin Pract.* Oct 1997;51(7):455–462.
9. Martin RJ, Cicutto LC, Smith HR, Ballard RD, Szefler SJ. Airways inflammation in nocturnal asthma. *Am Rev Respir Dis.* Feb 1991;143(2):351–357.
10. Sullivan CE, Zamel N, Kozar LF, Murphy E, Phillipson EA. Regulation of airway smooth muscle tone in sleeping dogs. *Am Rev Respir Dis.* Jan 1979;119(1):87–99.
11. National Asthma Education and Prevention Program. Expert panel report 3 (EPR-3): guidelines for the diagnosis and management of asthma-summary report 2007. *J Allergy Clin Immunol.* Nov 2007;120(suppl 5):S94–S138.

A 16-year-old boy with intractable seizure disorder and snoring

Lourdes M. DelRosso

CASE PRESENTATION

A 16-year-old boy with static encephalopathy of unknown etiology and intractable epilepsy presented for evaluation of snoring. He had multiple types of seizures including generalized tonic-clonic seizures, staring events, and episodes of extreme laughter alternating with periods of quiescence. He had a vagus nerve stimulator (VNS) implanted 6 months previously. He experienced mild cough after VNS activation that subsequently resolved. The family reported a mild improvement in the frequency and duration of seizures since VNS activation but noted snoring since then. The patient went to bed at 9:30 PM and woke up at 7 AM. He did not have nocturnal awakenings. The family reported soft snoring without gasping or witnessed apneas. He did not take naps during the day. He did not have any other medical problems. His past surgical history included tonsillectomy and adenoidectomy at age 4. His medications included lamotrigine, phenobarbital, and levetiracetam. There had been no change in medications over the last year. Review of systems was negative.

PHYSICAL EXAMINATION

The patient was in a wheelchair and was developmentally delayed. Vital signs were normal. Oral exam revealed an oropharynx that was Mallampati grade II and tonsil size 1+. He did not have a high-arched palate, his tongue did not deviate laterally, and there were no lingual fasciculations or atrophy. His lungs were clear to auscultation. There was truncal hypotonia and contractures of the arms and legs. The remainder of the exam was noncontributory.

LABORATORY AND SLEEP FINDINGS

Polysomnography revealed a sleep efficiency of 85% and an arousal index of 7/h. The obstructive apnea–hypopnea index (AHI) was 6/h. The central AHI was 0/h, and the SpO_2 nadir was 91%. End-tidal CO_2 was <50 torr for 100% of total sleep time. The periodic leg movements index (PLMI) was 0/h. A representative epoch is seen in Figure 78-1.

QUESTION

What is the pathophysiology of the hypopneas seen in Figure 78-1?

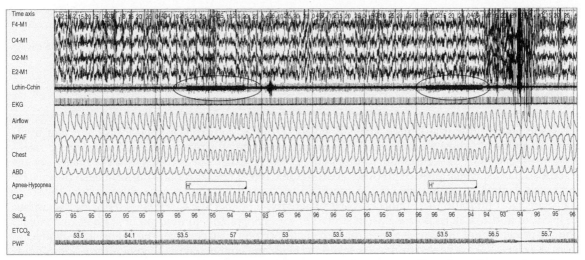

FIGURE 78-1 ■ **Three hundred–second epoch showing representative hypopneas.** Note the artifact on the chin electromyogram caused by the VNS stimulator (*encircled*).

ANSWER

VNS may affect breathing during sleep, by its effect on the upper-airway musculature or by its effect on the central control of breathing.

DISCUSSION

VNS was approved by the United States Food and Drug Administration in 1997 for adjuvant treatment of multidrug-resistant epilepsy. VNS has proven to be effective in seizure reduction by retrograde stimulation of the central nervous system (CNS). Afferent fibers connect to the nucleus of the tractus solitarius, which projects to other areas of the CNS. Three mechanisms have been postulated: increased gamma-aminobutyric acid in the CNS, decreased norepinephrine release from the locus coeruleus, and inhibition of abnormal cortical activity. The VNS surgery consists of two incisions: an incision in the neck to isolate a 3-cm stretch of vagus nerve and an incision in the anterior axillary line for placement of the device generator. A coiled electrode is placed over the vagus nerve, and leads from the electrode are passed from the neck to the chest and connected to the generator.[1] Anterograde stimulation can affect areas innervated by vagal efferent nerves (the recurrent laryngeal nerve) and produce hoarseness (reported in up to 66% of patients), coughing (45%), pharyngeal irritation (35%), and dyspnea (25%).[2] Figure 78-2 shows the local anatomy and nerves related to the left vagus nerve.

About one third of patients develop mild obstructive sleep apnea after VNS implantation, and a small number of patients develop severe obstructive apnea.[3] Apneas, hypopneas, desaturation, and tachypnea have been reported to occur exclusively during VNS activation but not when the VNS is inactive. VNS may affect breathing either by its effect on the upper-airway musculature or by its effect on central control of breathing.[2] Vagal efferent nerves alter neuromuscular signals to the upper-airway musculature of the pharynx and larynx, resulting in airway narrowing and obstruction. Vagal projections to the brainstem can also affect the rate and depth of respiration.[4] The severity of airway

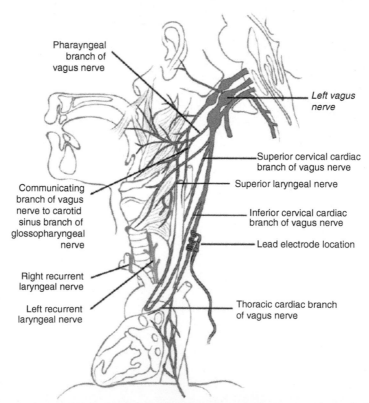

FIGURE 78-2 ■ **Local anatomy and nerves related to the left vagus nerve with attached VNS device wires.** (Copyright Grill MF, Ng YT. Dramatic first words spoken in 2 children after vagus nerve stimulation. *Semin Pediatr Neurol.* Mar 2010;17(1):54-57, p. 55.)

obstruction is related to the frequency of the VNS. Obstructive events occur most often at a frequency of 30 Hz, less at 20 Hz, and are minimal at 10 Hz.

Treatment of obstructive sleep apnea syndrome (OSAS) in patients with VNS needs to be individualized, but options include continuous positive airway pressure (CPAP) therapy, changing the VNS settings, or discontinuing the VNS. Our patient was successfully treated with CPAP therapy.

CLINICAL PEARLS

1. Patients with VNS should be screened for OSAS because about one third of patients will develop OSAS.
2. OSAS in patients with VNS can be treated with CPAP, changing the VNS settings, or discontinuing the VNS.

REFERENCES

1. Ghanem T, Early SV. Vagal nerve stimulator implantation: an otolaryngologist's perspective. *Otolaryngol Head Neck Surg.* Jul 2006;135(1):46–51.
2. Hsieh T, Chen M, McAfee A, Kifle Y. Sleep-related breathing disorder in children with vagal nerve stimulators. *Pediatr Neurol.* Feb 2008;38(2):99–103.
3. Parhizgar F, Nugent K, Raj R. Obstructive sleep apnea and respiratory complications associated with vagus nerve stimulators. *J Clin Sleep Med.* Aug 15. 2011;7(4):401–407.
4. Ebben MR, Sethi NK, Conte M, Pollak CP, Labar D. Vagus nerve stimulation, sleep apnea, and CPAP titration. *J Clin Sleep Med.* Oct 15 2008;4(5):471–473.

A 15-year-old girl with Lennox-Gastaut syndrome and breathing pauses

Lourdes M. DelRosso

CASE PRESENTATION

A 15-year-old girl with mitochondrial encephalomyopathy because of RMND1 mutation, Lennox-Gastaut syndrome, profound global developmental delay, and neuromuscular scoliosis presented for evaluation of witnessed breathing pauses at night. Her parents reported soft snoring but denied gasping. Seizures occurred daily, both during the day and night, at an average of six seizures a day. The majority of seizures were myoclonic, but some were tonic; her parents did not notice breathing pauses during the seizures. Medications included levetiracetam, clobazam, phenobarbital, and phenytoin.

PHYSICAL EXAM

The patient was wheelchair bound and severely developmentally delayed. She did not have an adenoid facies; oropharynx was Mallampati class II; and tonsil size was 2+. There was evidence of global hypotonia, muscle wasting, and kyphoscoliosis.

LABORATORY AND SLEEP FINDINGS

Video electroencephalogram (EEG) showed a disorganized background with lack of normal sleep architecture, mixed focal and generalized discharges, one tonic seizure, and two myoclonic seizures. Polysomnography showed poor sleep efficiency with a total sleep time of 258 minutes, total recording time of 410 minutes, and sleep efficiency 63%. The arousal index was 46/h. Sleep-stage distribution was normal. There were no significant central apneas. The obstructive apnea–hypopnea index was only 0.7/h. There were three apneic events, all similar to the one shown in Figures 79-1 and 79-2, and associated with desaturation to 75% (see Fig. 79-1). There were nine myoclonic seizures during wakefulness, seen on the video as arm shaking.

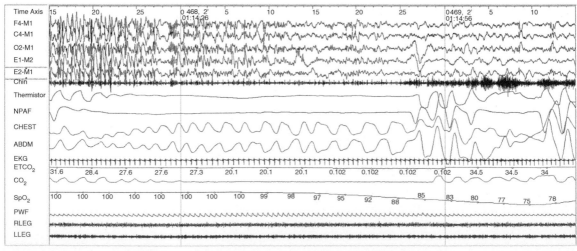

FIGURE 79-1 ■ **Sixty-second epoch showing an obstructive apnea.**

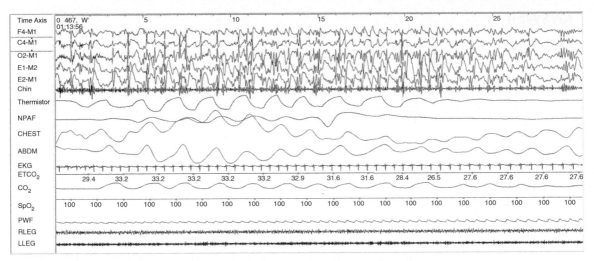

FIGURE 79-2 ■ Same event in a 30-second epoch.

QUESTION

What is the cause of the prolonged apnea and desaturation seen in Figures 79-1 and 79-2?

ANSWER

Nocturnal seizures. Notice in Figure 79-1 (60-second epoch) that the obstructive apnea was preceded by high-voltage rhythmic EEG activity. In Figure 79-2 (30-second epoch) we see numerous spike and wave complexes consistent with ictal activity. Video monitoring during the apnea also revealed myoclonic activity (arm shaking). Seizures may be associated with cardiopulmonary events including ictal and postictal apnea (obstructive or central), tachypnea, tachycardia, bradycardia, and hypoxemia.

DISCUSSION

An epilepsy syndrome is defined as the signs and symptoms unique to an epileptic condition. Some epileptic syndromes manifest most commonly during sleep (Table 79-1). Lennox-Gastaut syndrome is a severe form of epilepsy with onset usually before 8 years of age. The prevalence in the general population is approximately 0.25 in 1000 children, but it is seen in up to 10% of children with epilepsy and in up to 17% in children with both intellectual disability and epilepsy. Various seizure types may be present, but the most common are tonic seizures. Tonic seizures usually present with body stiffening, eye rolling, pupil dilation, and changes in breathing patterns, with 90% occurring during sleep. Myoclonic seizures consist of repetitive muscle jerks; absence seizures typically present with staring spells; and atonic seizures are characterized by sudden loss of muscle tone. The majority of affected children have developmental and intellectual disability, with the degree of disability inversely proportional to the age of seizure onset. Up to 80% of children with Lennox-Gastaut syndrome will continue to have seizures into adulthood. Many conditions have been associated with Lennox-Gastaut syndrome, the most common being infectious processes, inherited metabolic conditions, perinatal asphyxia, and head trauma; however, the etiology remains unknown in up to one third of patients. About 20% of patients with infantile spasms develops Lennox-Gastaut syndrome. The diagnosis is usually made using history and awake-sleep EEG.[1, 2]

Seizures have been associated with cardiopulmonary events; ictal and postictal apnea, tachypnea, tachycardia, bradycardia, and hypoxemia may occur. Central or obstructive apneas may precede the seizure, occur during the seizure, or be the only clinical manifestation of the seizure. Patients who

TABLE 79-1. Pediatric epilepsy syndromes with sleep predominance[6, 7]		
Epilepsy Syndrome	**Age Onset**	**Manifestation**
Juvenile myoclonic epilepsy	10-12 yr	Multiple seizure types: • Generalized tonic-clonic • Absence seizures • Myoclonic jerks
Benign childhood epilepsy with centro-temporal spikes (BECTS)	7-9 yr	Common at sleep onset Face twitching Drooling
Benign focal epilepsy with occipital spikes of Panayiotopoulos	4-5 yr	2/3 occur at night Unilateral clonic seizures Tonic head and eye deviation
Landau-Kleffner syndrome	3-7 yr	Focal motor seizure: eye blinking or automatisms Language regression
Infantile spams or West syndrome	3-18 mo	Epileptic spasms Hypsarrhythmia Intellectual disability
Autosomal dominant nocturnal frontal lobe epilepsy (ADNFLE)	9-11 yr	Lifelong but not progressive Clusters of nocturnal motor seizures Tonic-dystonic features Retained awareness is common

are younger, have temporal lobe epilepsy, or have symptomatic generalized seizures are at higher risk of ictal apnea. Patients with longer seizures are at higher risk of ictal apnea, bradycardia, or postictal desaturation. Ictal apneas can potentially contribute to sudden unexpected death in epilepsy (SUDEP), which incidentally occurs more often during sleep. Patients with generalized seizures, poorly controlled seizures, male gender, and need for multiple antiepileptic drugs are at higher risk of SUDEP.[3, 4] The mechanism of ictal apnea is not completely understood, but it may be secondary to brainstem respiratory control dysfunction during the seizure.[5]

Our patient demonstrated nocturnal seizures with associated apnea. The neurology team was contacted to evaluate further and optimize seizure management.

CLINICAL PEARLS

1. All types of seizures can occur during sleep.
2. Some seizures occur predominantly during sleep.
3. Seizures during sleep can be associated with obstructive or central apnea.
4. SUDEP occurs more often during sleep.

REFERENCES

1. Archer JS, Warren AE, Jackson GD, Abbott DF. Conceptualizing Lennox-Gastaut syndrome as a secondary network epilepsy. *Front Neurol.* 2014;5:225.
2. Camfield PR. Definition and natural history of Lennox-Gastaut syndrome. *Epilepsia.* Aug 2011;52(suppl 5):3–9.
3. Vendrame M, Jackson S, Syed S, Kothare SV, Auerbach SH. Central sleep apnea and complex sleep apnea in patients with epilepsy. *Sleep Breath.* Mar 2014;18(1):119–124.
4. Singh K, Katz ES, Zarowski M, et al. Cardiopulmonary complications during pediatric seizures: a prelude to understanding SUDEP. *Epilepsia.* Jun 2013;54(6):1083–1091.
5. DelRosso L, Hoque R. Central apnea at electroencephalographic seizure onset. *Sleep Med.* Dec 2013;14(12):1426–1427.
6. Bazil CW. Nocturnal seizures. *Semin Neurol.* Sep 2004;24(3):293–300.
7. Muthugovindan D, Hartman AL. Pediatric epilepsy syndromes. *Neurologist.* Jul 2010;16(4):223–237.

A 2-year-old girl with abnormal nocturnal events

Lourdes M. DelRosso

CASE PRESENTATION

A 2-year-old girl was referred for evaluation of abnormal nocturnal behaviors. Her mother reported witnessing episodes of right-arm jerking for a few seconds that occurred repetitively during sleep. Her mother also reported restless sleep and frequent awakenings. The child had a past medical history of congenital cytomegalovirus infection, global developmental delay, hypertonia, and deafness.

PHYSICAL EXAM

The patient's weight was at the 31st percentile; height at the 62th percentile; and head circumference at the 1st percentile (microcephalic). She had truncal hypotonia and hypertonia of her extremities. Deep tendon reflexes were increased (3+) bilaterally. The remainder of the exam was noncontributory.

LABORATORY AND SLEEP FINDINGS

Brain magnetic resonance imaging (MRI) revealed extensive bilateral frontoparietotemporal polymicrogyria. Multiple tiny cystic structures consistent with cytomegalovirus infection were noted.

On polysomnography (PSG), the total sleep time (TST) was 418 minutes; total recording time 505 minutes; and sleep efficiency 83%. Differentiation between NREM stages was not possible. NREM constituted 86% of TST. There were no respiratory events. Excerpts of the electroencephalogram (EEG) are shown in Figures 80-1 and 80-2. Clinical seizure activity was not seen on video monitoring.

QUESTION

What is the diagnosis in this patient?

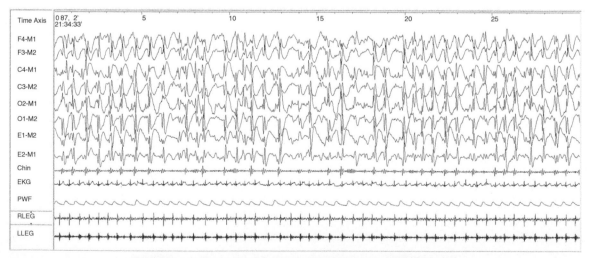

FIGURE 80-1 ■ Thirty-second epoch representative of NREM sleep.

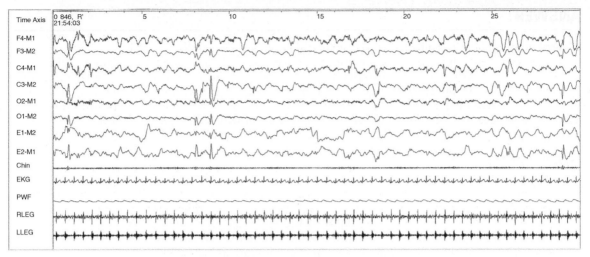

FIGURE 80-2 ■ **Thirty-second epoch during REM sleep.**

ANSWER

Electric status epilepticus during sleep (ESES). PSG revealed a generalized slow background while the patient was awake, with occasional epileptiform discharges. With sleep onset, a continuous spike-wave pattern appeared during NREM sleep (see Fig. 80-1), with attenuation of spike-and-wave discharges during REM (see Fig. 80-2). The diagnosis was confirmed by a full EEG montage, which revealed frequent independent bilateral central and frontal spike-wave discharges. These epileptiform discharges activated and became almost continuous in sleep, consistent with a diagnosis of ESES.

DISCUSSION

Congenital cytomegalovirus infection occurs in 0.2% to 2.5% of live births. Both primary and recurrent infection in the mother can be transmitted to the fetus, but primary infection has a higher rate of transmission (40% vs. 3%).[1] Further, 90% of affected infants are symptomatic at birth. The most common symptoms are jaundice, petechiae, hepatosplenomegaly, and microcephaly with severe developmental delays. Patients with congenital cytomegalovirus are at increased risk of seizures, with some patients having intractable epilepsy.[2]

ESES is a state of subclinical status epilepticus in children characterized by EEG findings of epileptic activity for more than 85% of NREM sleep. ESES has been described in different seizure types including generalized tonic-clonic, absence, and partial seizures.[3] Although there is not full consensus about whether ESES needs to be treated in the absence of clinical seizure activity, some studies that support treatment have revealed that children with ESES are at higher risk for behavioral and cognitive problems compared with controls.[4] ESES is rare in adults.[5]

In general, epileptic discharges increase during sleep. With sleep onset, the input from cholinergic, monoaminergic, and glutamatergic pathways decreases, producing hyperpolarization of the cortical and thalamocortical neurons. As this process continues, slow-wave activity becomes more prominent and synchronized, becoming more susceptible to spike-and-wave activity. Sleep has been shown to activate epileptiform discharges in patients with various epileptic syndromes.[6]

Our patient was referred for neurologic consultation, and treatment with levetiracetam was initiated based on the clinical presentation, as well as daytime episodes of arm stiffening consistent with seizures, her history of congenital cytomegalovirus infection, associated abnormal brain MRI findings, and ESES.

CLINICAL PEARLS

1. ESES can be present in various epileptic syndromes of childhood. It is rare in adulthood.
2. ESES is manifested in NREM sleep, as epileptiform discharges are attenuated during REM and wakefulness.
3. ESES is diagnosed by EEG when spike-and-wave activity exceeds 85% of NREM sleep.

REFERENCES

1. Leung AK, Sauve RS, Davies HD. Congenital cytomegalovirus infection. *J Natl Med Assoc*. Mar 2003;95(3):213–218.
2. Suzuki Y, Toribe Y, Mogami Y, Yanagihara K, Nishikawa M. Epilepsy in patients with congenital cytomegalovirus infection. *Brain Dev*. Jun 2008;30(6):420–424.
3. Yilmaz S, Serdaroglu G, Akcay A, Gokben S. Clinical characteristics and outcome of children with electrical status epilepticus during slow wave sleep. *J Pediatr Neurosci*. May 2014;9(2):105–109.
4. Degerliyurt A, Yalnizoglu D, Bakar EE, Topcu M, Turanli G. Electrical status epilepticus during sleep: a study of 22 patients. *Brain Dev*. Feb 2015;37(2):250–264.
5. Hoque R, DelRosso LM. Epileptiform discharges during slow wave sleep on polysomnogram. *J Clin Sleep Med*. Mar 15 2014;10(3):336–339.
6. Kotagal P, Yardi N. The relationship between sleep and epilepsy. *Semin Pediatr Neurol*. Jun 2008;15(2):42–49.

A 13-year-old boy with snoring and headaches

Lourdes M. DelRosso

CASE PRESENTATION

A 13-year-old boy presented for sleep evaluation because of snoring and persistent headaches. The headaches first appeared 3 months ago, when he started practicing wrestling. The headaches occurred approximately 3 times a week; they were localized at the back of the head and neck. They were not associated with an aura, nausea, vomiting, or paresthesia. The headaches occurred at various times of the day, usually after coughing, sneezing, or practicing wrestling. He tried acetaminophen and ibuprofen without relief. The patient reported a consistent bedtime routine with a total sleep time (TST) of 10 hours. He did not nap during the day. His parents reported loud snoring and witnessed apneas during sleep but no parasomnias or daytime sleepiness. There was no other past medical or surgical history. He did not take any medications. The review of systems was negative for weakness, hearing loss, visual problems, dizziness, or gait changes.

PHYSICAL EXAM

The physical exam revealed a cooperative boy in no distress. His weight and height were at the 25th percentile. His vital signs were within normal limits. The oropharynx was Mallampati class II, and his tonsils were size 1+. Cranial nerves II-XII were normal. His neck was not tender to palpation. Strength was 5/5 bilaterally in all extremities. Deep tendon reflexes were 2+ in the biceps, patella, and Achilles tendons bilaterally. Toes exhibited flexor response to plantar stimulation bilaterally. The finger-to-nose coordination test was normal bilaterally. Gait was normal.

LABORATORY AND SLEEP FINDINGS

A brain magnetic resonance imaging (MRI) scan was ordered (Fig. 81-1).

Nocturnal polysomnography (PSG) revealed a TST of 424 minutes; total recording time of 475 minutes; sleep efficiency 89%; and arousal index 9/h. The obstructive apnea–hypopnea index (AHI) was 16/h; central AHI was 1/h; and SpO_2 nadir was 85%. The end-tidal CO_2 was below 50 torr for 100% of the TST. The periodic leg movements index was 1/h.

A lateral neck x-ray showed a patent airway without adenoid hypertrophy and with small tonsils.

QUESTION

What is the diagnosis in this patient?

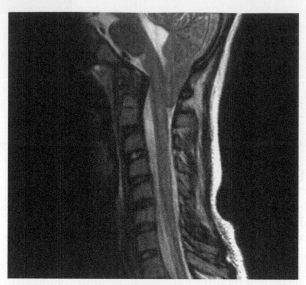

FIGURE 81-1 ■ Sagittal MRI of brain and cervical spine.

ANSWER

Chiari malformation type 1 and obstructive sleep apnea.

DISCUSSION

A Chiari malformation is an anomaly of the craniocervical junction. A Chiari malformation type I is the most common type. It is characterized by caudal displacement of the cerebellar tonsils below the foramen magnum. Syringomyelia is present in up to 75% of cases. Chiari type I can be asymptomatic or can present with headaches, weakness, or cranial nerve abnormalities.[1] A Chiari type II malformation is characterized by cerebellar vermis displacement and lumbar or sacrolumbar myelomeningocele (a type of spina bifida); Chiari type III has some of the features of Chiari type II, but it is also associated with occipital encephalocele; and Chiari type IV is characterized by cerebellar agenesis.

A Chiari malformation can result in compression of the cranial nerves that innervate the oropharynx (mainly cranial nerves IX-XII), producing obstructive apnea; compression and/or dysplasia of the brainstem respiratory nuclei can produce central apnea and/or alveolar hypoventilation. Studies have demonstrated a high prevalence of sleep-disordered breathing in patients with Chiari malformation with or without spina bifida. PSG in 83 children with Chiari type I or Chiari type II revealed a 42% prevalence of mild sleep-disordered breathing and 20% prevalence of moderate/severe sleep-disordered breathing; among the severe group, 71% had central apnea, and the remainder had obstructive apnea.[2] The sensory and motor level of the lesion correlated with the severity of AHI; patients with lesions at the thoracic or thoracolumbar functional lesion level (i.e., wheelchair-bound patients) were 9.8 times more likely to have moderate to severe sleep-disordered breathing.[2] Another study in 20 affected children revealed central sleep apnea in 25% of patients.[3] An MRI study in 22 children with Chiari type I showed that patients with significant crowding at the level of the foramen magnum had a higher probability of sleep-disordered breathing (both obstructive sleep apnea syndrome (OSAS) and central apnea).[1] Sleep-disordered breathing in children and adolescents with Chiari type I is independent of the size of cerebellar tonsil herniation, but it is associated with the presence of syringomyelia, hydrocephalus, and neurologic symptoms.[4] Respiratory arrest and nocturnal deaths have occurred in patients with Chiari malformation.[5] Other sleep-related symptoms found in patients with Chiari malformation include excessive daytime sleepiness, parasomnias, periodic leg movements of sleep, and insomnia.[5] Severe breath-holding spells may occur during wakefulness in infants and young children with Chiari malformations.

Patients with spina bifida myelomeningocele may also have muscle weakness and kyphoscoliosis, as well as swallowing dysfunction with resultant aspiration, leading to restrictive pulmonary disease and hypoventilation (worse in REM sleep because of muscle atonia). Pulmonary function tests revealed restrictive lung disease in 42% of patients and severe restriction in 16% of patients.[2, 6]

The physical exam in patients with cervicomedullary compression initially reveals upper motor neuron signs: generalized hyperreflexia, spasticity, and plantar extensor response. Later on, lower motor neuron signs develop: atrophy, weakness, fasciculations, and areflexia. Patients may present with dysphagia, lingual atrophy, and absent gag reflex. Patients with syringomyelia may present with cerebellar signs (ataxia).

Symptomatic Chiari malformation is often treated with ventriculoperitoneal shunts for decompression, or posterior fossa decompressive surgery. However, as breathing abnormalities may be due to brainstem dysplasia rather than compression, patients do not always improve after surgery. Other treatment options for sleep-disordered breathing in these patients include adenotonsillectomy, oxygen supplementation, and noninvasive or invasive ventilation.[7] Although headaches improve in the majority of patients after decompression surgery, some neurologic symptoms persist, and some may worsen after surgery.[8-10]

Our patient underwent cervicomedullary decompression with resolution of headaches and OSAS. Follow-up PSG revealed an AHI of 1.5/h.

CLINICAL PEARLS

1. Patients with Chiari malformation may present with headaches, snoring, and witnessed apnea.
2. Central sleep apnea or hypoventilation and obstructive sleep apnea are commonly found in patients with cervicomedullary compression secondary to Chiari malformation.
3. Patients with Chiari malformation or spina bifida should be screened for sleep-disordered breathing.

REFERENCES

1. Khatwa U, Ramgopal S, Mylavarapu A, et al. MRI findings and sleep apnea in children with Chiari I malformation. *Pediatr Neurol*. Apr 2013;48(4):299–307.
2. Waters KA, Forbes P, Morielli A, et al. Sleep-disordered breathing in children with myelomeningocele. *J Pediatr*. Apr 1998;132(4):672–681.
3. Dauvilliers Y, Stal V, Abril B, et al. Chiari malformation and sleep related breathing disorders. *J Neurol Neurosurg Psychiatry*. Dec 2007;78(12):1344–1348.
4. Losurdo A, Dittoni S, Testani E, et al. Sleep disordered breathing in children and adolescents with Chiari malformation type I. *J Clin Sleep Med*. Apr 15 2013;9(4):371–377.
5. Ferre Maso A, Poca MA, de la Calzada MD, Solana E, Romero Tomas O, Sahuquillo J. Sleep disturbance: a forgotten syndrome in patients with Chiari I malformation. *Neurologia*. Jun 2014;29(5):294–304.
6. Kirk V, Kahn A, Brouillette RT. Diagnostic approach to obstructive sleep apnea in children. *Sleep Med Rev*. Nov 1998;2(4):255–269.
7. Kirk VG, Morielli A, Gozal D, et al. Treatment of sleep-disordered breathing in children with myelomeningocele. *Pediatr Pulmonol*. Dec 2000;30(6):445–452.
8. Botelho RV, Bittencourt LR, Rotta JM, Tufik S. The effects of posterior fossa decompressive surgery in adult patients with Chiari malformation and sleep apnea. *J Neurosurg*. Apr 2010;112(4):800–807.
9. Gagnadoux F, Meslier N, Svab I, Menei P, Racineux JL. Sleep-disordered breathing in patients with Chiari malformation: improvement after surgery. *Neurology*. Jan 10 2006;66(1):136–138.
10. Chotai S, Medhkour A. Surgical outcomes after posterior fossa decompression with and without duraplasty in Chiari malformation-I. *Clin Neurol Neurosurg*. Oct 2014;125:182–188.

A 13-year-old boy with facial weakness and severe obstructive sleep apnea

Lourdes M. DelRosso

CASE PRESENTATION

A 13-year-old boy presented for follow-up of severe obstructive sleep apnea (OSA) diagnosed by polysomnography (PSG) a year before the visit. The PSG revealed an apnea–hypopnea index (AHI) of 45/h; SpO_2 nadir of 83%; and no evidence of hypoventilation. He underwent tonsillectomy and adenoidectomy (T&A). The parents denied loud snoring, witnessed apneas, or gasping after the surgery. The family was referred for repeat PSG because of the severity of the OSA before tonsillectomy. The patient denied nocturnal enuresis. He reported going to bed at 10 PM and falling asleep within 15 minutes. He reported waking up refreshed at 6:45 AM. He did not endorse daytime sleepiness, parasomnias, symptoms of restless legs, hypnagogic hallucinations, sleep paralysis, or cataplexy.

The patient had been diagnosed with facioscapulohumeral dystrophy (FSHD) at the age of 6 years by genetic testing after winging of his scapulae and upper-extremity weakness was noted on routine physical exam. His family history includes a father with FSHD (diagnosed at age 25), OSA, hypertension, and hypercholesterolemia, and paternal grandfather with FSHD diagnosed at age 50. Review of systems was positive for mild facial weakness and upper-extremity weakness and negative for swallowing difficulties or gastroesophageal reflux.

PHYSICAL EXAM

Physical exam revealed a well-developed, cooperative boy. Vital signs included weight 89.6 kg (99th percentile); height 163.1 cm (59th percentile); pulse 96 and blood pressure 128/65 mm Hg. His pupils were equal in size and reactive to light. Extraocular movements were intact without nystagmus. He was able to raise his eyebrows bilaterally but unable to close his eyes tightly. He was unable to puff his cheeks, and the corners of his mouth did not go up when smiling. Oral exam revealed a Mallampati II oropharynx, surgically absent tonsils, and midline located uvula. He did not have a high-arched palate and exhibited symmetrical palate elevation. Thoracic exam revealed normal muscle bulk with scapular winging on the right. Muscle strength was 4/5 for biceps and triceps bilaterally. The remainder of the cardiovascular and neurologic exam was normal.

LABORATORY AND SLEEP FINDINGS

Initial PSG (Fig. 82-1) revealed a total sleep time (TST) 280 minutes, total recording time (TRT) 459 minutes; sleep efficiency 61%; and arousal index 21. The AHI was 45/h; the nadir was SpO_2 83%; and the $ETCO_2$ was above 50 torr for 3% of the study. The periodic leg movements index (PLMI) was 0. A repeat PSG a year after T&A (Fig. 82-2) revealed a TST of 463 minutes; TRT 542 minutes; sleep efficiency 86%; and an arousal index of 8. The AHI was 15/h; the nadir SpO_2 was 86%; and the $ETCO_2$ was below 50 torr throughout the study. The PLMI was 0.

QUESTION

Are patients with FSHD at increased risk of sleep disorders?

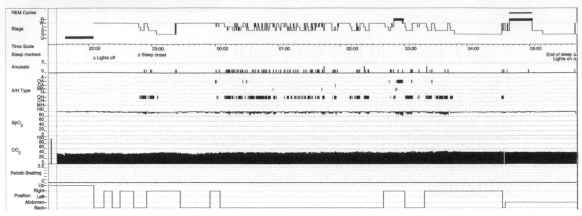

FIGURE 82-1 ■ Hypnogram before T&A shows severe OSA with sleep fragmentation.

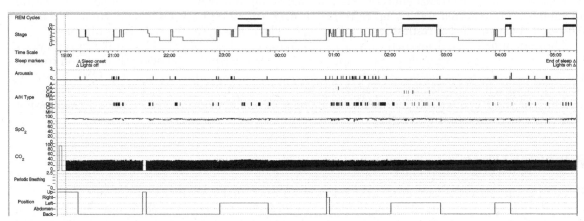

FIGURE 82-2 ■ Hypnogram after T&A shows residual severe OSA with improved sleep continuity.

ANSWER

Patients with FSHD are at increased risk of sleep disorders. These include sleep disruption, excessive daytime sleepiness, hypoventilation, and OSA.

DISCUSSION

FSHD is an autosomal dominant disorder with various degrees of severity. It affects approximately 1 in 20,000 people and is the third most common muscular dystrophy after Duchenne dystrophy and myotonic dystrophy. Symptoms are commonly noticed by the second decade of life. Although facial weakness heralds the condition, the most common presenting symptom is arm weakness manifested as difficulty raising the arm above the shoulder. Weakness of the lower extremities is usually absent or very minimal, but, when present, usually starts with the distal muscles of the lower extremity (foot-drop). Weakness of the abdominal and back muscles can be present and is usually manifested on physical exam by a distended abdomen or lumbar lordosis. Molecular genetic testing diagnoses FSHD, with 95% of affected patients having a deletion on chromosome 4q35.[1]

Common physical findings include asymmetric muscle weakness of the face (Fig. 82-3), pouting of the lips secondary to preserved strength of the orbicularis oris in contrast to other facial muscles (Tapir sign), and asymmetric winging of the scapula. The symptoms are usually slowly progressive and range from minimal weakness to severe impairment. FSHD usually spares bulbar, cardiac, and extraocular muscles. The most severe forms of FSHD present with symptom onset during infancy; therefore, prognosis is inversely related to age of onset. Approximately 10% of patients have respiratory involvement. Predictors of respiratory failure in patients with FSHD are the presence of kyphoscoliosis, wheelchair dependence, and severe muscle weakness.[2]

Sleep disturbances resemble those found in other muscular dystrophies and include sleep disruption, excessive daytime sleepiness, chronic hypoventilation, and OSA. Sleep-disordered breathing can be found in asymptomatic patients, and it is not correlated with disease severity. There are no predictors of OSA because patients with FSHD usually do not present with snoring; however, weight gain

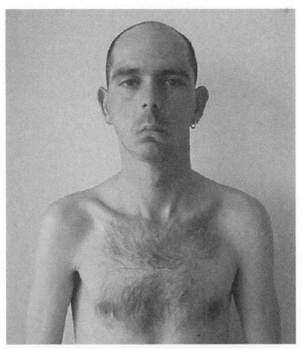

FIGURE 82-3 ■ Prominent pouting appearance of the lips ("tapir sign") and wasting of the facial, shoulder, and upper-arm muscles in a sporadic case of FSHD. (Copyright from Rupprecht, S. et. al; Alveolar hypoventilation as an early symptom of muscle weakneass in facioscapulohumeral muscular; *Sleep Med.* Vol 10, Issue 5, 2009, page 592–593.)

can increase the risk of OSA in these patients.[3] Muscle weakness and mouth opening may make continuous positive airway pressure (CPAP) use challenging.[4]

There is currently no treatment for FSHD, and management usually consists of strengthening exercises and supportive measures.

CLINICAL PEARLS

1. Patients with FSHD are at high risk for sleep-disordered breathing independent of disease severity and presence of snoring.
2. CPAP therapy can be challenging because of air leaks secondary to facial weakness.
3. Predictors of respiratory failure in patients with FSHD are kyphoscoliosis, wheelchair dependence, and severe muscle weakness.

REFERENCES

1. Statland J, Tawil R. Facioscapulohumeral muscular dystrophy. *Neurol Clin*. Aug 2014;32(3):721–728. ix.
2. Della Marca G, Frusciante R, Vollono C, et al. Sleep quality in facioscapulohumeral muscular dystrophy. *J Neurol Sci*. Dec 15 2007;263(1-2):49–53.
3. Della Marca G, Frusciante R, Dittoni S, et al. Sleep disordered breathing in facioscapulohumeral muscular dystrophy. *J Neurol Sci*. Oct 15 2009;285(1-2):54–58.
4. Della Marca G, Frusciante R, Vollono C, Dittoni S, Tonali PA, Ricci E. Mouth leaks may complicate positive airway pressure treatment of OSAS in facioscapulohumeral muscular dystrophy. *Sleep Med*. Jan 2009;10(1):147–149.

A 13-year-old girl with medulloblastoma and breathing pauses

Lourdes M. DelRosso

CASE PRESENTATION

A 13-year-old girl with a history of medulloblastoma of the cerebellum, status post surgical resection, chemotherapy, and radiation, presented with snoring and witnessed apneas. The parents reported that the symptoms started after the surgery to resect the tumor. She denied symptoms of insomnia, restless legs, or daytime sleepiness. She did not have any other past medical or surgical history. Review of systems was positive for blurred vision, right facial-nerve paralysis, and speech delay. Medications included artificial tears.

PHYSICAL EXAM

The girl was sitting in a wheelchair, alert and in no distress. Her vital signs were within normal range. Her weight was at the 50th percentile and her height at the 75th percentile. She exhibited slow, uncoordinated eye movements bilaterally. She had a right facial-nerve palsy. She did not have a high-arched palate; oropharyngeal Mallampati grade was II, and tonsil size was 1+. Her tongue did not deviate laterally and did not have fasciculations or atrophy. Her lungs were clear to auscultation. There was truncal hypotonia and an ataxic gait.

LABORATORY AND SLEEP FINDINGS

Polysomnography (PSG) revealed a total sleep time (TST) of 339 minutes; total recording time 501 minutes; sleep efficiency 68%; and an arousal index of 6.8/h. The obstructive apnea–hypopnea index (AHI) was 0.4/h. The central AHI was 39.2/h; periodic breathing was seen for 40% of the TST; and the SpO_2 nadir was 80%. End-tidal CO_2 was >50 torr for 10% of TST. The periodic leg movements index was 0/h. A representative epoch is seen in Figure 83-1.

Magnetic resonance imaging (MRI) revealed postsurgical changes, as demonstrated in Figure 83-2.

QUESTION

What is the pathophysiology of the breathing disorder seen in this patient?

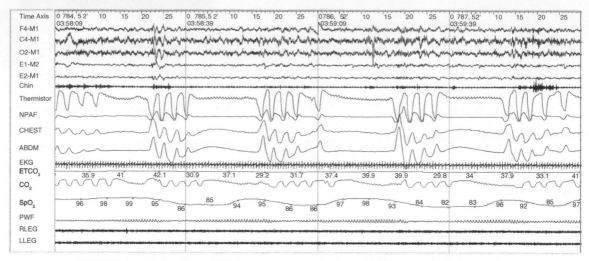

FIGURE 83-1 ■ Two-minute PSG fragment showing central apneas (periodic breathing).

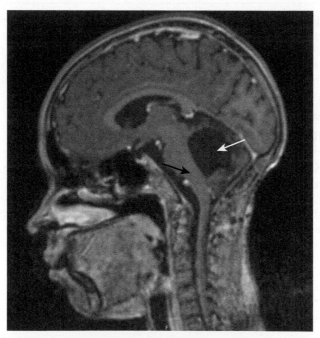

FIGURE 83-2 ■ Sagittal brain MRI demonstrates postsurgical changes after suboccipital craniotomy, with a postresection cavity in the cerebellum (*white arrow*). The *black arrow* points at the medulla.

ANSWER

The central apneas and periodic breathing are likely secondary to damage of the medullary respiratory centers by tumor infiltration or damage during surgical resection.

DISCUSSION

Of newly diagnosed pediatric tumors, 25% occur in the central nervous system. Both the tumor and the treatment can affect sleep, depending on the size, type, and location of the tumor. Tumors that affect the hypothalamus (e.g., craniopharyngioma and suprasellar germinoma) can affect the sleep-wake patterns and produce fragmented sleep, increased daytime sleepiness, obesity, and secondary narcolepsy.[1, 2] Tumors located in the frontal or temporal lobe can induce epileptic syndromes (electric status epilepticus of sleep), parasomnias, and abnormal nocturnal behaviors.[1, 3] A case report of a germ cell tumor involving the pineal gland showed decreased melatonin production with a clinical presentation of insomnia; melatonin supplementation improved the symptoms.[4]

Medulloblastoma and brainstem gliomas can cause central and obstructive apnea by compression of the respiratory nuclei or cranial nerves that innervate the tongue and pharynx. Some of the medullary nuclei involved in breathing include the dorsal respiratory nucleus (inspiration), the ventral respiratory nucleus (inspiration and expiration), the pre-Botzinger complex (respiratory pacemaker), and the nucleus of the tractus solitarius (vagal afferents) (Fig. 83-3). Cranial nerves that innervate the tongue and pharyngeal muscles emerge from nuclei in the medulla (hypoglossal nucleus and nucleus ambiguous). Damage to these nuclei by tumor compression or as a complication of surgical resection can affect breathing, producing either central or obstructive apnea.[5-8] Patients treated for central nervous system tumors may also present with more daytime sleepiness compared with patients treated for other malignancies.[9, 10]

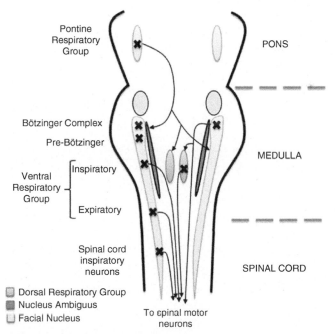

FIGURE 83-3 ■ **Brainstem centers that control breathing.** (From Sowho M, Amatoury J, Kirkness JP, Patil SP. Sleep and respiratory physiology in adults. *Clin Chest Med.* Sep 2014;35(3):469-481, figure 1, p. 471.)

CLINICAL PEARLS

1. Of newly diagnosed pediatric tumors, 25% occur in the central nervous system.
2. Brainstem tumors can cause central and obstructive apnea by compression of the respiratory nuclei or cranial nerves that innervate the tongue and pharynx.
3. Tumors that affect the hypothalamus can affect the sleep-wake patterns and produce fragmented sleep, increased daytime sleepiness, obesity, and secondary narcolepsy.

REFERENCES

1. Prashad PS, Marcus CL, Brown LW, et al. Brain tumor presenting as somnambulism in an adolescent. *Pediatr Neurol*. Sep 2013;49(3):209–212.
2. Marcus CL, Trescher WH, Halbower AC, Lutz J. Secondary narcolepsy in children with brain tumors. *Sleep*. Jun 15 2002;25(4):435–439.
3. Mikati MA, El-Bitar MK, Najjar MW, et al. A child with refractory complex partial seizures, right temporal ganglioglioma, contralateral continuous electrical status epilepticus, and a secondary Landau-Kleffner autistic syndrome. *Epilepsy Behav*. Feb 2009;14(2):411–417.
4. Etzioni A, Luboshitzky R, Tiosano D, Ben-Harush M, Goldsher D, Lavie P. Melatonin replacement corrects sleep disturbances in a child with pineal tumor. *Neurology*. Jan 1996;46(1):261–263.
5. Sowho M, Amatoury J, Kirkness JP, Patil SP. Sleep and respiratory physiology in adults. *Clin Chest Med*. Sep 2014;35(3): 469–481.
6. Ito K, Murofushi T, Mizuno M, Semba T. Pediatric brain stem gliomas with the predominant symptom of sleep apnea. *Int J Pediatr Otorhinolaryngol*. Sep 1996;37(1):53–64.
7. Greenough G, Sateia M, Fadul CE. Obstructive sleep apnea syndrome in a patient with medulloblastoma. *Neuro Oncol*. Oct 1999;1(4):289–291.
8. Delrosso LM, Hoque R, Gonzalez-Toledo E. Two-year-old with post-surgical hypoglossal nerve injury and obstructive sleep apnea. *J Clin Sleep Med*. Jan 15 2014;10(1):97–98.
9. Verberne LM, Maurice-Stam H, Grootenhuis MA, Van Santen HM, Schouten-Van Meeteren AY. Sleep disorders in children after treatment for a CNS tumour. *J Sleep Res*. Aug 2012;21(4):461–469.
10. Rosen GM, Bendel AE, Neglia JP, Moertel CL, Mahowald M. Sleep in children with neoplasms of the central nervous system: case review of 14 children. *Pediatrics*. Jul 2003;112(1 Pt 1):e46–e54.

An 11-year-old with Rett syndrome and cyanotic spells

Suzanne E. Beck

CASE PRESENTATION

An 11-year-old girl with Rett syndrome was evaluated because of intermittent cyanotic spells. These episodes of cyanosis occurred following breath-holding spells, which tended to occur during the day, during periods of agitation, or during periods of restless sleep, especially early in the night when she had frequent awakenings. Her bedtime routine was prolonged because of fears and anxiety around bedtime, and she took naps during the day. In addition, her parents noted that she had bruxism and often had fits of screaming or laughing during the night that preceded breath-holding and cyanotic spells. Episodes usually lasted 30 seconds to 2 minutes and self-resolved. There was no loss of consciousness or seizure activity during the spells. Past medical history revealed that she was born after a full-term gestation and was neurodevelopmentally normal until the age of 9 to 12 months, when her development and head-circumference growth slowed. Subsequently, she lost developmental milestones and communication skills, developed hypotonia and motor apraxia, and was diagnosed with Rett syndrome at age 5 years. She had epilepsy, which was well controlled on her current medication regimen. She had a feeding gastrostomy. Review of systems was negative for recent seizures, coughing, congestion with feeds, or anemia. Medications included clobazam, levocarnitine, valproic acid, diazepam p.r.n., and multivitamins.

PHYSICAL EXAM

Vital signs: respiratory rate 15 breaths/min; heart rate 80 beats/min; blood pressure 103/76 mm Hg; SpO_2 98% room air; weight 30.6 kg (8th percentile); and length 132 cm (5th percentile).

She was nonverbal, made little eye contact, and was in no apparent distress. She demonstrated stereotypical hand-wringing movements. She was able to ambulate with assistance. Eye movements and fundi were normal. She had awake bruxism and some drooling. Tonsils were 2+. There was mild scoliosis. Lungs were clear. Heart sounds were normal. A gastrostomy tube was in place. She had decreased muscle tone and was diffusely hyperreflexic. Physical exam was otherwise unremarkable.

LABORATORY AND SLEEP FINDINGS

Polysomnography (PSG) revealed a total sleep time (TST) of 472 minutes; SE 88%; N1 30 min (6.4%); N2 197 min (42%); N3 185 min (39%); REM 59 minutes (13%); arousal index 28.5/h; obstructive apnea–hypopnea index 2.1/h; central apnea index 1.7/h; maximum length of central apnea 99 seconds; and mean duration of central apnea 42 seconds (representative central apnea shown in Fig. 84-1). SpO_2 was <90% for 5% TST; SpO_2 nadir was 48%; mean SpO_2 97%; mean $ETCO_2$ awake 27 Torr; and mean $ETCO_2$ asleep 48 Torr. Electroencephalogram (EEG) showed a definite, although slow, posterior dominant frequency during arousal at 7 Hz with an anterior-posterior gradient. REM and non-REM sleep were identified, but there was a lack of usual sleep architectural findings, such as spindles, vertex waves, and K-complexes. Throughout the recording, there were no focal, lateralizing, or epileptiform features. There were no EEG changes before, during, or following the apneas associated with severe desaturation.

QUESTION

Are these findings typically associated with Rett syndrome?

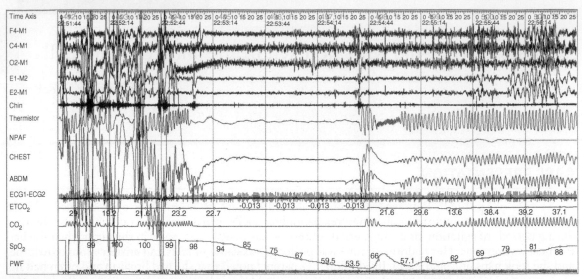

FIGURE 84-1 ■ Illustrative 300-second epoch showing profound desaturation during N1 sleep following a 99-second breath hold (central apnea) that began after a period of hyperventilation during wake. Note hyperventilation with profound hypocapnia (transcutaneous CO_2 17 Torr) preceding the prolonged central apnea (duration 99 seconds), followed by profound desaturation (SpO_2 nadir 48%) and then spontaneous recovery of SpO_2 and PCO_2. The patient experienced similar episodes during the night.

ANSWER

Sleep problems are common in individuals with Rett syndrome and are identified in over 80% of patients. They include decreased night sleep, increased excessive daytime and total sleep which may worsen with age, nighttime laughter, teeth grinding, night screaming, and nighttime seizures. Abnormal breathing patterns while awake are one of the hallmark features of Rett syndrome. Patients with Rett syndrome have characteristic breathing abnormalities while awake: periods of hyperventilation, alternating with breath holds or central apneas. The PSG findings of periods of hyperventilation during wakefulness followed by breath holding (central apnea) and desaturation as she transitioned into sleep were attributed to the patient's diagnosis of Rett syndrome.

DISCUSSION

Rett syndrome, first described by Andreas Rett in 1966, is a rare neurodevelopmental genetic disorder associated with cognitive and physical impairments most often because of a de novo mutation of the *MECP2* gene located on the X chromosome,[1] but it is a clinical diagnosis because not all patients with the mutation have the disorder, and some patients with Rett syndrome do not have a known mutation. Because it is X linked, classic Rett syndrome primarily affects females, with a prevalence of approximately 1 in 10,000 female births; it rarely affects males.[2] Rett syndrome is characterized by severe cognitive and physical impairments, autistic features, hypotonia, motor apraxia, sleep problems, and breathing abnormalities.[2] Revised diagnostic criteria for classic Rett syndrome require a period of apparently normal psychomotor development in the first 6 months of life, followed by a period of regression (which is not due to brain injury secondary to trauma, neurometabolic disease, or severe infection), and it involves partial or complete loss of acquired purposeful hand skills and language, social withdrawal, gait abnormalities, and the development of stereotypic hand movements, followed by stabilization or even some degree of recovery.[3] Importantly, the symptoms of Rett syndrome usually do not appear until later in infancy or early childhood, after a period of apparently normal development, and may sometimes be misdiagnosed as autism, cerebral palsy, or nonspecific developmental delays.

Sleep problems in individuals with Rett syndrome vary with age and mutation type.[4] A longitudinal survey of 300 Rett syndrome patients enrolled in a population-based registry in Australia found sleep problems in over 80% of the population.[4] Daytime napping, nighttime laughter, teeth grinding, screaming during the night, and nighttime seizures were the problems most frequently reported.[4] The prevalence of nighttime laughter decreased with age, and the prevalence of nighttime seizures and daytime napping increased with age.[4] The prevalence of sleep problems was highest in cases with a large deletion of the *MECP2* gene and in those with the p.R294X or p.R306C mutations.[4] Another study of 20 females with classic Rett syndrome showed that patients with Rett syndrome had less nighttime sleep and more daytime sleep than peers, and that the girls commonly had delayed sleep onset and increased night waking.[4] The authors of this study speculated that the aberrant sleep patterns seen in this population may reflect a disturbance of circadian rhythm resulting from progressive central nervous system damage, which may be unrelated to underlying EEG findings. Some of the dysfunctional sleep patterns of girls with Rett syndrome may be amenable to behavioral treatments.[5] Melatonin may also be useful in improving the duration of night sleep.[6]

Abnormal breathing while awake is one of the hallmark features of Rett syndrome. Girls with Rett syndrome have characteristic breath holds or central apneas alternating with periods of hyperventilation while awake (reviewed in Ramirez[7]). A PSG study of 30 girls with Rett syndrome (median age 7 years) found that 67% of the girls showed the classic pattern of hyperventilation followed by central apnea and/or breath holding with desaturation during wakefulness.[8] Compared with controls, the girls with Rett syndrome had no increase in the number of central or obstructive apneas during sleep, no differences in end-tidal CO_2 levels during sleep, and only slightly lower oxyhemoglobin saturation during REM sleep. The complexity of the breathing phenotype in Rett syndrome may be explained by underlying genotype-phenotype relationships—specifically, the types of mutation and degree of X-chromosome inactivation.[1] The mechanism for the hyperventilation-central apnea is unclear. It is thought that patients with Rett syndrome have normal brainstem control of ventilation but that the disordered breathing seen during wakefulness is due to an abnormality of the cortical influence on ventilation. It has been speculated that the hyperventilation is one of the Rett syndrome stereotypies, similar to the hand-wringing and body rocking seen in these patients, or that the hyperventilation produces some sort of pleasurable sensation. Hyperventilation results in hypocapnia and alkalosis, thus reducing the drive to breathe. This results in a central apnea, which results in oxyhemoglobin desaturation and CO_2 accumulation. The resultant hypoxemia, along with normalization of CO_2 levels, is a stimulus to resume breathing.

Our patient had a classic presentation of Rett syndrome, with apparently normal development until age 9 months, after which she developed at a slower rate, with a decrease in head-circumference growth. She subsequently lost communication skills and later developed characteristic hand-wringing and apraxia. She developed sleep problems associated with Rett syndrome, namely frequent night waking and screaming, and laughing during the night. In addition, she developed characteristic irregular breathing during wakefulness, with bouts of hyperventilation, breath holding, and cyanosis, which were exacerbated by her underlying anxiety. These events were captured on PSG (see Fig. 84-1), demonstrating that the periods of prolonged central apnea with profound desaturation during light sleep were actually preceded by bouts of hyperpnea-induced hypocapnia during arousals or wakefulness.

Treatment of these events is difficult. Noninvasive ventilation is not helpful because most of the events occur during wakefulness; further, noninvasive ventilation would exacerbate the hyperventilation. Supplemental oxygen was considered. However, this can suppress the hypoxic ventilatory drive and may therefore lengthen the breath-holding spells. Case reports have described the administration of exogenous supplemental carbon dioxide,[9] but this is impractical to administer episodically, and it can be a safety hazard in the home. Because our patient's episodes resolved spontaneously, our approach was to implement a behavior plan for her caregivers to recognize situations that typically precipitated agitation or anxiety. This included a bedtime routine with calming activities aimed to allay sleep-associated fears in hopes of decreasing periods of agitation and hyperventilation. The family was counseled that these breath-holding spells seem to run a benign course in children with Rett syndrome. Our patient continued to have similar episodes, but they were less frequent and less severe.

CLINICAL PEARLS

1. The classic breathing abnormality in patients with Rett syndrome occurs during wakefulness and is characterized by rapid shallow breathing (causing hyperventilation), followed by central apnea-breath holding, often followed by desaturation and cyanosis.
2. Sleep problems are very common in Rett syndrome and can be unusual: nighttime laughter, night screaming, nighttime seizures, and severe bruxism. These may vary with mutation type and age.
3. Children with Rett syndrome have markedly impaired sleep-wake patterns (delayed sleep onset, more night waking, and excessive daytime sleep), which may worsen over time but may be amenable to behavioral modification and melatonin.

REFERENCES

1. Amir RE, Van den Veyver IB, Wan M, Tran CQ, Francke U, Zoghbi HY. Rett syndrome is caused by mutations in X-linked MECP2, encoding methyl-CpG-binding protein 2. *Nat Genet.* Oct 1999;23(2):185–188.
2. Hagberg B. Clinical manifestations and stages of Rett syndrome. *Ment Retard Dev Disabil Res Rev.* 2002;8(2):61–65.
3. Neul JL, Kaufmann WE, Glaze DG, et al. Rett syndrome: revised diagnostic criteria and nomenclature. *Ann Neurol.* Dec 2010;68(6):944–950.
4. Young D, Nagarajan L, de Klerk N, Jacoby P, Ellaway C, Leonard H. Sleep problems in Rett syndrome. *Brain Dev.* Nov 2007;29(10):609–616.
5. Piazza CC, Fisher W, Moser H. Behavioral treatment of sleep dysfunction in patients with the Rett syndrome. *Brain Dev.* Jul 1991;13(4):232–237.
6. Appleton RE, Jones AP, Gamble C, et al. The use of Melatonin in children with neurodevelopmental disorders and impaired sleep: a randomised, double-blind, placebo-controlled, parallel study (MENDS). *Health Technol Assess.* 2012;16(40): i-239.
7. Ramirez JM, Ward CS, Neul JL. Breathing challenges in Rett syndrome: lessons learned from humans and animal models. *Respir Physiol Neurobiol.* Nov 1 2013;189(2):280–287.
8. Marcus CL, Carroll JL, McColley SA, et al. Polysomnographic characteristics of patients with Rett syndrome. *J Pediatr.* Aug 1994;125(2):218–224.
9. Smeets EE, Julu PO, van Waardenburg D, et al. Management of a severe forceful breather with Rett syndrome using carbogen. *Brain Dev.* Nov 2006;28(10):625–632.

An 11-year-old boy with morning headaches

Lourdes M. DelRosso

CASE PRESENTATION

An 11-year-old boy presented for evaluation of morning headaches that started 3 months before presentation. The headaches, which occurred several times a week, were frontal, bilateral, and resolved soon after waking. There were no associated symptoms of nausea, dizziness, or visual changes. His bedtime was 10 PM. His mother did not notice nocturnal awakenings. On weekdays, his mother woke him up at 6:30 AM to go to school; on weekends, he slept until 9 AM. He snored loudly. He denied symptoms of restless legs. The family denied parasomnias. He had no daytime sleepiness. There were no other past surgical or medical problems. His review of systems was negative for depression and anxiety. He did not take any medications.

PHYSICAL EXAM

Physical exam revealed an obese, cooperative boy in no distress. His vital signs were within normal limits. Weight was at the 95th percentile, height at the 40th percentile, and body mass index greater than the 95th percentile. He had an adenoid facies. The oropharyngeal Mallampati grade was III, and tonsil size was 4+. His lungs were clear to auscultation. Neurologic exam was normal.

LABORATORY AND SLEEP FINDINGS

Magnetic resonance imaging of the brain was normal. Polysomnography (PSG) showed normal sleep efficiency and stage distribution. The obstructive apnea–hypopnea index was 30/h. SpO_2 nadir was 62%. The peak end-tidal CO_2 was 62 mm Hg, and CO_2 was >50 mm Hg for 10% of total sleep time (Fig. 85-1).

QUESTION

What is the diagnosis in this patient?

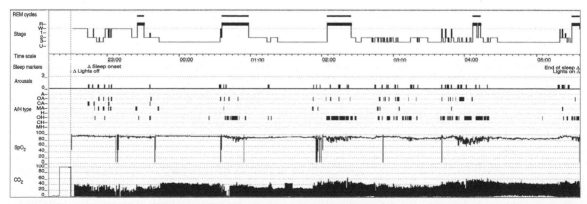

FIGURE 85-1 ■ Hypnogram reveals severe obstructive sleep apnea associated with severe desaturation and hypercapnia.

ANSWER

Headache secondary to severe obstructive sleep apnea.

DISCUSSION

Headache is a common complaint in children. The prevalence of headaches increases with age; headaches are rare before 4 years of age, with an overall prevalence of 19% in children aged 5 years; the prevalence of occasional headaches increases to 51% in children aged 7 years.[1] The prevalence of migraines in children is 10%.[2] Headaches affect more boys than girls before puberty and more girls than boys after puberty.[3] Headaches in children are commonly associated with comorbidities including depression, anxiety, attention-deficit/hyperactivity disorder, atopy (asthma and eczema), and sleep disorders.[4]

The relationship between sleep and headache is complex: primary headaches (migraine and tension headaches) can occur during or after sleep; headaches can contribute to sleep disruption, insomnia, and restless sleep; and headaches can occur secondary to sleep disorders (obstructive sleep apnea syndrome [OSAS] and insufficient sleep). Children with migraines have been found to have a higher prevalence of parasomnias (sleep talking, bruxism, and nightmares), shorter sleep duration, prolonged sleep latency, and increased number of nocturnal awakenings.[5] A study of 70 children with migraine and 135 children with nonmigraine headache revealed that poor sleep or insufficient sleep was the most common headache trigger in both groups.[6] The second most common trigger was emotional distress.

Morning headaches may occur in patients with severe OSAS. The pathophysiology may be secondary to hypercapnia, hypoxemia, altered cerebral blood flow, or increased intracranial pressure. Although morning headaches have been described in children with OSAS,[7] detailed studies on headache secondary to OSAS in children are lacking. Morning headaches may also be secondary to insufficient sleep. The headache is usually dull and frontal and can occur in individuals with or without a prior history of headaches.[8]

The *International Classification of Sleep Disorders*, third edition (ICSD-3) describes sleep-related headaches as a group of headaches that occur during sleep or upon awakening from sleep. Among these are migraine headaches, cluster headaches, chronic paroxysmal hemicranias, and hypnic headaches. Cluster headaches are rare in children, with a prevalence of 0.1%.[9] The most striking feature is the circadian pattern of the headache. When cluster headaches occur at night, they tend to occur during the first REM cycle. Chronic paroxysmal hemicrania occurs mainly in adults but has been reported in children. It typically presents with severe unilateral pain, conjunctival erythema, photophobia, and vomiting; the dramatic response to indomethacin aids in the diagnosis.[10] Hypnic headaches occur exclusively during REM sleep, are mainly seen in the elderly, and have rarely been described in children.[11]

Nocturnal PSG is not indicated in the evaluation of headaches unless sleep disordered breathing is suspected, as it was in our patient. OSAS in our patient was treated with tonsillectomy and adenoidectomy. The headaches resolved after the surgery.

CLINICAL PEARLS

1. Headaches are common in children.
2. Primary headaches (migraine and tension headache) may disrupt sleep (with multiple nocturnal awakenings, prolonged sleep latency, and parasomnias).
3. Morning headaches can be a symptom of obstructive sleep apnea. OSAS should be suspected if the child snores or has other symptoms of OSAS, and the headaches occur only upon awakening and improve soon after the child awakens.

REFERENCES

1. Wober-Bingol C. Epidemiology of migraine and headache in children and adolescents. *Curr Pain Headache Rep.* Jun 2013;17(6):341.
2. Dosi C, Figura M, Ferri R, Bruni O. Sleep and headache. *Semin Pediatr Neurol.* Jun 2015;22(2):105–112.
3. Parisi P, Vanacore N, Belcastro V, et al. Clinical guidelines in pediatric headache: evaluation of quality using the AGREE II instrument. *J Headache Pain.* 2014;15:57.

4. Bellini B, Arruda M, Cescut A, et al. Headache and comorbidity in children and adolescents. *J Headache Pain*. 2013;14:79.
5. Bellini B, Panunzi S, Bruni O, Guidetti V. Headache and sleep in children. *Curr Pain Headache Rep*. Jun 2013;17(6):335.
6. Bruni O, Russo PM, Ferri R, Novelli L, Galli F, Guidetti V. Relationships between headache and sleep in a non-clinical population of children and adolescents. *Sleep Med*. Jul 2008;9(5):542–548.
7. Guilleminault C, Pelayo R. Sleep-disordered breathing in children. *Ann Med*. Aug 1998;30(4):350–356.
8. Palma JA, Urrestarazu E, Iriarte J. Sleep loss as risk factor for neurologic disorders: a review. *Sleep Med*. Mar 2013;14(3):229–236.
9. Lampl C. Childhood-onset cluster headache. *Pediatr Neurol*. Aug 2002;27(2):138–140.
10. Tarantino S, Vollono C, Capuano A, Vigevano F, Valeriani M. Chronic paroxysmal hemicrania in paediatric age: report of two cases. *J Headache Pain*. Apr 2011;12(2):263–267.
11. Silva-Neto RP, Almeida KJ. Hypnic headache in childhood: a literature review. *J Neurol Sci*. Sep 15 2015;356(1-2):45–48. Epub Jun 24 2015.

An 11-year-old boy with history of concussion and insomnia

Lourdes M. DelRosso

CLINICAL PRESENTATION

An 11-year-old boy presented for evaluation of sleep disturbances after a second concussion. He was kicked in the head during a soccer game 6 months before presentation. He did not experience loss of consciousness but was confused for 5 minutes, with subsequent headache and nausea. It took him several weeks before he felt back to normal, and he took a month off of school. He had a second concussion 3 months before presentation. He was hit in the back of the head with a soccer ball. He did not lose consciousness but had significant headache and confusion for 15 to 20 minutes. He was subsequently evaluated by a neurologist, a sports medicine physician, and a physical therapist.

Two weeks after the second concussion, he developed sleep problems, mainly difficulty falling asleep and frequent nocturnal awakenings. He went to bed at 9:30 PM. It took him at least an hour to fall asleep. During this time, he lay in bed tossing and turning. He was finally asleep by 11 PM. He had 3 to 4 nocturnal awakenings of various durations. During these awakenings, he stayed in his bed trying to fall asleep again. He woke up at 6:30 AM. He did not take naps during the day.

The family denied snoring. The child denied an urge to move the legs at bedtime, enuresis, excessive daytime sleepiness, cataplexy, hypnagogic hallucinations, and sleep paralysis. There was no history of sleepwalking, nightmares, or night terrors. Daytime symptoms included difficulty concentrating in class and academic decline (his grades dropped from As and Bs to Cs). The review of systems was negative for headaches, depression, or anxiety.

PHYSICAL EXAM

The physical exam revealed a friendly and cooperative boy in no distress. Vital signs were within normal range. Physical and neurologic exam were normal.

LABORATORY AND SLEEP FINDINGS

Magnetic resonance imaging of the brain: normal.

QUESTION

What is the diagnosis in this patient?

ANSWER

Insomnia secondary to postconcussion syndrome.

DISCUSSION

Approximately 1.5 million Americans per year suffer closed head injuries with loss of consciousness, with 20% of these injuries being sports related.[1] Head injuries represent 2.5% of all pediatric visits to the emergency department.[1] The majority of head injuries are classified as mild head trauma (loss of consciousness and/or confusion and disorientation lasting <30 minutes).[2] The constellation of symptoms after mild head trauma is called "postconcussion syndrome." The symptoms of postconcussion syndrome include headaches, dizziness, inattention, memory disturbance, sleep problems, learning and concentration difficulties, fatigue, emotional instability, mood swings, anxiety, and fears.[2] When the symptoms include nightmares, the diagnosis of posttraumatic stress disorder is suspected.[3]

A study of 280 patients (ages 11 to 22 years) demonstrated that the most common symptoms seen immediately after mild head trauma included headache, fatigue, dizziness, and taking longer to think.[4] Symptoms that were not initially present but developed at follow-up (at least a week later) included sleep disturbance, frustration, forgetfulness, and fatigue. The majority of cognitive deficits resolved in 3 months, but sleep disturbance was among the symptoms that persisted the longest. When symptoms persist, it is important to differentiate between symptoms related to the concussion pathophysiology, symptoms related to a preconcussion condition, or symptoms related to a secondary process after the concussion (depression or anxiety). Usually, symptoms secondary to the concussion improve with rest and are exacerbated by activity, but when symptoms no longer improve with rest, they may represent manifestations of a superimposed psychological diagnosis.[5]

A study of 19 adolescents who suffered mild head trauma 3 years earlier and 16 age-matched controls revealed that the patients who suffered mild head trauma complained of disrupted sleep. The sleep complaints were validated using polysomnography and actigraphy. The results demonstrated similar sleep latencies between both groups but decreased sleep efficiency in the mild head trauma group. The findings met criteria for chronic insomnia.[6] Another study of 98 adolescents who experienced mild head trauma 0.5 to 6 years before the study and 80 controls (matched for age, sex, socioeconomic status, and weight) demonstrated an increased prevalence of sleep complaints in the head trauma group (28% vs. 11%). The sleep complaints included difficulties falling asleep, frequent awakenings, early morning awakenings, nonrestorative sleep, and daytime sleepiness.[3]

Mechanisms responsible for postconcussion syndrome include structural changes (edema and axonal damage), physiologic changes (altered autonomic regulation), and metabolic disarray (cerebral glucose metabolism and blood flow). If a second head trauma occurs before healing from the first injury, the second impact can produce rapid brain edema and longer (or permanent) impairment. This is referred to as second impact syndrome.[5]

Management of sleep complaints in patients with postconcussion syndrome includes education on sleep hygiene (avoidance of electronics and caffeine, consistent bedtime routine, and avoidance of naps), behavioral sleep interventions for insomnia, and evaluation of possible comorbidities (depression, anxiety). Melatonin and antidepressants have been used anecdotally.[7] Our patient was evaluated by a sleep behavioral psychologist who recommended sleep restriction, with a bedtime of 11 PM and rise time of 6:30 AM. The behavioral treatment was combined with melatonin 1 mg at 9 PM. As the sleep efficiency improved, the bedtime was moved earlier over the course of a few days to 9:30 PM, and melatonin administration was moved earlier as well.

CLINICAL PEARLS

1. The symptoms of postconcussion syndrome include headaches, dizziness, inattention, memory disturbance, and sleep problems, among others.
2. Mechanisms responsible for postconcussion syndrome include structural changes, physiologic changes, and metabolic disarray.
3. Management of sleep complaints in patients with postconcussion syndrome includes education on sleep hygiene, behavioral sleep interventions for insomnia, and evaluation of possible comorbidities.

REFERENCES

1. Meehan WP 3rd, Mannix R. Pediatric concussions in United States emergency departments in the years 2002 to 2006. *J Pediatr*. Dec 2010;157(6):889–893.
2. Necajauskaite O, Endziniene M, Jureniene K. The prevalence, course and clinical features of post-concussion syndrome in children. *Medicina (Kaunas)*. 2005;41(6):457–464.
3. Pillar G, Averbooch E, Katz N, Peled N, Kaufman Y, Shahar E. Prevalence and risk of sleep disturbances in adolescents after minor head injury. *Pediatr Neurol*. Aug 2003;29(2):131–135.
4. Eisenberg MA, Meehan WP 3rd, Mannix R. Duration and course of post-concussive symptoms. *Pediatrics*. Jun 2014; 133(6):999–1006.
5. Leddy JJ, Sandhu H, Sodhi V, Baker JG, Willer B. Rehabilitation of concussion and post-concussion syndrome. *Sports Health*. Mar 2012;4(2):147–154.
6. Kaufman Y, Tzischinsky O, Epstein R, Etzioni A, Lavie P, Pillar G. Long-term sleep disturbances in adolescents after minor head injury. *Pediatr Neurol*. Feb 2001;24(2):129–134.
7. Meehan WP 3rd. Medical therapies for concussion. *Clin Sports Med*. Jan 2011;30(1):115–124. ix.

A 16-year-old girl with panic attacks and multiple nocturnal awakenings

Lourdes M. DelRosso

CASE PRESENTATION

A 16-year-old girl presented for evaluation of multiple nocturnal awakenings. She reported going to bed at 10 PM but she felt keyed up and unable to relax. She denied use of electronics or television. She stated that she fell asleep at around midnight, only to wake up 30 to 60 minutes later. She reported watching the clock and worrying about school and homework during each awakening. She would fall asleep within 30 to 60 minutes after each awakening. These awakenings occurred 2 to 4 times a night. Her parents woke her up at 6 AM on school days. Her schedule did not vary significantly during the weekends. She reported feeling fatigued in the morning. Once at school, she would not doze off but reported difficulty concentrating. She denied taking naps during the day. She denied snoring, restless legs, excessive sleepiness, bruxism, or parasomnias.

The patient was recently diagnosed with generalized anxiety disorder. Review of systems was positive for headaches and negative for depression or recent weight changes. She did not have any other past medical or surgical history. She did not take any medications or drugs.

PHYSICAL EXAM

The patient was cooperative and in no distress. Her vital signs were within normal limits.

Her weight was at the 34th percentile and her height at the 9th percentile. The physical exam was unremarkable.

QUESTION

What is the diagnosis in this patient?

ANSWER

Insomnia secondary to generalized anxiety disorder.

DISCUSSION

Anxiety disorder is common in children, with a prevalence of 20%. Studies have shown that childhood anxiety does not remit spontaneously but persists into adulthood and may be complicated by substance abuse, comorbid depression, and suicidal ideation. The *Diagnostic and Statistical Manual of Mental Disorders*, fifth edition (DSM-V) criteria for generalized anxiety disorder in children include excessive anxiety or worry for at least 6 months, difficulty controlling the worry, and one of the following (three are required in adults): restlessness, feeling on edge or feeling keyed up, being easily fatigued, irritability, muscle tension, difficulty concentrating, or difficulty falling or staying asleep. The anxiety must affect one area of functioning, must not be attributed to drugs or medications, and must not be better explained by another medical or mental disorder.[1]

Up to 90% of children with generalized anxiety disorder experience insomnia symptoms, either by parental report or by self-report. Sleep complaints in children with anxiety vary with age. Younger children usually present with bedtime resistance, refusal to sleep alone, nightmares, and parasomnias, whereas older children and adolescents present with difficulty falling asleep and multiple nocturnal awakenings. Children with anxiety do not present with excessive daytime sleepiness, likely because they have hyperarousability related to the anxiety.[2] Polysomnography (PSG) has shown prolonged sleep onset latency, decreased REM onset latency, decreased sleep efficiency, increased REM percentage, and preserved slow-wave sleep; however, these findings have not been duplicated when the PSG was performed at home.[3,4]

Cognitive behavioral therapy improves anxiety symptoms and sleep complaints. The most common recommended techniques target inconsistent bedtime schedules and sleep associations (parental presence). Scheduled "worry times" in the afternoon can help decrease bedtime concerns and worries. Other techniques include systematic desensitization (relaxation and imagery) and reinforcement (a point system).[5] There is very little evidence regarding pharmacologic treatment of anxiety in children.

CLINICAL PEARLS

1. Of children with generalized anxiety disorder, 90% experience insomnia symptoms.
2. Children with anxiety do not usually present with excessive daytime sleepiness.
3. Cognitive behavioral therapy is successful in treating anxiety symptoms and sleep disturbances in children with generalized anxiety disorder.

REFERENCES

1. American Psychiatric Association. *Desk Reference to the Diagnostic Criteria from DSM-5*. Washington, DC: American Psychiatric Publishing; 2013.
2. Alfano CA, Pina AA, Zerr AA, Villalta IK. Pre-sleep arousal and sleep problems of anxiety-disordered youth. *Child Psychiatry Hum Dev*. Apr 2010;41(2):156–167.
3. Alfano CA, Reynolds K, Scott N, Dahl RE, Mellman TA. Polysomnographic sleep patterns of non-depressed, non-medicated children with generalized anxiety disorder. *J Affect Disord*. May 2013;147(1-3):379–384.
4. Patriquin MA, Mellman TA, Glaze DG, Alfano CA. Polysomnographic sleep characteristics of generally-anxious and healthy children assessed in the home environment. *J Affect Disord*. Jun 2014;161:79–83.
5. Ducasse D, Denis H. [Pathological nighttime fears in children: clinical specificities and effective therapeutics]. *Encephale*. Sep 2015;41(4):323–331. Epub Nov 4 2014.

A 12-year-old girl with fatigue and difficulty falling asleep

Lourdes M. DelRosso

CASE PRESENTATION

A 12-year-old girl presented for evaluation of difficulty falling asleep that began 2 months ago. The patient went to bed at 10 PM but was not able to fall asleep for 1 to 2 hours. She would turn the lights and her electronic devices off and lie down in bed. Once asleep, she did not wake during the night. She woke up at 7 AM. Her schedule was the same on weekends. During the day, she felt fatigued but did not doze off and did not take naps. The Epworth sleepiness score modified for children was 5. She denied symptoms of restless legs syndrome, snoring, daytime sleepiness, nightmares, hypnagogic hallucinations, or sleep paralysis. Her parents reported that during the day, she spent most of the time lying in bed. She used to enjoy dancing and ballet but stopped attending the school practices 3 months ago. Her grades had dropped from As and Bs to Cs. She had difficulty concentrating during classes. She denied depression, anxiety, or suicidal ideation. Her review of systems was positive for a 2-kg weight loss in the last month and negative for unexplained fevers, abdominal pain, or headaches. Her past medical and surgical history was negative. She did not take any medications.

PHYSICAL EXAM

Physical exam revealed a well-appearing girl with flat affect. Her vital signs were within normal limits. Her weight was at the 26th percentile and her height at the 40th percentile. The exam was otherwise unremarkable.

LABORATORY AND SLEEP FINDINGS

Thyroid-stimulating hormone, complete blood count, and metabolic panel were within normal limits. Her sleep diary is shown in Figure 88-1.

QUESTION

What is the diagnosis in this patient?

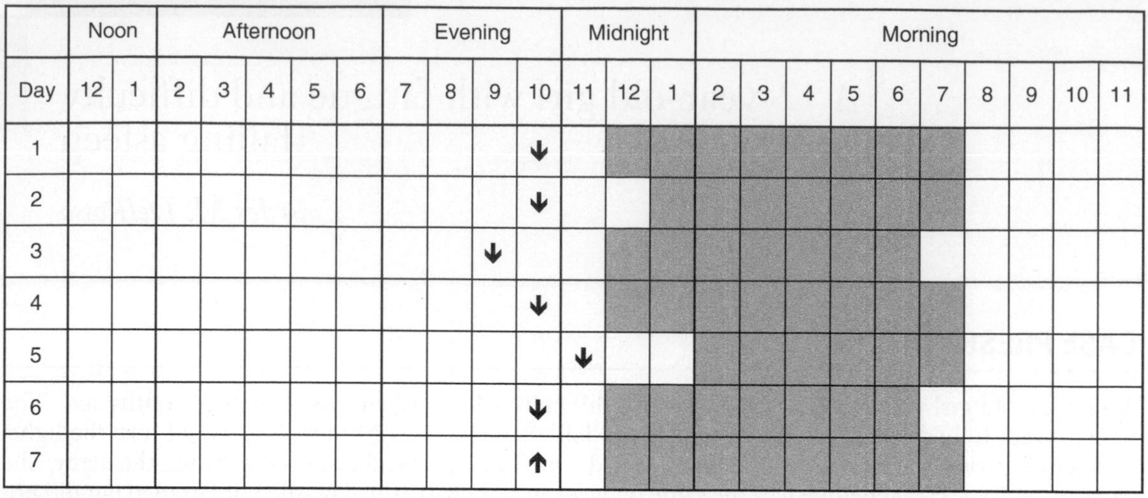

Day	Noon		Afternoon					Evening				Midnight			Morning										
	12	1	2	3	4	5	6	7	8	9	10	11	12	1	2	3	4	5	6	7	8	9	10	11
1											↓		▓	▓	▓	▓	▓	▓	▓	▓				
2											↓		▓		▓	▓	▓	▓	▓	▓				
3										↓		▓	▓	▓	▓	▓	▓	▓	▓					
4											↓		▓	▓	▓	▓	▓	▓	▓					
5												↓		▓	▓	▓	▓	▓	▓	▓				
6											↓		▓	▓	▓	▓	▓	▓	▓					
7											↑		▓	▓	▓	▓	▓	▓	▓	▓				

FIGURE 88-1 ■ **Patient's 1-week sleep diary.** *Arrow* indicates her bedtime, and *shadowed areas* indicate time asleep.

ANSWER

Our patient fits criteria for major depressive disorder (MDD). Sleep diaries are consistent with the patient's reported sleep history. Our patient's delayed sleep onset is consistent with insomnia secondary to MDD. When the patient goes to bed later (day 5), her sleep onset is still delayed by 2 hours. In addition, when she is allowed to sleep on weekends, her sleep duration does not improve (wake-up time is still 7 AM). These two features rule out delayed sleep-wake phase disorder.

DISCUSSION

MDD occurs in 2% of children and 8% of adolescents. Up to 53% of children with MDD report symptoms of insomnia; up to 10% report hypersomnia; and another 10% report both insomnia and hypersomnia symptoms.[1] The *Diagnostic and Statistical Manual of Mental Disorders*, fifth edition (DSM-5) criteria[2] for MDD include five of the following symptoms for at least 2 weeks: depressed mood, loss of interest and pleasure in activities, presence of insomnia or hypersomnia nearly every day, significant weight loss or weight gain, psychomotor retardation or agitation, diminished ability to think or concentrate, loss of energy, feelings of worthlessness, and suicidal thoughts. The relationship between sleep and depression is not clear in terms of cause and effect. Given the uncertainty with cause and effect, insomnia associated with depression is termed "comorbid" rather than secondary insomnia. Among adolescents diagnosed with MDD, 90% complain of sleep difficulties and 75% report having had sleep disturbances before the diagnosis of MDD; these associations may contribute to create a vicious cycle whereby lack of sleep leads to depressive symptoms and depression leads to difficulty sleeping. The presence of sleep disturbances has also been associated with more severe degrees of depression and reports of suicidal ideation.[3] Polysomnography (PSG) (which is not typically performed for patients with MDD) has revealed prolonged sleep latency in children with MDD, but studies have not shown consistent differences in sleep architecture or a shortened REM latency or increased REM density as has been seen in adults.[4,5] Young patients with MDD typically report more sleep-onset than sleep-maintenance insomnia. The major differential diagnosis of a patient with sleep-onset insomnia is the delayed sleep-wake phase disorder[6] (a circadian-rhythm sleep-wake disorder). These patients also do not complain of sleep-maintenance insomnia. However, when allowed to wake up on their own schedule, they typically sleep until late in the morning or early afternoon. When allowed to sleep on their own schedule, they feel refreshed in contrast to patients with depression, who report unrefreshing sleep and fatigue.

The treatment of MDD in children and adolescents includes cognitive behavioral therapy, pharmacological therapy, or a combination of both. Approximately 50% of patients who respond to therapy (i.e., no longer meet DSM-5 depression criteria) continue having residual symptoms, of which sleep disturbance is the most common. Patients with residual symptoms may be at increased risk for relapse of depression. Simultaneous management of both depression and insomnia or hypersomnia is therefore recommended.[7]

Our patient fit DSM-5 diagnostic criteria for depression and was referred for psychiatric evaluation and management. Behavioral therapy for sleep symptoms was initiated.

CLINICAL PEARLS

1. Insomnia symptoms are common in children and adolescents with MDD. Sleep-onset insomnia complaints are often more prominent than are sleep-maintenance complaints.
2. PSG in depressed children typically does not show the REM changes seen in adults with depression (although PSG is not usually clinically indicated).
3. Simultaneous management of both depression and insomnia is recommended.
4. The delayed sleep-wake phase disorder (a circadian-rhythm sleep-wake disorder) also causes sleep-onset insomnia but is characterized by unrestricted wake-up times (on the weekend) typically in the late morning or early afternoon. Patients with this disorder awaken feeling refreshed if allowed to sleep on their own schedule.

REFERENCES

1. Kotagal S, Broomall E. Sleep in children with autism spectrum disorder. *Pediatr Neurol.* Oct 2012;47(4):242–251.
2. American Psychiatric Association. *Diagnostic and Statistical Manual of Mental Disorders.* 5th ed. Arlington, VA: American Psychiatric Association; 2013.
3. Rao U. Sleep disturbances in pediatric depression. *Asian J Psychiatr.* Dec 2011;4(4):234–247.
4. Forbes EE, Bertocci MA, Gregory AM, et al. Objective sleep in pediatric anxiety disorders and major depressive disorder. *J Am Acad Child Adolesc Psychiatry.* Feb 2008;47(2):148–155.
5. Augustinavicius JL, Zanjani A, Zakzanis KK, Shapiro CM. Polysomnographic features of early-onset depression: a meta-analysis. *J Affect Disord.* Apr 2014;158:11–18.
6. American Academy of Sleep Medicine. *Internation Classification of Sleep Disorders.* 3rd ed. Darien, IL: American Academy of Sleep Medicine; 2014.
7. Kennard B, Silva S, Vitiello B, et al. Remission and residual symptoms after short-term treatment in the Treatment of Adolescents with Depression Study (TADS). *J Am Acad Child Adolesc Psychiatry.* Dec 2006;45(12):1404–1411.

An 8-year-old boy with attention-deficit/hyperactivity disorder and multiple nocturnal awakenings

Lourdes M. DelRosso

CASE PRESENTATION

An 8-year-old boy with attention-deficit/hyperactivity disorder (ADHD) presented for evaluation of frequent nocturnal awakenings. The patient had a bedtime routine that started at 8 PM. His routine included reading a book while in bed in his bedroom. Most nights while in bed, he felt the urge to move his legs. He would not get up from bed but would move his legs until he fell asleep at around 9 PM. He would usually wake up at 1 AM and go to his mother's room. His mother allowed him to sleep in her bed for the rest of the night. She reported that he kicked his legs while asleep. He would wake up once more at around 4 AM to use the bathroom. He usually woke up for the day at 6:45 AM. He did not nap during the day. The parents denied snoring, excessive daytime sleepiness, or parasomnias. The patient did not have any other medical or surgical history. His medications included methylphenidate ER 30 mg in the morning. His review of systems was negative for anxiety and depression. Physical exam was unremarkable.

LABORATORY AND SLEEP FINDINGS

Ferritin level was 17 ng/mL (normal range is 10 to 70 ng/mL).

QUESTION

What is the next step in the management of the sleep complaints in this patient?

ANSWER

The patient can benefit from iron supplementation for restless leg syndrome (RLS) and behavioral sleep interventions to address the nocturnal awakenings.

DISCUSSION

ADHD is a neurodevelopmental condition characterized by inattention, hyperactivity, and impulsivity. ADHD occurs in up to 7.5% of school-aged children. Sleep problems are reported in up to 50% of children with ADHD.[1] The most common sleep complaint in children with ADHD is difficulty initiating and maintaining sleep. The pathophysiology of the sleep problems is multifactorial. Some of the proposed mechanisms address the intrinsic pathophysiology of ADHD and include altered arousal pathways, alterations in the cortical and brainstem circuits that control wake and sleep, and alteration in the neurotransmitters that control attention and sleep.[2] Other contributing factors include stimulant medications, severity of ADHD symptoms, and the presence of both internalizing and externalizing comorbidities. Internalizing comorbidities include mood disorders such as depression and anxiety, and externalizing comorbidities include conduct disorders and oppositional defiant disorders.[3] A study of 195 children with ADHD, ages 5 to 13 years old, demonstrated that most sleep problems in affected children appeared to be transient, but in 10% of the participants, the problems persisted for longer than 12 months. Predictors for both transient and persistent sleep problems were the co-occurrence of internalizing and externalizing comorbidities and severity of ADHD symptoms. Predictors for persistent sleep problems alone were the use of ADHD medications and the presence of externalizing comorbidities.[4] The use of stimulant medication has been shown to interfere with sleep by increasing restlessness, nocturia, movements during sleep, and parasomnias.[5]

RLS and periodic leg movements of sleep (PLMS) are commonly found in children and adults with ADHD. These conditions are hypothesized to be manifestations of a common central nervous system process. Iron deficiency can lead to dopaminergic dysfunction, which has been associated with ADHD, RLS, and PLMS. Rhythmic movement disorders, head banging, and body rocking have also been found frequently in patients with ADHD.[6]

Management of sleep problems in children with ADHD includes sleep hygiene and behavioral intervention, which consist of establishing a consistent bedtime routine, limit setting, a behavioral reward system (e.g., sticker chart), setting times for returning to check on the child during the night, and relaxation strategies. Accurate identification and management of RLS has been shown to improve both nocturnal and diurnal hyperactivity. Other medical and psychiatric comorbidities should be addressed. The child with ADHD will benefit from a multidisciplinary team that includes a pediatrician, psychiatrist, sleep specialist, and psychologist.[7,8]

In the current patient, the ferritin is within normal limits; however, levels of >45 to 50 (some use 70 ng/mL) should be the goal in patients with RLS. The patient was started on iron supplementation. Behavioral interventions to address the nocturnal awakenings were also pursued.

CLINICAL PEARLS

1. Children with ADHD have difficulty initiating and maintaining sleep.
2. RLS, PLMS, and rhythmic movement disorders are commonly found in patients with ADHD.
3. Treatment of sleep disorders in patients with ADHD includes behavioral modifications and management of comorbidities.

REFERENCES

1. Kotagal S, Broomall E. Sleep in children with autism spectrum disorder. *Pediatr Neurol*. Oct 2012;47(4):242–251.
2. Owens J, Gruber R, Brown T, et al. Future research directions in sleep and ADHD: report of a consensus working group. *J Atten Disord*. Oct 2013;17(7):550–564.
3. Lycett K, Sciberras E, Mensah FK, Hiscock H. Behavioral sleep problems and internalizing and externalizing comorbidities in children with attention-deficit/hyperactivity disorder. *Eur Child Adolesc Psychiatry*. Jan 2015;24(1):31–40.
4. Lycett K, Mensah FK, Hiscock H, Sciberras E. A prospective study of sleep problems in children with ADHD. *Sleep Med*. Nov 2014;15(11):1354–1361.
5. Mick E, Biederman J, Jetton J, Faraone SV. Sleep disturbances associated with attention deficit hyperactivity disorder: the impact of psychiatric comorbidity and pharmacotherapy. *J Child Adolesc Psychopharmacol. Fall*. 2000;10(3):223–231.

6. Walters AS, Silvestri R, Zucconi M, Chandrashekariah R, Konofal E. Review of the possible relationship and hypothetical links between attention deficit hyperactivity disorder (ADHD) and the simple sleep related movement disorders, parasomnias, hypersomnias, and circadian rhythm disorders. *J Clin Sleep Med*. Dec 15 2008;4(6):591–600.
7. Sciberras E, Fulton M, Efron D, Oberklaid F, Hiscock H. Managing sleep problems in school aged children with ADHD: a pilot randomised controlled trial. *Sleep Med*. Oct 2011;12(9):932–935.
8. Walters AS, Mandelbaum DE, Lewin DS, Kugler S, England SJ, Miller M. Dopaminergic therapy in children with restless legs/periodic limb movements in sleep and ADHD. Dopaminergic Therapy Study Group. *Pediatr Neurol*. Mar 2000; 22(3):182–186.

A 13-year-old boy with autism spectrum disorder and difficulty falling asleep

Lourdes M. DelRosso

CASE PRESENTATION

The patient is a 13-year-old boy with autism spectrum disorder referred for evaluation of difficulty falling asleep. The parents brought a sleep diary (Fig. 90-1). The parents stated that the child has never had a regular sleep schedule. The patient usually went to sleep between 12 AM and 4 AM and woke up between 4 AM and 11 AM. The patient did not have a consistent bed routine and usually watched television before going to bed. He slept in his own room in his own bed and did not require parental intervention to fall asleep. He usually woke up once a night and watched television until he fell asleep (after 1 to 3 hours). The parents expressed concern that some nights he slept for only 4 hours. During the day he was irritable but he would not doze off or take naps. He was homeschooled. He did not have any other medical problems and did not take any medications. His past surgical history included tonsillectomy and adenoidectomy at age 4 for snoring. The review of systems was negative for current snoring, enuresis, leg discomfort, excessive daytime sleepiness, parasomnias, and anxiety.

PHYSICAL EXAM

The child was watching a program on his electronic device throughout the interview and exam. His vital signs were within normal limits. His weight was at the 59th percentile, and his height was at the 64th percentile. His physical exam was unremarkable.

QUESTION

What interventions would you recommend for this child?

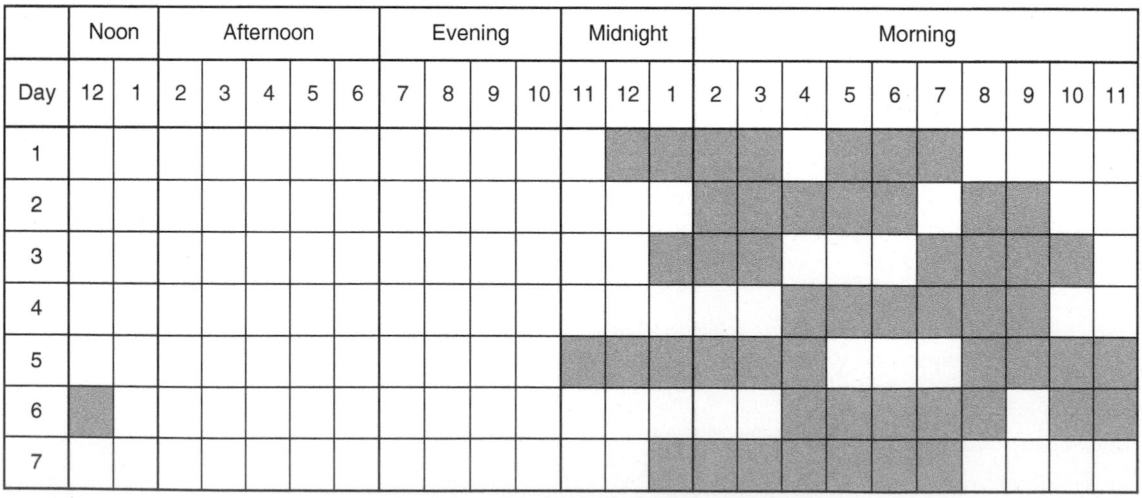

Day	Noon 12	1	Afternoon 2	3	4	5	6	Evening 7	8	9	10	Midnight 11	12	1	Morning 2	3	4	5	6	7	8	9	10	11
1												■	■		■	■		■	■					
2												■	■		■	■	■		■	■		■		
3											■	■			■	■	■		■	■	■		■	
4												■	■	■	■	■		■	■	■		■		
5										■	■	■			■	■	■		■	■	■		■	
6	■												■	■	■	■		■	■	■	■		■	■
7											■	■	■		■	■	■		■	■				

FIGURE 90-1 ■ The patient's 1-week sleep diary.

ANSWER

Children with autism spectrum disorder and sleep onset difficulties may benefit from behavioral sleep interventions and melatonin.

DISCUSSION

Autism spectrum disorder encompasses a group of disorders with varied degrees of severity and manifestations. The core characteristics of autism spectrum disorder are impairment in social and communication skills (verbal and nonverbal), repetitive behaviors, and hyper- or hyposensitivities to stimuli such as pain, sound, or light. Studies have suggested a strong genetic and environmental influence, with siblings of affected children having a higher risk. Autism spectrum disorder has a prevalence of 1 in 68 children, and it affects more boys than girls.

Sleep disturbances are common among children with autism, with a prevalence between 40% and 80%. It is unknown whether sleep problems are correlated with the severity of cognitive impairment.[1] Children with sleep problems, however, have demonstrated more behavioral problems compared with children with autism spectrum disorder who do not have sleep problems. The most common sleep complaints are difficulty with sleep onset and frequent nocturnal awakenings. The etiology of the sleep problems in children with autism is likely multifactorial. A circadian entrainment disruption has been proposed as one possible mechanism.[2] In fact, it has been speculated that repetitive stereotypic behaviors represent an attempt to compensate for lack of daily rhythmicity. The majority of studies have confirmed decreased levels of nocturnal melatonin production and improvement in sleep latency and sleep efficiency with melatonin administration.[3,4] γ-Aminobutyric acid, a sleep promoter neurotransmitter that normally inhibits the wake-promoting neurotransmitters located in the brainstem, may also be affected in autism, thus leading to insomnia.[5] Other contributing factors to the sleep disturbances in patients with autism include hyperarousability, sensory over-responsivity, and anxiety.[6]

Paroxysmal nocturnal behaviors, NREM parasomnias (sleep walking, confusional arousals, and night terrors), rhythmic movement disorders, and periodic leg movements occur frequently in children with autism spectrum disorder and may be secondary to increased arousability.[7] It is important to differentiate these nocturnal behaviors from seizure disorders, which affect approximately 15% of children with autism spectrum disorder. Polysomnography (PSG) findings have not been consistent among affected children, but, in general, a prolonged sleep latency and frequent nocturnal awakenings have been identified in the majority of studies. PSG is not indicated for evaluation of sleep patterns in children with autism unless sleep-disordered breathing is suspected. Sleep diaries and actigraphy are often useful.[5]

There is no cure for autism. Although some of the symptoms may improve with intervention, various degrees of impairment remain through the lifespan. Early intervention has been shown to result in improvement in language, cognition, and behavior, with mixed results on sleep quality. For sleep complaints, behavioral interventions are usually the first approach and are no different from those used with typically developing children (e.g., sleep hygiene, graduated extinction, and consistent bedtime routines). Melatonin supplementation has been shown to decrease sleep latency and improve sleep efficiency. Other medications have not been thoroughly studied. Weighted blankets, commonly used for calming and relaxing purposes, have not been shown to result in a statistically significant difference in total sleep time, sleep latency, or sleep efficiency.[5,8]

CLINICAL PEARLS

1. The most common sleep complaints in children with autism spectrum disorder are difficulty with sleep onset and frequent nocturnal awakenings.
2. Paroxysmal nocturnal behaviors, NREM parasomnias, rhythmic movement disorders, and periodic leg movements occur frequently in children with autism spectrum disorder.
3. Behavioral interventions and melatonin can be helpful with sleep latency and sleep continuity.

REFERENCES

1. Sikora DM, Johnson K, Clemons T, Katz T. The relationship between sleep problems and daytime behavior in children of different ages with autism spectrum disorders. *Pediatrics*. Nov 2012;130(suppl 2):S83–S90.
2. Cohen S, Conduit R, Lockley SW, Rajaratnam SM, Cornish KM. The relationship between sleep and behavior in autism spectrum disorder (ASD): a review. *J Neurodev Disord*. 2014;6(1):44.
3. Tordjman S, Najjar I, Bellissant E, et al. Advances in the research of melatonin in autism spectrum disorders: literature review and new perspectives. *Int J Mol Sci*. 2013;14(10):20508–20542.
4. Rossignol DA, Frye RE. Melatonin in autism spectrum disorders. *Curr Clin Pharmacol*. 2014;9(4):326–334.
5. Johnson KP, Giannotti F, Cortesi F. Sleep patterns in autism spectrum disorders. *Child Adolesc Psychiatr Clin N Am*. Oct 2009;18(4):917–928.
6. Mazurek MO, Petroski GF. Sleep problems in children with autism spectrum disorder: examining the contributions of sensory over-responsivity and anxiety. *Sleep Med*. Feb 2015;16(2):270–279. Epub Nov 28 2014.
7. Ming X, Sun YM, Nachajon RV, Brimacombe M, Walters AS. Prevalence of parasomnia in autistic children with sleep disorders. *Clin Med Pediatr*. 2009;3:1–10.
8. Gringras P, Green D, Wright B, et al. Weighted blankets and sleep in autistic children–a randomized controlled trial. *Pediatrics*. Aug 2014;134(2):298–306.

CASE 91

A 13-year-old girl with excessive daytime sleepiness

Lourdes M. DelRosso

CASE PRESENTATION

A 13-year-old girl presented with excessive daytime sleepiness that started a year ago. She went to bed at 9 PM and awoke at 6 AM, without nocturnal awakenings. She did not take naps during the day, but she reported dozing off during classes and car rides. She did not snore and denied symptoms of restless legs, sleep paralysis, cataplexy, or hypnagogic hallucinations. Her past medical history included allergic rhinitis and migraines. Review of systems was negative for depression and anxiety. Her medications included gabapentin 600 mg 3 times a day for migraine prophylaxis, cetirizine 10 mg a day for allergic rhinitis, and fluticasone nasal spray.

PHYSICAL EXAM

Physical exam revealed a sleepy girl in no distress. Her vital signs were within normal limits, her weight was at the 55th percentile, and her height was at the 20th percentile. Her physical exam was normal.

LABORATORY AND SLEEP FINDINGS

Magnetic resonance imaging of the brain done previously to evaluate headaches was normal.
Actigraphy is shown in Figure 91-1.

QUESTION

What is the diagnosis in this child?

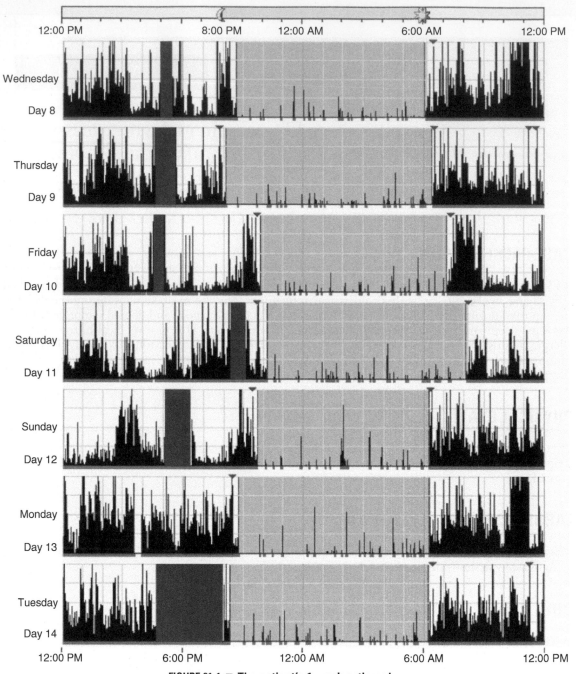

FIGURE 91-1 ■ The patient's 1-week actigraphy.

ANSWER

Excessive sleepiness is likely secondary to medication effect (gabapentin and cetirizine). Actigraphy reveals adequate sleep time with a bedtime between 8 PM and 10 PM, a wake-up time between 6 AM and 8 AM, and total sleep at night averaging 9 hours a night, without daytime naps.

DISCUSSION

Excessive daytime sleepiness is one of the most common complaints in the pediatric sleep medicine clinic. The *International Classification of Sleep Disorders*, third edition (ICSD-3) criteria for central disorders of hypersomnolence require that sleepiness not be better explained by the effect of medications. Sleepiness is a common side effect of many medications used in pediatrics: alpha$_2$-blockers (clonidine), anticonvulsants (including gabapentin), antihistamines, antipsychotics, antidepressants, and benzodiazepines.[1]

The sleep-wake cycles are regulated by various neurotransmitters. Sleep-promoting neurotransmitters include adenosine, γ-aminobutyric acid (GABA), galanin, and melatonin. Wake-promoting neurotransmitters include hypocretin, norepinephrine, histamine, serotonin, dopamine, and acetylcholine (Table 91-1).[2] Agonists of sleep-promoting neurotransmitters or antagonists of the wake-promoting neurotransmitters will generally produce sleepiness. Some of these medications have been successfully used to manage insomnia. Long-acting medications or those used during the day may produce excessive daytime sleepiness.

Excessive daytime sleepiness is also a common side effect reported by patients taking anticonvulsants. Polysomnography studies have revealed that some of these drugs may disrupt sleep by decreasing N3 and increasing N1 and arousals in the absence of seizures (phenytoin and valproic acid). The sleep architecture changes may be responsible for the sleepiness reported.[3] Other studies have shown decreased sleep latency with gabapentin, phenytoin, phenobarbital, clobazam, and carbamazepine. Multiple Sleep Latency Test studies have been conflicting. Although sleepiness has been reported with topiramate and zonisamide, studies have not shown evidence of decreased sleep latency, which may indicate that patients who report subjective daytime sleepiness may not have objective findings.[4]

New-generation antihistamines reduce sleep latency and increase daytime sleepiness. Sedation has been reported with desloratadine, cetirizine, and levocetirizine.[5, 6] Cetirizine was stopped in our patient, and gabapentin was titrated down with resolution of daytime sleepiness. The patient is following with neurology for alternative treatments for migraines.

TABLE 91-1.   Neurotransmitters of sleep and wake

Sleep Promoter		Wake Promoter	
Neurotransmitter	Location	Neurotransmitter	Location
GABA	Ventrolateral preoptic nucleus	Histamine	Tuberomammillary nucleus
Adenosine	Basal forebrain and cortex	Serotonin	Raphe nucleus
Galanin	Hypothalamus	Cholinergic	Pedunculopontine tegmentum Laterodorsal tegmentum
Melatonin	Pineal gland	Dopamine	Ventral periaqueductal gray
		Norepinephrine	Locus ceruleus
		Hypocretin	Lateral hypothalamus

CLINICAL PEARLS

1. Medication side effects are a common cause of daytime sleepiness.
2. Common medications that cause sleepiness include alpha$_2$-blockers, anticonvulsants, antihistamines, antipsychotics, antidepressants, and benzodiazepines.
3. If medication effect is suspected, a nonsedating alternative can be used or the medication can be titrated down to the lowest effective dose.

REFERENCES

1. Pagel JF. Excessive daytime sleepiness. *Am Fam Physician*. Mar 1 2009;79(5):391–396.
2. Krystal AD, Benca RM, Kilduff TS. Understanding the sleep-wake cycle: sleep, insomnia, and the orexin system. *J Clin Psychiatry*. 2013;74(suppl 1):3–20.
3. Legros B, Bazil CW. Effects of antiepileptic drugs on sleep architecture: a pilot study. *Sleep Med*. Jan 2003;4(1):51–55.
4. Jain SV, Glauser TA. Effects of epilepsy treatments on sleep architecture and daytime sleepiness: an evidence-based review of objective sleep metrics. *Epilepsia*. Jan 2014;55(1):26–37.
5. Tzanetos DB, Fahrenholz JM, Scott T, Buchholz K. Comparison of the sedating effects of levocetirizine and cetirizine: a randomized, double-blind, placebo-controlled trial. *Ann Allergy Asthma Immunol*. Dec 2011;107(6):517–522.
6. Ozdemir PG, Karadag AS, Selvi Y, et al. Assessment of the effects of antihistamine drugs on mood, sleep quality, sleepiness, and dream anxiety. *Int J Psychiatry Clin Pract*. Aug 2014;18(3):161–168.

A 12-year-old girl with narcolepsy and motor tics

Lourdes M. DelRosso

CASE PRESENTATION

A 12-year-old with narcolepsy type 2 presented for routine follow-up of treatment for narcolepsy. The patient was diagnosed with narcolepsy type 2 1 year before presentation. The parents reported onset of motor tics (eye blinking and facial grimacing) soon after she began treatment with methylphenidate about 8 months before the current clinic visit. A presumptive diagnosis of Tourette syndrome was considered, and the patient was started on haloperidol. Her bedtime was 10 PM and wake-up time was 7 AM. She took a 15-minute nap at noon and fell asleep on the ride home at 3 PM. The family denied snoring, sleepwalking, dream enactment, symptoms of restless legs, cataplexy, hypnagogic hallucinations, or sleep paralysis. Her medications included methylphenidate 30 mg at 6:30 AM and 30 mg at 1 PM and haloperidol 5 mg 3 times a day. Review of systems was negative for weight gain. The modified pediatric Epworth Sleepiness Scale was 11/24.

PHYSICAL EXAM

Physical exam revealed a sleepy girl in no distress. Her vital signs were within normal limits. The cardiovascular and neurologic exam was normal. The patient was noted to have repeated episodes of facial grimacing while remaining attentive and responding to questions. The neurologic examination was otherwise normal.

QUESTIONS

1. What is the likely cause of the tics?
2. Does the patient meet criteria for Tourette syndrome?

ANSWERS

1. Tics can occur with stimulant medication.
2. The patient does not meet criteria for Tourette syndrome because the tics were entirely motor (no vocalizations) and the duration was less than 1 year.

DISCUSSION

Tourette syndrome is a disorder characterized by the presence of tics. The *Diagnostic and Statistical Manual of Mental Disorders*, fifth edition (DSM-V), classifies Tourette syndrome under neurodevelopmental disorders. The diagnostic criteria include the presence of multiple motor tics and at least one vocal tic (vocalization) for at least a year. The vocalizations are sometimes called phonic tics. The pathophysiology of Tourette syndrome suggests an abnormality in dopamine neurotransmission. Increase in dopamine release has been reported in the putamen, striatum, and thalamocortical circuits of patients with Tourette syndrome.[1] Tics usually appear before 18 years of age and are more common in males. Our patient does not fit criteria for Tourette syndrome because her tics were not phonic and were present for less than a year.

Tics are brief stereotypic, repetitive, and involuntary movements or vocalizations. Tics can be simple or complex. Simple motor tics are usually brief and repetitive movements such as blinking. Simple vocal tics are inarticulate sounds such as grunting or throat clearing. Complex motor tics are sequential movements that may appear purposeful such as bending, and complex vocal tics consist of words or sentences.[2] Perhaps the most dramatic and disabling tics include motor movements that result in self-harm such as punching oneself in the face or vocal tics including coprolalia (uttering socially inappropriate words such as swearing) or echolalia (repeating the words or phrases of others). However, coprolalia is only present in a small number (10% to 15%) of individuals with Tourette syndrome.

Tics that last less than a year are considered transient and are relatively common in children. Motor or phonic (but not both) tics present for longer than a year are considered chronic. Chronic motor tics have a prevalence of up to 40 in 1000 children between 6 and 18 years of age, and chronic vocal tics have a prevalence of 8 in 1000 children of the same age range.[3] Secondary tics can be caused by a variety of conditions, including autism spectrum disorders, RETT syndrome, some genetic disorders (Fragile X syndrome and Lesch-Nyhan syndrome, among others), acute brain lesions, and following infections and medications (Table 92-1).[3] Higher doses of stimulants have shown a reversible increase in tic severity. A study on 12 adults with Tourette syndrome demonstrated increased tic activity after amphetamine administration.[4] Stimulants are commonly used to treat attention-deficit/hyperactivity disorder (ADHD) and excessive sleepiness in patients with narcolepsy, via a complex orchestration of neurotransmitters. Methylphenidate,

---

TABLE 92-1.   Tic-inducing or Tic-exacerbating agents[3]

- Amphetamines
- Cocaine
- Heroin
- Methylphenidate
- Pemoline
- Antipsychotics (D2 blockers)[a]
  - Fluphenazine
  - Perphenazine
  - Thiothixene
- Antidepressants
- Antiepiliptics
  - Carbamazepine
  - Phenytoin
  - Phenobarbital
  - Lamotrigine
- Levodopa

[a]Although most antipsychotics can be helpful for motor tics, those listed in the table have been rarely reported to cause tardive tics.

Copyright "Tic Disorders" Martino and Mink, *Continuum* 2013, 19(5), page 1297.

for example, releases presynaptic dopamine and norepinephrine stores and reduces the uptake of catecholamines. In a study of 555 children diagnosed with ADHD, 8% of patients treated with various stimulants developed tics without any specific relationship to dose or duration of treatment.[5]

Polysomnography in 18 children with tic disorders demonstrated difficulty with sleep onset and decreased sleep efficiency in proportion to tic severity.[6] Tics persist in all stages of sleep. Patients with tic disorders can experience non–tic-related movements during sleep that may disturb sleep and contribute to the increased arousal index and decreased sleep efficiency.[7]

In patients with narcolepsy or ADHD, it is recommended to document the presence, type, and severity of tics before initiation of treatment with stimulants. Low-dose and short-acting medications are recommended.[8] Management of tics should be individualized to the patient's needs, diagnosis, and coexistence of psychiatric conditions.

Because of the close association between the onset of tics and start of methylphenidate, the tics were believed to be due to this medication. Haloperidol and methylphenidate were titrated down and eventually discontinued. Modafinil was initiated. The tics resolved and were attributed to methylphenidate.

CLINICAL PEARLS

1. Tics can be associated with medications including stimulants used for treatment of narcolepsy or ADHD.
2. Patients with tic disorders have disturbed sleep with decreased sleep efficiency.
3. Tourette syndrome is characterized by multiple motor tics and at least one vocal tic for at least 1 year.

REFERENCES

1. Steeves TD, Ko JH, Kideckel DM, et al. Extrastriatal dopaminergic dysfunction in tourette syndrome. *Ann Neurol*. Feb 2010;67(2):170–181.
2. Shprecher D, Kurlan R. The management of tics. *Mov Disord*. Jan 15 2009;24(1):15–24.
3. Martino D, Mink JW. Tic disorders. *Continuum (Minneap Minn)*. Oct 2013;19(5 Movement Disorders):1287–1311.
4. Denys D, de Vries F, Cath D, et al. Dopaminergic activity in Tourette syndrome and obsessive-compulsive disorder. *Eur Neuropsychopharmacol*. Nov 2013;23(11):1423–1431.
5. Varley CK, Vincent J, Varley P, Calderon R. Emergence of tics in children with attention deficit hyperactivity disorder treated with stimulant medications. *Compr Psychiatry*. May-Jun 2001;42(3):228–233.
6. Kirov R, Kinkelbur J, Banaschewski T, Rothenberger A. Sleep patterns in children with attention-deficit/hyperactivity disorder, tic disorder, and comorbidity. *J Child Psychol Psychiatry*. Jun 2007;48(6):561–570.
7. Kostanecka-Endress T, Banaschewski T, Kinkelbur J, et al. Disturbed sleep in children with Tourette syndrome: a polysomnographic study. *J Psychosom Res*. Jul 2003;55(1):23–29.
8. Rizzo R, Gulisano M, Cali PV, Curatolo P. Tourette syndrome and comorbid ADHD: current pharmacological treatment options. *Eur J Paediatr Neurol*. Sep 2013;17(5):421–428.

A 15-year-old girl with narcolepsy type 1 needs sedation for dental work

Angele Arthur and Lourdes M. DelRosso

CASE PRESENTATION

A 15-year-old girl with past medical history of narcolepsy type 1 presented to the clinic requesting authorization for the use of nitrous oxide (laughing gas) anesthesia during dental work. Her parents report good control of daytime sleepiness and cataplexy. She went to bed at 10 PM and woke up at 7 AM. She took one 20-minute nap daily at 1 PM. Cataplexy, consisting of generalized muscle weakness, was elicited by laughter, and it occurred once every 2 weeks. She denied sleep paralysis or hypnagogic hallucinations. She did not have any other medical problems. Review of systems was negative. Her daily medications included modafinil 100 mg twice a day and protriptyline 5 mg thrice a day.

PHYSICAL EXAM

Vitals signs were within normal limits. The physical and neurologic exam was unremarkable.

QUESTION

Will laughing gas produce cataplexy in this patient?

ANSWER

Nitrous oxide anesthesia should be safe for dental procedures in pediatric patients with narcolepsy. The dentist should be aware of the patient's diagnosis, symptoms, and current medications (see Discussion section).

DISCUSSION

Nitrous oxide has been used as an inhaled anesthetic for over 150 years. Its short action and analgesic and anxiolytic properties make it an attractive choice for pediatric dentistry. It is popularly known as "laughing gas" because of its euphoric effects. Nitrous oxide appears to have multiple mechanisms of action. Inhibition of N-methyl-D-aspartate receptors with a limited effect on γ-aminobutyric acid[1] may be responsible for the anesthetic properties. The antinociceptive properties appear to be mediated by activation of mesolimbic dopaminergic neurons.[2] Adverse events have been shown to be related to the length of exposure, and include oxygen desaturation, diaphoresis, agitation, nausea, and vomiting.[3] Nitrous oxide affects vitamin B_{12} metabolism and has been linked to neurologic and hematologic conditions in patients with vitamin B_{12} deficiency.[4] Contraindications for the use of nitrous oxide may include chronic obstructive pulmonary disease, severe emotional disturbance, drug dependency, treatment with bleomycin sulfate, methylenetetrahydrofolate reductase deficiency, and first trimester of pregnancy.[5] Although rare, death from nitrous oxide intoxication has been reported in either accidental or abuse-related cases.[6]

Patients with narcolepsy pose specific concerns for prolonged hypersomnia, cataplexy episodes, and sleep paralysis upon emergence from anesthesia, independent of discontinuation of medications.[7] Chronic stimulant use in these patients may also place them at increased risk of cardiovascular complications related to anesthesia. However, studies have not shown evidence of an increased risk of perioperative complications in adult patients with narcolepsy treated with amphetamines.[8,9]

Our patient had a successful dental intervention with nitrous oxide-oxygen inhalation without any adverse events.

CLINICAL PEARLS

1. Patients with narcolepsy must inform their treating dentist about their diagnosis.
2. The dentist must be aware of the potential for emergence of narcolepsy symptoms.
3. Use of sedatives should be avoided.

REFERENCES

1. Emmanouil DE, Quock RM. Advances in understanding the actions of nitrous oxide. *Anesth Prog.* 2007;54(1):9–18.
2. Koyanagi S, Himukashi S, Mukaida K, Shichino T, Fukuda K. Dopamine D2-like receptor in the nucleus accumbens is involved in the antinociceptive effect of nitrous oxide. *Anesth Analg.* 2008;106(6):1904–1909.
3. Zier JL, Liu M. Safety of high-concentration nitrous oxide by nasal mask for pediatric procedural sedation: experience with 7802 cases. *Pediatr Emerg Care.* 2011;27(12):1107–1112.
4. Krajewski W, Kucharska M, Pilacik B, et al. Impaired vitamin B12 metabolic status in healthcare workers occupationally exposed to nitrous oxide. *Br J Anaesth.* 2007;99(6):812–818.
5. *Guidelines on Use of Nitrous Oxide for Pediatric Dental Patients.* Chicago, IL: American Academy of Pediatric Dentistry; 2009.
6. Potocka-Banas B, Majdanik S, Dutkiewicz G, Borowiak K, Janus T. Death caused by addictive inhalation of nitrous oxide. *Hum Exp Toxicol.* 2011;30(11):1875–1877.
7. Gomez-Garrido M, Torcal E, Nevado E, Ibarra M, Cuesta J. Inhalation anesthesia in Gelineau syndrome (cataplexy-cataplexy). *Revista espanola de anestesiologia y reanimacion.* 2002;49(6):338–339.
8. Fischer SP, Schmiesing CA, Guta CG, Brock-Utne JG. General anesthesia and chronic amphetamine use: should the drug be stopped preoperatively? *Anesth Analg.* 2006;103(1):203–206. table of contents.
9. Burrow B, Burkle C, Warner DO, Chini EN. Postoperative outcome of patients with narcolepsy. A retrospective analysis. *J Clin Anesth.* 2005;17(1):21–25.

A 14-year-old boy with short stature and snoring

Lourdes M. DelRosso

CASE PRESENTATION

A 14-year-old boy was referred for evaluation of snoring during the past year. The family denied witnessed apneas or gasping for air. He reported morning headaches, nocturnal diaphoresis, and daytime fatigue. He went to bed at 10 PM and woke up at 7 AM feeling tired. He did not doze off in school but dozed off on the bus ride home. He denied cataplexy, hypnagogic hallucinations, sleep paralysis, symptoms of restless legs, and parasomnias. His past medical history was significant for growth-hormone deficiency. His growth was slow in early childhood. He was always the shortest child in his class. Height was below the 3rd percentile when his growth was evaluated at 9 years of age, and growth-hormone supplementation was initiated. His medications included somatropin 0.049 μg/kg/day.

PHYSICAL EXAM

The patient is shown in Figures 94-1 and 94-2. He appeared alert and cooperative. His vital signs were within normal range, his weight was at the 61st percentile, and his height was at the 17th percentile. He did not have an adenoid facies. The oropharynx was Mallampati class IV, and tonsils were size 1+. He had a large tongue. The remainder of the physical exam was normal.

LABORATORY AND SLEEP FINDINGS

Magnetic resonance imaging of the brain was normal (no pituitary abnormality).

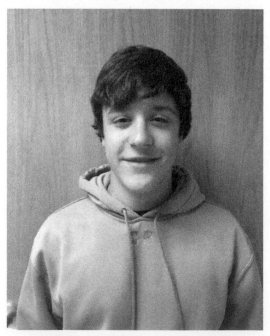

FIGURE 94-1 ■ Frontal view of the patient.

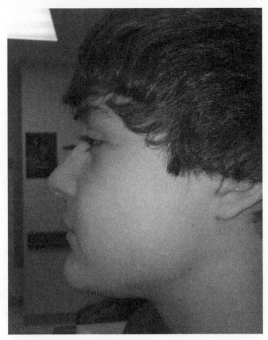

FIGURE 94-2 ■ Lateral view of the patient.

Polysomnography revealed a total recording time of 480 minutes, with a total sleep time (TST) of 361 minutes. Sleep efficiency was 75%. Sleep onset latency was 20 minutes. Arousal index was 11/h. The obstructive apnea–hypopnea index (AHI) was 4.7/h. The central AHI was 0/h. SpO_2 nadir was 88%. The end-tidal CO_2 was <50 torr for 100% of TST. The periodic leg movements index was 0/h.

Lateral x-ray of the neck soft tissue did not reveal adenoid hypertrophy.

QUESTION

What physical findings in this patient can be attributed to growth-hormone supplementation?

ANSWER

The patient has a large mandible and macroglossia. Both features have been described in patients with growth-hormone supplementation.

DISCUSSION

Growth hormone is approved for the treatment of idiopathic short stature (height below 2 standard deviations for age), growth-hormone deficiency, Turner syndrome, Prader-Willi syndrome, chronic renal failure, and being born small for gestational age. The dose varies from 0.02 to 0.067 mg/kg/day. The most common side effects of treatment are headaches, eosinophilia, hypothyroidism, and injection-site reactions.[1,2]

    Children with idiopathic short stature have small facial features and micrognathia. When supplemented, growth hormone results in accelerated growth beyond normal limits in mandibular length and total anterior face height.[3] Growth hormone can also stimulate tonsillar and adenoidal hypertrophy and macroglossia. Studies on the effects of growth-hormone supplementation in the sleep and breathing patterns of children with idiopathic short statures are lacking. For growth-hormone supplementation in Prader-Willi patients, see Clinical Pearls in Case 58: A 3-year-old girl with Prader-Willi syndrome and obesity. Patients with growth-hormone excess such as in acromegaly are at increased risk of obstructive sleep apnea (up to 81% prevalence); the pathophysiology is thought to be related to enlarged tongue and pharyngeal tissues and facial bone growth.[4]

    Our patient had mild obstructive sleep apnea without adenoidal or tonsillar hypertrophy. Continuous positive airway pressure (CPAP) was initiated and titrated to 5 cm H_2O. The patient had excellent adherence to CPAP. His morning headaches and daytime sleepiness improved. The patient continues growth-hormone supplementation.

CLINICAL PEARLS

1. Growth-hormone supplementation is approved for the treatment of idiopathic short stature, growth-hormone deficiency, Turner syndrome, Prader-Willi syndrome, chronic renal failure, and being born small for gestational age.
2. Side effects of growth-hormone supplementation include headaches and hypothyroidism, macroglossia, and large mandible.
3. Patients on growth-hormone supplementation should be screened for snoring and obstructive sleep apnea.

REFERENCES

1. Watson SE, Rogol AD. Recent updates on recombinant human growth hormone outcomes and adverse events. *Curr Opin Endocrinol Diabetes Obes*. Feb 2013;20(1):39–43.
2. Tabatabaei-Malazy O, Mohajeri-Tehrani MR, Heshmat R, et al. Efficacy and safety of Samtropin recombinant human growth hormone: a double-blind randomized clinical trial. *J Diabetes Metab Disord*. 2014;13(1):115.
3. Kjellberg H, Wikland KA. A longitudinal study of craniofacial growth in idiopathic short stature and growth hormone-deficient boys treated with growth hormone. *Eur J Orthod*. Jun 2007;29(3):243–250.
4. Hernandez-Gordillo D, Ortega-Gomez Mdel R, Galicia-Polo L, et al. Sleep apnea in patients with acromegaly. Frequency, characterization and positive pressure titration. *Open Respir Med J*. 2012;6:28–33.

A 17-year-old boy with both insomnia and excessive daytime sleepiness

Lourdes M. DelRosso

CASE PRESENTATION

A 17-year-old male presented with difficulty falling asleep at night and excessive sleepiness during the day for the last 6 months. The symptoms started without any apparent precipitating factor. The patient went to bed at 10 PM but was not able to fall asleep until 1 AM. After 15 minutes in bed, he usually left the bedroom and went outside to "breathe fresh air and relax." Once asleep, he reported restless sleep and frequent awakenings. The family denied snoring, sleep walking, dream enactment, symptoms of restless legs, cataplexy, hypnagogic hallucinations, or sleep paralysis. The patient woke up at 10 AM. He felt sleepy during the day. He dozed off in school and during car rides but did not take scheduled naps. Epworth sleepiness score was 13. There were no other past medical problems. His review of systems was negative for depression and anxiety. He denied taking any medications, herbal products, or recreational drugs. Physical exam was normal.

LABORATORY AND SLEEP FINDINGS

A nocturnal polysomnography (PSG) revealed total sleep time (TST) of 470 minutes; total recording time (TRT) 601 minutes; sleep efficiency 78%, sleep latency 90 minutes; and REM latency 50 minutes. The apnea–hypopnea index was 0.5/h. The periodic leg movements index was 2/h.

Multiple Sleep Latency Test (MSLT) data are presented in Table 95-1.

Urine toxicology the morning of the MSLT was positive for cannabis.

QUESTION

What is the diagnosis in this patient?

TABLE 95-1. **Multiple Sleep Latency Test results**

	Nap 1 (min)	Nap 2 (min)	Nap 3 (min)	Nap 4 (min)	Nap 5 (min)
Sleep latency	4	5	8	11	15
REM latency	10	3	-		-

ANSWER

The patient's excessive daytime sleepiness was attributed to "hypersomnia because of a medication or substance." The patient likely had delayed sleep-wake phase disorder as well. The patient's MSLT was invalidated because of the positive drug screen.

DISCUSSION

The differential diagnosis of excessive sleepiness in a teenager is vast, and a detailed history and physical are of utmost importance. As seen in previous chapters, insufficient sleep syndrome, inadequate sleep hygiene, delayed sleep-wake phase disorder, and sleep disorders such as narcolepsy, Kleine-Levin syndrome, and obstructive sleep apnea syndrome are included in the differential diagnosis. In the Clinical Pearls section we discuss another important cause of excessive sleepiness in the teenager: drug use.

Cannabis is the most common recreational drug used in the world, with increasing numbers of users among adolescents. Cannabis use among adolescents has been associated with cognitive deficits, memory, attention, and sleep disturbances. These deficits have also been found in adults; however, they tend to persist after abstinence in teenagers.[1]

The main active component found in cannabis is tetrahydrocannabinol (THC). This substance acts on two main receptors: CB1, found in the central nervous system, and CB2, found in immune cells and peripheral tissues. THC interacts with other neurotransmitters such as dopamine, adenosine, and hypocretin. CB1 and hypocretin 1 and 2 receptors are widely expressed in the hypothalamus, amygdala, frontal cortex, and ventral tegmental area and seem to have antagonistic effects in the sleep-wake cycle.[2] Studies have shown that cannabis may have an effect on sleep architecture (lower TST, reduced slow-wave sleep, and increased N2 sleep) and on subjective sleep quality.[3] One study found MSLT results consistent with narcolepsy in male teenagers with urine drug screens positive for THC.[4] The American Academy of Sleep Medicine (AASM) practice parameters for the clinical use of the MSLT state that test results are influenced by physiologic, psychological, and test protocol variables, and recommends drug screening the morning of the MSLT.[5]

Cannabis discontinuation has been associated with prolonged sleep latency, decreased sleep efficiency, and less TST. These findings may be secondary to the effect of cannabis on CB1 receptors on the various areas of the brain discussed previously. The degree of sleep disturbance after cannabis discontinuation may be a contributing factor for cannabis use relapse in some patients. The sleep symptoms should be addressed with appropriate behavioral or pharmacologic options.[6]

In this patient, the PSG was remarkable for a long sleep latency (not consistent with narcolepsy). Although the MSLT met criteria for narcolepsy, this was felt secondary to his chronic cannabis use. The long sleep latency would be consistent with the delayed sleep phase syndrome. Of note, circadian disorders (e.g., delayed sleep period) can be associated with a positive MSLT. If only the first or second naps of an MSLT have sleep-onset REM (SOREMP) this may suggest a circadian effect. Carskadon et al. [7] found one SOREMP in 48% and two SOREMPs in 16% of a group of normal adolescents with early school start times.

The patient admitted using cannabis to help him relax at night and help him fall asleep. He was referred to a drug program to stop cannabis use and was enrolled in behavioral sleep therapy to address possible sleep side effects of cannabis discontinuation.

CLINICAL PEARLS

1. Urine drug toxicology the morning of the MSLT is recommended by the AASM to evaluate for hypersomnia related to medication or drug use.
2. Cannabis use and withdrawal have been associated with sleepiness, abnormal sleep perception, and abnormal sleep architecture.
3. Concomitant behavioral sleep intervention is recommended during cannabis discontinuation to avoid relapse because of sleep disturbances.

REFERENCES

1. Lubman DI, Cheetham A, Yucel M. Cannabis and adolescent brain development. *Pharmacol Ther*. Apr 2015;148:1–16.
2. Flores A, Maldonado R, Berrendero F. Cannabinoid-hypocretin cross-talk in the central nervous system: what we know so far. *Front Neurosci*. 2013;7:256.
3. Gates PJ, Albertella L, Copeland J. The effects of cannabinoid administration on sleep: a systematic review of human studies. *Sleep Med Rev*. Dec 2014;18(6):477–487.
4. Dzodzomenyo S, Stolfi A, Splaingard D, Earley E, Onadeko O, Splaingard M. Urine toxicology screen in multiple sleep latency test: the correlation of positive tetrahydrocannabinol, drug negative patients, and narcolepsy. *J Clin Sleep Med*. Feb 15 2015;11(2):93–99.
5. Littner MR, Kushida C, Wise M, et al. Practice parameters for clinical use of the multiple sleep latency test and the maintenance of wakefulness test. *Sleep*. Jan 2005;28(1):113–121.
6. Bolla KI, Lesage SR, Gamaldo CE, et al. Sleep disturbance in heavy marijuana users. *Sleep*. Jun 2008;31(6):901–908.
7. Carskadon MA, Wolfson AR, Acebo C, Tzischinsky O, Seifer R. Adolescent sleep patterns, circadian timing, and sleepiness at a transition to early school days. *Sleep*. 1998 Dec 15;21(8):871–881.

A 10-year-old with acute pancreatitis and snoring

Lourdes M. DelRosso

CASE PRESENTATION

A 10-year-old obese boy was referred for inpatient bedside polysomnography (PSG) for loud snoring and nocturnal desaturations. The patient was hospitalized for acute pancreatitis. His past medical and surgical history were negative. His only medication was morphine for abdominal pain.

PHYSICAL EXAM

Physical exam revealed an alert and cooperative obese boy. His vital signs were within the normal range. His height was at the 40th percentile, and his weight was at the 99th percentile. He did not have an adenoid facies. The oropharynx was Mallampati grade III. Tonsils were 1+. He did not have micrognathia or retrognathia. The remainder of the exam was normal (the patient had recently received a dose of morphine for abdominal pain).

LABORATORY AND SLEEP FINDINGS

Complete blood count and comprehensive chemistry panel were within the normal range. Amylase was elevated.

QUESTION

You receive an order for a bedside PSG in this patient. What do you do recommend?

ANSWER

Opioids cause respiratory depression. The patient is not at his baseline. You recommend waiting until the morphine is discontinued before proceeding with the PSG.

DISCUSSION

Opioids are commonly used in clinical settings for pain relief. Respiratory depression is a common side effect and is manifested by slow, irregular breathing; central apnea; hypercapnia; and hypoxemia. Therefore, a polysomnogram performed while the patient is receiving narcotics may show abnormalities that would not otherwise be present. The mechanism of respiratory depression is multifactorial. Opioid receptors are present in the respiratory control centers including the Pre-Botzinger complex in the ventrolateral medulla, which is active during inspiration. Opioid effects on the Kolliker-Fuse and parabrachial nuclei in the pons lead to irregular respirations.[1] Incidentally, the Kolliker-Fuse nuclei is also involved in control of airway patency and may contribute to difficulty swallowing, another side effect of opioids.[2] Hypoxic and hypercapnic responses mediated in the brainstem are decreased in the presence of opioids.[1]

Although opioids are commonly used in children, it is important to remember that children may respond differently than adults do. A series of deaths in children who were given codeine after adenotonsillectomy[3,4] led to the addition of a black-box warning by the U.S. Food and Drug Administration contraindicating codeine for pain control in children with obstructive sleep apnea syndrome (OSAS) after adenotonsillectomy. The mechanisms of severe respiratory depression in these children were attributed to increased conversion of codeine to morphine by ultrarapid codeine metabolism in patients with a genetic duplication in the CYP2D6 allele (a member of the cytochrome P450 oxidase system). This mutation is present in up to 10% of individuals of European descent and in up to 30% of individuals of northern African descent.[5] In addition, children with more severe OSAS-related hypoxemia have an increased sensitivity to the analgesic effects of opiates and, therefore, require lower doses.[6] Other opioids such as oral morphine or oxycodone should be used with caution, and when possible, nonopioid analgesia should be considered.

Our patient's PSG was performed after the morphine was discontinued.

CLINICAL PEARLS

1. Opioids produce respiratory depression by their effect on the central control of breathing.
2. The respiratory depressive effect of opioids may alter the PSG results. Patients who are on opioids for temporary control of pain should be studied when at baseline. Patients on chronic opioids should be studied on their maintenance dose.
3. Codeine is contraindicated for pain control after tonsillectomy and/or adenoidectomy.

REFERENCES

1. Pattinson KT. Opioids and the control of respiration. *Br J Anaesth*. Jun 2008;100(6):747–758.
2. Levitt ES, Abdala AP, Paton JF, Bissonnette JM, Williams JT. μ Opioid receptor activation hyperpolarizes respiratory-controlling Kölliker-Fuse neurons and suppresses post-inspiratory drive. *J Physiol*. Oct 1 2015;593(19):4453–4469.
3. Ciszkowski C, Madadi P, Phillips MS, Lauwers AE, Koren G. Codeine, ultrarapid-metabolism genotype, and postoperative death. *N Engl J Med*. Aug 20 2009;361(8):827–828.
4. Kelly LE, Rieder M, van den Anker J, et al. More codeine fatalities after tonsillectomy in North American children. *Pediatrics*. May 2012;129(5):e1343–e1347.
5. Williams DG, Patel A, Howard RF. Pharmacogenetics of codeine metabolism in an urban population of children and its implications for analgesic reliability. *Br J Anaesth*. Dec 2002;89(6):839–845.
6. Brown KA, Laferriere A, Lakheeram I, Moss IR. Recurrent hypoxemia in children is associated with increased analgesic sensitivity to opiates. *Anesthesiology*. Oct 2006;105(4):665–669.

Common Abbreviation List

AASM	American Academy of Sleep Medicine
AHI	apnea hypopnea index
ASV	adaptive servo-ventilation
AVAPS	average volume assured pressure support
BMI	body mass index
BP	blood pressure
BPAP	bilevel positive airway pressure
CA	central apnea
CBT	cognitive behavioral therapy
CCHS	congenital central hypoventilation syndrome
CFlow	positive pressure device airflow
CPAP	continuous positive airway pressure
CSA	central sleep apnea
EDS	excessive daytime sleepiness
EEG	electroencephalogram
EMG	electromyogram
EOG	electro-oculagram
ESS	Epworth Sleepiness Scale
ETCO$_2$	end-tidal CO$_2$
GERD	gastroesophageal reflux disease
GH	growth hormone
GABA	gamma aminobutyric acid
HR	heart rate
ICSD-3	International Classification of Sleep Disorders, 3rd Edition
MRI	magnetic resonance imaging
MSLT	multiple sleep latency test
NPAF	nasal pressure transducer air flow
NREM	non-REM sleep
OA	obstructive apnea
OSAS	obstructive sleep apnea syndrome
PDR	posterior dominant rhythm
PFT	pulmonary function test
PLMD	period limb movement disorder
PLMS	period limb movements in sleep
PSG	polysomnogram
PWF	pulse waveform
REM	rapid eye movement sleep
RLS	restless legs syndrome
SpO$_2$	arterial oxygen saturation
SDB	sleep-disordered breathing
SE	sleep efficiency
SL	sleep latency
SOREMP	sleep onset REM period
SWS	slow wave sleep
T&A	tonsillectomy and adenoidectomy
TCO$_2$	transcutaneous capnography
TRT	total recording time
TST	total sleep time
WASO	wake after sleep onset

Thematic Table of Contents

INDEX

Note: Page numbers followed by "b", "f" and "t" indicate boxes, figures and tables respectively.